The Brain and Emotion

The Brain and Emotion

Edmund T. Rolls

Department of Experimental Psychology
University of Oxford,
Oxford OX1 3UD, England

OXFORD NEW YORK TOKYO
OXFORD UNIVERSITY PRESS
1999

Oxford University Press, Great Clarendon Street, Oxford OX2 6DP
Oxford New York
Athens Auckland Bangkok Bogota Bombay Buenos Aires Calcutta
Cape Town Chennai Dar es Salaam Delhi Florence Hong Kong Istanbul
Karachi Kuala Lumpur Madrid Melbourne Mexico City Mumbai
Nairobi Paris São Paolo Singapore Taipei Tokyo Toronto Warsaw
and associated companies in
Berlin Ibadan

Oxford is a trade mark of Oxford University Press

Published in the United States
by Oxford University Press Inc., New York

A catalogue record for this book is available from the British Library

Library of Congress Cataloging in Publication Data
(Data available)

ISBN 0 19 852464 1   1001466262

Typeset by Technical Typesetting Ireland in Belfast
Printed in Great Britain by
Bookcraft (Bath) Ltd
Midsomer Norton, Avon

Preface

What are emotions? Why do we have emotions? What are the rules by which emotion operates? What are the brain mechanisms of emotion, and how can disorders of emotion be understood? Why does it feel like something to have an emotion?

What motivates us to work for particular rewards such as food when we are hungry, or water when we are thirsty? How do these motivational control systems operate to ensure that we eat approximately the correct amount of food to maintain our body weight or to replenish our thirst? What factors account for the overeating and obesity which some humans show?

Why is the brain built to have reward, and punishment, systems, rather than in some other way? Raising this issue of brain design and why we have reward and punishment systems, and emotion and motivation, produces a fascinating answer based on how genes can direct our behaviour to increase their fitness. How does the brain produce behaviour by using reward, and punishment, mechanisms? These are some of the questions considered in this book.

The brain mechanisms of both emotion and motivation are considered together in this book. The examples of motivated behaviour described are hunger, thirst, and sexual behaviour. The reason that both emotion and motivation are described here is that both involve rewards and punishments as the fundamental solution of the brain to interfacing sensory systems to action selection and execution systems. Computing the reward and punishment value of sensory stimuli, and then using selection between different rewards and avoidance of punishments in a common reward-based currency appears to be the fundamental solution that brains use in order to produce appropriate behaviour. The behaviour selected can be thought of as appropriate in the sense that it is based on the sensory systems and reward decoding that our genes specify (through the process of natural selection) in order to maximize their fitness (reproductive potential). Having reward and punishment systems is the solution that evolution has developed to produce appropriate behaviour. Emotion and motivation are considered together because they are the types of behaviour in which rewards and punishments operate.

The book provides a modern neuroscience-based approach to information processing in the brain, and deals especially with the information processing involved in emotion, motivation, and reward. The book links this analysis of the brain mechanisms of emotion and motivation to the wider context of what emotions are, what their functions are, how emotions evolved, and the larger issue of why emotional and motivational feelings and consciousness might arise in a system organized like the brain.

This book is thus intended to uncover some of the most important and fundamental aspects and principles of brain function and design. The book is also intended to show that the way in which the brain functions in motivation and emotion can be seen to be the result of natural selection operating to select genes which optimize our behaviour by building into us the appropriate reward and punishment systems, and the appropriate rules for the operation of these systems.

The material in this text is copyright E. T. Rolls. Part of the material presented in the book reflects work done over many years in collaboration with many colleagues, whose tremendous contribution is warmly appreciated. The contribution of many will be evident from the references cited in the text. They include Larry Abbott (Brandeis University), Gordon C. Baylis (University of South Carolina), Alain Berthoz (CNRS, Paris), Steven J. Cooper (University of Durham), James G. Gibbs (Cornell Medical Centre), Michael Hasselmo (Harvard), Raymond P. Kesner (University of Utah), Christiana M. Leonard (University of Florida, Gainesville), Yasushi Miyashita (University of Tokyo), the late Gordon J. Mogenson (University of Western Ontario), Francisco Mora (Universidad Complutense, Madrid), Vanit Nalwa (New Delhi), Hiroaki Niki (University of Tokyo), Stefano Panzeri (University of Oxford, and International School of Physics, Trieste), Nestor Parga (Theoretical Physics, Madrid), David Perrett (University of St. Andrews), Anthony G. Phillips (University of British Columbia), Barbara J. Rolls (Pennsylvania State University), Juliet H. Rolls (Cambridge University), Thomas R. Scott (University of Delaware), Steven J. Simpson (University of Oxford), Chantal Stern (Boston University), Simon J. Thorpe (CNRS, Toulouse), Alessandro Treves (International School of Advanced Studies, SISSA, Trieste), and T. R. Vidyasagar (Australian National University).

I am very grateful to my collaborators on the most recent research work, including: M. Booth, R. Bowtell, A. Browning, H. Critchley, S. Francis, P. Georges-François, F. McGlone, T. Milward, S. Panzeri, and Robert Robertson, who have agreed to include recent material in this book, at a time when part of it has not yet been published in research journals. In addition, I have benefited enormously from the discussions I have had with a large number of colleagues and friends, many of whom I hope will see areas of the text which they have been able to illuminate. Especial thanks are due to A. Treves, M. Stamp Dawkins, and M. Davies, for guiding me to new areas of scientific and philosophical enquiry. Much of the work described would not have been possible without financial support from a number of sources, particularly the Medical Research Council of the UK, the Human Frontier Science Program, the McDonnell-Pew Foundation for Cognitive Neuroscience, and the Commission of the European Communities.

Oxford   E. T. R.
April 1998

Contents

1 Introduction

1.1 Introduction

What motivates us to work for particular rewards such as food when we are hungry, or water when we are thirsty? How do these motivational control systems operate to ensure that we eat approximately the correct amount of food to maintain our body weight or to replenish our thirst? What factors account for the over-eating and obesity which some humans show? The issues of what motivation is, and how it is controlled, are introduced in this chapter.

What are emotions? Why do we have emotions? What are the rules by which emotion operates? What are the brain mechanisms of emotion, and how can disorders of emotion be understood? Why does it feel like something to have an emotion? This is the issue of consciousness. In fact, why do some aspects of what the brain does feel like something, whereas other aspects do not? Why is the brain built to have reward, and punishment, systems, rather than in some other way? This issue of brain design and why we have reward and punishment systems, and emotion and motivation, produces a fascinating answer based on how genes can direct our behaviour to increase their fitness. How does the brain produce behaviour by using reward, and punishment, mechanisms? These are some of the questions considered in this book.

The major approach taken is of understanding emotion and motivation, and their underlying reward and punishment systems, in terms of the brain mechanisms that implement them. Understanding the brain processing and mechanisms of behaviour is one way to ensure that we have the correct explanation for how the behaviour is produced. But at the same time, with issues such as emotion and motivation, and reward and punishment, it is interesting to open up the approach from 'how?' to 'why?', which is the type of question that can be approached from the perspectives of evolutionary biology and neural network engineering.

A major reason for investigating the actual brain mechanisms that underlie emotion and motivation, and reward and punishment, is not only to understand how our own brains work, but also to have the basis for understanding and treating medical disorders of these systems. It is because of the intended relevance to humans that emphasis is placed on research in non-human primates. It turns out that many of the brain systems that are involved in emotion and motivation have undergone considerable development in primates. For example, the temporal lobe has undergone great development in primates, and several systems in the temporal lobe are either involved in emotion (e.g. the amygdala), or provide some of the main sensory inputs to brain systems involved in emotion and motivation. The prefrontal cortex has also undergone great development in primates, and one part of it, the orbitofrontal cortex, is very little developed in rodents, yet is one of the major brain areas involved in emotion and motivation in primates including humans. The development of some of these brain areas has been so great in primates that even evolutionarily old systems such as the taste system appear to have been rewired, compared with that of rodents, to place much more emphasis on cortical processing, taking place in areas such as the orbitofrontal cortex (see Chapter 2). The principle of the stage of sensory processing at which reward value is extracted and made explicit in the representation may even have changed between rodents and primates, in, for example, the taste system (see Chapter 2). In primates, there has also been great development of the visual system, and this itself has had important implications for the types of sensory stimuli that are processed by brain systems involved in emotion and motivation. One example is the importance of face identity and face expression decoding, which are both important in primate emotional behaviour, and indeed provide an important part of the foundation for much primate social behaviour. These are among the reasons why emphasis is placed on brain systems in primates, including humans, in the approach taken here. The overall medically relevant aim of the research described in this book is to provide a foundation for understanding the brain mechanisms of emotion and motivation, and thus their disorders including depression, anxiety, and addiction in humans.

When considering brain mechanisms involved in emotion in primates, recent findings with the human brain-imaging approaches are described. These approaches including functional magnetic resonance imaging (fMRI) to measure changes in brain oxygenation level locally (using a signal from deoxyhaemoglobin) to provide an index of local brain activity, as well as positron emission tomography (PET) studies to estimate local regional cerebral blood flow, again to provide an index of local brain activity. It is, however, important to note that these approaches provide rather coarse approaches to brain function, in that the spatial resolution is seldom better than 2 mm, so that the picture given is one of 'blobs on the brain', which give some indication of what is happening where in the brain, and what types of dissociation of functions are possible. However, because there are tens of millions of neurons in the areas that can be resolved, such imaging techniques give rather little evidence on *how* the brain works. For this, one needs to know what information is represented in each brain area at the level at which information is exchanged between the computing elements of the brain, the neurons. One also needs to know how the representation of information changes from stage to stage of the processing in the brain, to understand how the system works. It turns out that one can read this information from the brain by recording the activity of single neurons, or groups of single neurons. The reason that this is an effective procedure for understanding what is represented is that each neuron has one information output channel, the firing of its action potentials, so that one can measure the full richness of the information being represented in a region by measuring the firing of its neurons. This can reveal fundamental evidence crucial for understanding how the brain operates. For example, neuronal recording can reveal all the information represented in an area even if parts of it are encoded by relatively small numbers, perhaps a few percent, of its neurons. (This is impossible with brain-imaging techniques, which also are susceptible to the interpretation problem that whatever causes the largest activation is interpreted as 'what' is being encoded in a region). Neuronal recording also provides evidence for the level at which it is appropriate to build computational models of brain function, the neuronal network level.

Such neuronal network computational models consider how populations of neurons with the connections found in a given brain area, and with biologically plausible properties such as local learning rules for altering the strengths of synaptic connections between neurons, actually could perform useful computation to implement the functions being performed by that area. This approach should not really be considered as a metaphor for brain operation, but as a theory of how each part of the brain operates. The neuronal network computational theory, and any model or simulation based on it, may of course be simplified to some extent to make it tractable, but nevertheless the point is that the neuron-level approach, coupled with neuronal network models, together provide some of the fundamental elements for understanding how the brain actually works. For this reason, emphasis is also placed in this book on what is known about what is being processed in each brain area as shown by recordings from neurons. Such evidence, in terms of building theories and models of how the brain functions, can never be replaced by brain imaging evidence, although these approaches do complement each other very effectively. The approach to brain function in terms of computations performed by neuronal networks in different brain areas is the subject of the book 'Neural Networks and Brain Function' by Rolls and Treves (1998). (When Rolls is the first-named author of a reference this is always E. T. Rolls unless indicated otherwise.) The reader is referred to that for a more comprehensive account of this biologically plausible approach to brain function. In this book, the neurophysiological evidence on which the full computational account of brain mechanisms of emotion and motivation must be based is described, but the way in which the neuronal networks might perform these functions is reserved mainly for the Appendix, and is provided more comprehensively in the book by Rolls and Treves (1998). The intention is that Rolls and Treves (1998) and this book taken together provide a foundation for understanding the operation and functions of a wide range of interconnected brain systems.

1.2 Definitions of reward, punishment, classical conditioning, stimulus–reinforcement association, instrumental learning

Short descriptions and definitions of the above terms are given as they will be referred to throughout this book.

A **reward** is something for which an animal will work. A **punishment** is something an animal will work to escape or avoid. In order to exclude simple reflex-like behaviour, the concept invoked here by the term work is to perform an arbitrary behaviour (called an **operant response**) in order to obtain the reward or avoid the punishment. An example of an operant response might be pressing a lever in a Skinner box, or putting money in a vending machine to obtain food. Thus **motivated behaviour** is present when an animal (including of course a human) will perform an arbitrary operant response to obtain a reward or to escape from or avoid a punishment. This definition implies that learned responses are important in demonstrating motivated behaviour, and indeed two types of learning, classical conditioning and instrumental learning, that are important in motivated behaviour, will be described next.

A fundamental operation of most nervous systems is to learn to associate a first stimulus with a second which occurs at about the same time, and to retrieve from memory the second stimulus (or its consequences) when the first is presented. The first stimulus might be the sight of an object (which happens to be a new food, or to signify that food is about to be delivered), and the second stimulus the taste of food. After the association has been learned, the sight of food would enable its taste to be retrieved. In **classical conditioning**, the taste of food (the **unconditioned stimulus**) might elicit an unconditioned response of salivation, and if the sight of the food is paired with its taste, then the sight of that food would by learning come to produce salivation, and would become a **conditioned stimulus** for the **conditioned response** of salivation. Classical conditioning is usually of autonomic responses, of which salivation, a response studied by Pavlov, is an example. The fundamental property though of classical conditioning is that the conditioned stimulus and the unconditioned stimulus are paired (optimally with the conditioned stimulus just before the unconditioned stimulus), and there is no voluntary or instrumental response that the animal can make to influence the pairing. However, it is the case that usually the unconditioned stimuli in classical conditioning can act as rewards or punishments, that is, as we will see in a moment, they are usually reinforcers.

An identical operational procedure, of pairing the sight of an object with a reward or punishment, may lead to other outputs or states than only autonomic. For example, if a tone is paired with footshock, then the emotional state of fear will be produced by the tone. The state of fear may have a number of consequences, including motivating the animal to escape from the tone and if possible avoid the shock. Thus we can think of emotional states as being learned by a process that is like classical conditioning (Weiskrantz, 1968). It is convenient to think of this type of learning as involving association to primary or unlearned reinforcers (such as pain), as this type of learning appears to be performed by particular brain systems, as described in Chapter 4. We call this learning **stimulus–reinforcement association** learning. (This is the term that has been used in the literature. A more accurate term might actually be stimulus–reinforcer association learning, because the learning is of an association between one stimulus and another stimulus which is a reinforcer.) The conditioned stimulus can be called a secondary reinforcer. If the association is between a third stimulus and a stimulus which is already a secondary reinforcer, the brain systems involved may be different to those involved in learning associations to primary reinforcers (see Chapter 4). (Note that stimulus–reinforcement association learning is to be clearly distinguished from stimulus–response, S–R, or habit learning, in which the association is to a response, and in which other brain systems are implicated—see Rolls and Treves 1998, Chapter 9.)

Another type of learning is **instrumental learning**, in which what the animal does alters the outcome. An example might be learning to press a lever when a tone sounds in order to avoid a shock. Here the arbitrary instrumental response of pressing the lever is instrumental in affecting whether the shock will be given. In this type of learning, **instrumental reinforcers** are stimuli which if their occurrence, termination, or omission is made contingent upon the making of a response, alter the probability of the future emission of that response (as a result of the contingency on the response). Some stimuli are unlearned instrumental reinforcers (e.g. the taste of food if the animal is hungry, or pain); while others may become reinforcing by learning, because of their association with such primary reinforcers, thereby becoming 'secondary reinforcers'. The type of learning that enables previously neutral stimuli to develop instrumentally reinforcing properties may thus be called 'stimulus-reinforcement association', and probably actually occurs via a process like that of classical conditioning as described above. It is a form of pattern association between two stimuli, one of which is a primary reinforcer, and the other of which becomes a secondary reinforcer (see Rolls and Treves 1998). If a reinforcer increases the probability of emission of a response on which it is contingent, it is said to be a 'positive reinforcer' or 'reward'; if it reduces the probability of such a response it is a 'negative reinforcer' or 'punisher'. (It is strictly the operation performed by punishers that is referred to as punishment.) For example, fear is an emotional state which might be produced by a sound that has previously been associated with an electric shock. Shock in this example is the primary negative reinforcer, and fear is the emotional state which occurs to the tone stimulus as a result of the learning of the stimulus (i.e. tone) -reinforcer (i.e. shock) association. The tone in this example is a conditioned stimulus because of classical conditioning, and has secondary reinforcing properties in that responses will be made to escape from it and thus avoid the primary reinforcer of shock.

The converse reinforcement contingencies produce the opposite effects on behaviour. The omission or termination of a positive reinforcer ('extinction' and 'time out' respectively, sometimes described as 'punishing'), reduce the probability of responses. Responses followed by the omission or termination of a negative reinforcer (or punisher) increase in probability, this pair of reinforcement operations being termed 'active avoidance' and 'escape' respectively. A further discussion of some of the terminology and processes involved in animal learning is provided by J. Gray (1975, Chapter 4); Mackintosh (1983, pp. 19–21); Dickinson (1980); and Pearce (1996).

1.3 Reward, punishment, emotion, and motivation

It may be useful to make it clear why the brain mechanisms of both emotion and motivation (with the examples of motivated behaviour considered being hunger, thirst, and sexual behaviour) are being considered together in this book. The reason is that for both emotion and motivation, rewards and punishments are assessed in order to provide the goals for behaviour. Operation of the brain to evaluate rewards and punishers is the fundamental solution of the brain to interfacing sensory systems to action selection and execution systems. Computing the reward and punishment value of sensory stimuli, and then using selection between different rewards and avoidance of punishments in a common reward-based currency appears to be the fundamental design that brains use in order to produce appropriate behaviour (see Chapter 10). The behaviour selected can be thought of as appropriate in the sense that it is based on the sensory systems and reward decoding that our genes specify (through the process of natural selection) in order to maximize their fitness (reproductive potential). Having reward and punishment systems is the solution that evolution has developed to produce appropriate behaviour. It happens that motivational and emotional behaviour are the types of behaviour in which rewards and punishers operate. (An unimportant distinction here is that motivated behaviour often refers to behaviour where the initiating stimulus is internal, for example cellular dehydration producing thirst; whereas emotional behaviour often refers to behaviour where the initiating stimulus is external, for example a painful stimulus on the leg.)

Considering both emotional and motivational behaviour in this book means that we can look for the principles that underlie the decoding of many types of rewarding and punishing stimulus. We can also see to some extent how the common currency of reward works to enable different rewards to be compared, and in particular how the reward value of all the different potential rewards that our genes specify is kept within a comparable range, so that we select different behaviours as appropriate. That is, we can examine many of the different ways in which the reward value of different sensory stimuli is modulated, both by internal signals as physiological needs are satisfied, and in addition to some extent by sensory-specific satiety (the mechanism by which repeating one reward causes it gradually to decrease its reward value somewhat, assisting the selection of other rewards in the environment).

However, perhaps the most important reason for treating reward and punishment systems, and the brain systems dealing with rewards and punishers, together is that we can develop an overall theory of how this set of issues, which might sometimes appear mysterious, is actually at the heart of brain design. Much of sensory processing, at least through the brain systems that are concerned with object identification (whether by sight, sound, smell, taste, or touch), can be seen to have the goal of enabling the correct reward value to be decoded and represented *after* the object has been identified. This means for example that in vision, invariant representations of objects must be formed, and encoded in an appropriate way for the brain to decode their reward value in a pattern associator in which the same object has been associated with a primary (unlearned) reinforcer. The actual motivational and emotional parts of the processing, the parts where the reward or punishment value is made explicit in the representation, should indeed no longer be seen as mysterious or perhaps superfluous aspects of brain processing. Instead, they are at the heart of which behavioural actions are selected, and how they are selected. Moreover, a large part of the brain's action and motor systems can be seen as having the goal in systems design of producing behaviour that will obtain the rewards decoded from sensory (and memory) inputs by the motivational and emotional systems of the brain. In particular, the implication is that the action systems for implicit behaviour have as part of their design principle the property that they will perform actions to optimize the output of the reward and punishment systems involved in motivation and emotion. Put another way, the brain systems involved in motivation and emotion must pass reward or punishment signals to the action systems, which must be built to attempt to obtain and maximize the reward signals being received; to switch behaviour from one reward to another as the reward values being received alter; and to switch behaviour also if signals indicating possible punishment are received (see Chapters 4, 6, and 10).

This book is thus intended to uncover some of the most important and fundamental aspects and principles of brain function and design. The book is also intended to show that the way in which the brain works in motivation and emotion can be seen to be the result of natural selection operating to select genes which optimize our behaviour by building into us the appropriate reward and punishment systems, and the appropriate rules for the operation of these systems.

The plan of the book is that we consider in Chapter 2 the control of food intake, for research in this area provides fundamental evidence about how rewards are processed in the taste, olfactory, and visual systems, and how the brain alters the reward value that sensory stimuli have by internal signals. Further evidence on the role of internal signals in modulating the reward value of sensory stimuli to produce motivated behaviour is left until Chapter 7, when brain mechanisms for thirst are described. Before that, in Chapters 3 and 4, we start on the major issue of emotion, and its brain mechanisms. A theory of emotion and its functions is described in Chapter 3 to provide a basis for a systematic understanding of the brain mechanisms of emotion described in Chapter 4. In Chapter 5, the issue of brain systems involved in reward is pursued further through an analysis of the mechanisms of reward produced by brain stimulation. In Chapter 6, the pharmacology of brain-stimulation reward is considered, and this leads towards an understanding of some of the brain mechanisms involved in drug addiction. Considering these issues leads us in Chapter 6 to a discussion of how reward systems interface to action selection and execution systems in brain systems such as the basal ganglia. In Chapter 8 we return to another example of motivated behaviour, sexual behaviour, and consider the brain reward systems that may be involved in this. In Chapter 9 the issues of emotional feelings, and of the brain processing involved in conscious feelings, are considered. In Chapter 10, many of the themes of the book are brought together in a consideration of why and how the brain is built to operate using reward and punishment systems, and of some of the broader implications of this design. The Appendix describes more formally the operation of some of the neuronal networks implicated in emotion and motivation.

2   The brain control of feeding and reward

2.1   Introduction

In this chapter and Chapter 7 we consider the rewards relevant to drives such as eating and drinking. In these cases there are internal signals which indicate that there is a need for food or water. The food or water are rewards, in that the organism will work to obtain the food or water. The signals that make the food or water rewarding originate internally. In the case of hunger, the internal signals reflect the state of energy balance, reflecting stimuli such as plasma glucose and gastric distension. In the case of thirst, the internal signals reflect the volumes of the cellular and extracellular fluids. In both cases the hunger and thirst operate to maintain the constancy of the internal milieu. The signals operate to alter the reward value which food or water has for the hungry or thirsty organism. The reward signals are conveyed primarily by the taste, smell, and sight of food or water. In this chapter we will consider where in information processing in these sensory systems the sensory stimulation produced by food (or, similarly, water) is decoded not just as a physical stimulus, but is coded in terms of its reward value. An important aspect of brain organization is that these two aspects of information processing are kept separate, at least in primates including humans. Another important aspect of brain organization for these types of reward is that the learning of which visual stimuli are food or water, or are associated with food or water, takes places in specialized parts for the brain for this type of learning. This learning takes place in the brain after analysis of what the stimulus is.

In this chapter reward systems related to the drive of hunger are considered, where the origin of the drive is of internal, homeostatic, origin. In Chapter 7, the systems that control thirst are described. These systems operate analogously to those involved in the control of feeding, although in the case of thirst the actual stimuli that initiate the thirst and drinking are relatively simple and prescribed, and so the precise way in which these signals control the motivated behaviour can be analysed quite precisely. For comparison, in Chapter 8 we consider the processing of rewards relevant to sexual behaviour, in which the conditions that initiate the drive are not simply homeostatic to maintain the internal milieu.

2.2   Peripheral signals for hunger and satiety

To understand how food intake is controlled, we first consider the functions of the different peripheral factors (i.e. factors outside the brain) such as taste, smell, and gastric distension, and the control signals, such as the amount of glucose in the blood. We focus particularly on which sensory inputs produce reward, and on which inputs act as hunger or satiety signals to modulate the reward value of the sensory inputs. Then we consider how the brain integrates these different signals, learns about which stimuli in the environment

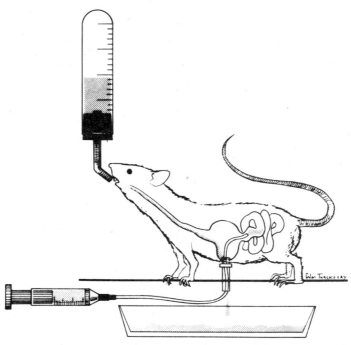

Fig. 2.1 Sham feeding preparation. Food can be tasted, smelled and ingested normally, but then it drains from the stomach so that gastric distension and other gastrointestinal factors are not produced. The diagram also shows a cannula entering the duodenum, so that the role of intestinal factors in eating can be studied by infusions of for example potential satiety–producing substances.

provide food, and how the brain initiates behaviour to obtain the correct variety and amount of food.

The functions of some different peripheral signals in the control of eating can be revealed with the sham feeding preparation shown in Fig. 2.1. In this situation, the animal can taste, smell, and eat the food normally, but the food drains from the stomach, so that no distension of the stomach occurs, and nor does any food enter the intestine for absorption. It is found that rats, monkeys, and humans will work to obtain food when they are sham feeding. This finding for primates is demonstrated in Fig. 2.2. This shows that it is the taste and smell of food which provide the immediate reward for food-motivated behaviour. Consistent with this, humans rate the taste and smell of food as being pleasant when they are hungry (see Section 2.3.1).

A second important aspect of sham feeding is that satiety (reduction of appetite) does not occur—instead rats and monkeys continue to eat for often more than an hour when they can taste and smell food normally, but food drains from the stomach, so that it does not accumulate in the stomach and enter the intestine (see, e.g., Fig. 2.2) (see classical literature reviewed by Grossman 1967; Gibbs, Maddison and Rolls 1981). We can conclude that taste and smell, and even swallowing food, do not produce satiety. There is an important psychological point here—reward itself does not produce satiety. Instead, the satiety for feeding is produced by food accumulating in the stomach, and entering the

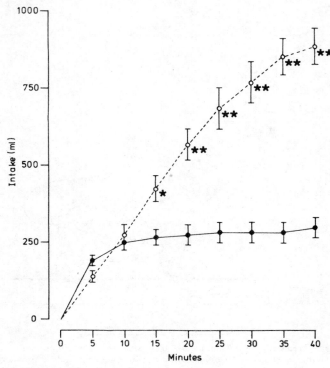

Fig. 2.2 Sham feeding in the monkey. The cumulative intakes of food with normal feeding (gastric cannula closed, closed circles), and with the gastric cannula open (open circles) allowing drainage of food from the stomach, are shown. The stars indicate significant differences between the open and closed gastric cannula conditions. (From Gibbs, Maddison and Rolls 1981.)

intestine. Evidence that gastric distension is an important satiety signal is that if an animal is allowed to eat to normal satiety, and then the food is drained through a cannula from the stomach, then the animal starts eating again immediately (Gibbs *et al.* 1981). Evidence that food entering the intestine can produce satiety is that small infusions of food into the duodenum (the first part of the intestine) reduce sham feeding (Gibbs *et al.* 1981). It is also interesting that food delivered directly into the stomach, or even glucose intravenously, is not very rewarding, in that animals learn only with difficulty to perform a response to obtain an intragastric or intravenous infusion of food or fluid (Nicolaidis and Rowland 1976, 1977, 1975). This emphasizes the point that the taste, smell, and sight of food are what normally provide the reward, and correspondingly the pleasant sensation, associated with eating.

These findings are summarized in Table 2.1.

Important conclusions about reward and its relation to hunger and satiety signals follow from what has just been described. First, reward and satiety are different processes. Second, reward is produced by oropharyngeal sensory signals such as the taste and smell of food. Third, satiety is produced by gastric, intestinal, and eventually other signals after the food is absorbed from the intestine. Fourth, hunger and satiety signals modulate the

Table 2.1
Summary of functions of peripheral signals in feeding

	Reinforcement	Satiety
Oropharyngeal factors	Yes	No (though contribute to sensory-specific satiety)
Gastric and intestinal factors	No	Yes

reward value of food (in that the taste and smell of food are rewarding when hunger signals are present and satiety signals are not present). In more general and psychological terminology, motivational state modulates the reward or reinforcement value of sensory stimuli. Fifth, given that reward and satiety are produced by different peripheral signals, one function of brain (i.e. central) processes in the control of feeding is to bring together satiety and reward signals in such a way that satiety modulates the reward value of food.

One of the aims of this chapter is to show how the brain processes sensory stimuli which can produce rewards for animals, where in the brain the reward value of such sensory stimuli is represented, and where and how the motivational signals which reflect hunger modulate this processing as part of the reward-decoding process. Of crucial interest in understanding the rules of operation of this reward system will therefore be where and how in the brain gastric and other satiety signals are brought together with taste and smell signals of food, to produce a taste/smell reward signal which is modulated by satiety.

2.3 The control signals for hunger and satiety

There is a set of different signals that each plays a role in determining the level of hunger vs satiety. These signals must all be integrated by the brain, and must then modulate how rewarding the sensory inputs such as the sight, taste, and smell of food are. These signals that influence hunger and satiety are summarized next, taken to some extent in the order in which they are activated in a meal.

2.3.1 Sensory-specific satiety

During experiments on brain mechanisms of reward and satiety Rolls and colleagues observed that if a lateral hypothalamic neuron had ceased to respond to a food on which the monkey had been fed to satiety, then the neuron might still respond to a different food (see example in Fig. 2.10 and Section 2.4.1.2). This occurred for neurons with responses associated with the taste (Rolls 1981b; Rolls, Murzi *et al.* 1986) or sight (Rolls and Rolls 1982; Rolls, Murzi *et al.* 1986) of food. (When Rolls is the first-named author of a reference this is always E. T. Rolls unless indicated otherwise.) Corresponding to this neuronal specificity of the effects of feeding to satiety, the monkey rejected the food on which he had been fed to satiety, but accepted other foods which he had not been fed.

As a result of these neurophysiological and behavioural observations showing the specificity of satiety in the monkey, and following up also an experiment by LeMagnen

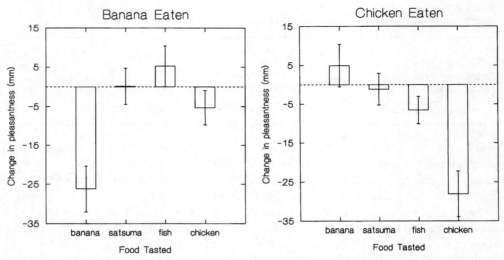

Fig. 2.3 Sensory-specific satiety for the flavour of a food: the changes in the pleasantness of the taste of four different foods after eating banana (left) or chicken (right) to satiety are shown. The change is shown as mm difference ($\pm$ the standard error of the mean, sem) on a 100 mm visual analogue rating scale marked at one end 'very pleasant' and at the other end 'very unpleasant'. (From Rolls and Rolls 1997.)

(1956) in which he had shown that rats drank more water if several tubes of water each had a different odour added to the water, we performed experiments to determine whether satiety in humans is specific to foods eaten. It was found that the pleasantness of the taste of food eaten to satiety decreased more than for foods that had not been eaten (B. Rolls, Rolls, Rowe and Sweeney 1981a). An example of the results of an experiment of this type are shown in Fig. 2.3. One implication of this finding is that if one food is eaten to satiety, appetite reduction for other foods is often incomplete, and this should mean that in humans also at least some of the other foods will be eaten. This has been confirmed by an experiment in which either sausages or cheese with crackers were eaten for lunch. The liking for the food eaten decreased more than for the food not eaten and, when an unexpected second course was offered, more was eaten if a subject had not been given that food in the first course than if he had been given that food in the first course (98% vs 40% of the first course intake eaten in the second courses, $P < 0.01$, B. Rolls *et al.* 1981a). A further implication of these findings is that if a variety of foods is available, the total amount consumed will be more than when only one food is offered repeatedly. This prediction has been confirmed in a study in which humans ate more when offered a variety of sandwich fillings than one filling or a variety of types of yoghurt which differed in taste, texture, and colour (B. Rolls, Rowe, Rolls, Kingston, Megson and Gunary 1981b). It has also been confirmed in a study in which humans were offered a relatively normal meal of four courses, and it was found that the change of food at each course significantly enhanced intake (B. Rolls, Van Duijenvoorde and Rolls 1984). Because sensory factors such as similarity of colour, shape, flavour, and texture are usually more important than metabolic equivalence in terms of protein, carbohydrate, and fat content in influencing how foods interact in this type of satiety, it has been termed 'sensory-specific satiety' (Rolls and Rolls 1977, 1982; B. Rolls, Rolls, Rowe and Sweeney 1981a; B. Rolls, Rowe, Rolls, Kingston, Megson and Gunary 1981b; B. Rolls, Rowe and Rolls 1982a,b; B. Rolls 1990). It should be noted that this effect is distinct from alliesthesia, in that alliesthesia is a change in the pleasantness of sensory inputs produced by internal signals (such as glucose in the gut) (see Cabanac and Duclaux 1970; Cabanac 1971; Cabanac and Fantino 1977), whereas sensory-specific satiety is a change in the pleasantness of sensory inputs which is accounted for at least partly by the external sensory stimulation received (such as the taste of a particular food), in that as shown above it is at least partly specific to the external sensory stimulation received.

The parallel between these studies of feeding in humans and of the neurophysiology of hypothalamic neurons in the monkey has been extended by the observations that in humans, sensory-specific satiety occurs for the sight (B. Rolls, Rowe and Rolls 1982a) and smell (Rolls and Rolls 1997) as well as for the taste and even texture (B. Rolls *et al.* 1982a) of food. Further, to complement the finding that in the hypothalamus neurons are found which respond differently to food and to water (see Fig. 2.11, Rolls and colleagues, unpublished observations), and that satiety with water can reduce the responsiveness of hypothalamic neurons which respond to water, it has been shown that in humans motivation-specific satiety can also be detected. For example, satiety with water reduces the pleasantness of the sight and taste of water but not of food (Rolls, Rolls and Rowe 1983a).

Some sensory-specific satiety can be produced just by tasting or even smelling a food for a few minutes, without swallowing any of it (Rolls and Rolls 1997; see Fig. 2.4). This shows that just the presence of neuronal activity produced by the taste or the smell of food is sufficient to reduce the firing of neurons which represent the pleasantness of the taste or smell of food. This can occur to some extent even without gastric and post-gastric factors such as gastric distension and intestinal stimulation by food. This indicates that this aspect of sensory-specific satiety can be produced by firing that is sustained for a few minutes in neurons in the pathway. Moreover, the decline in neuronal responsiveness must be at a late stage of the processing of the taste and probably the olfactory signals, in that just smelling the food for several minutes produces much more of a reduction in the pleasantness than in the intensity of the odour, and just tasting the food for several minutes produces much more of a decrease in the pleasantness than in the intensity of the taste (Rolls and Rolls 1997). It should be noticed that this decrease in the pleasantness of the sensory stimulation produced by a food only occurs if the sensory stimulation is repeated for several minutes. It has the adaptive value of changing the behaviour after a significant amount of that behaviour has been performed. In contrast, the reward value of sensory stimulation may increase over the first short period (of the order of a minute). This is called incentive motivation or the salted-nut phenomenon. It has the adaptive value that once a behaviour has been initiated, it will tend to continue for at least a little while. This is much more adaptive than continually switching behaviour, which has at least some cost in terms of efficiency, and might have a high cost if the different rewards are located far apart. The increase in the rate of behaviour, for example in the rate of feeding in the first part of a meal, probably reflects this effect. It was observed that this typical

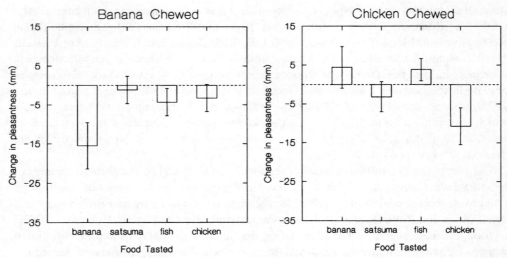

Fig. 2.4 The change in the pleasantness of the taste of four different foods after chewing banana (left) or chicken (right) for five minutes. Conventions as in Fig. 2.3. (From Rolls and Rolls 1997.)

increase in the rate of working for a reward early on in a meal was not found in rats with amygdala lesions (Rolls and Rolls 1973), and this implies that part of the mechanism for the increasing hedonic value of a food reward is implemented, at least in the rat, in the amygdala. Associated with this lack of increase in the rate of feeding early on in the meal, in the rat the meal pattern was disturbed. Instead of short rapid meals following by a bout of drinking and then other activity, the rats had long periods in which slow feeding and drinking were interspersed. This emphasizes the suggested function of the reward facilitation normally seen at the start of a period of rewarding sensory stimulation.

The enhanced eating when a variety of foods is available, as a result of the operation of sensory-specific satiety, may have been advantageous in evolution in ensuring that different foods with important different nutrients were consumed, but today in humans, when a wide variety of foods is readily available, it may be a factor which can lead to overeating and obesity. In a test of this in the rat, it has been found that variety itself can lead to obesity (B. Rolls *et al.* 1983; see further B. Rolls and Hetherington 1989).

Advances in understanding the neurophysiological mechanisms of sensory-specific satiety are being made in analyses of information processing in the taste and olfactory systems, as described below.

In addition to the sensory-specific satiety described above which operates primarily during the meal (see above) and during the post-meal period (B. Rolls, Van Duijenvoorde and Rolls 1984), there is now evidence for a long-term form of sensory-specific satiety (Rolls and de Waal 1985). This was shown in a study in an Ethiopian refugee camp, in which it was found that refugees who had been in the camp for 6 months found the taste of their three regular foods less pleasant than that of three comparable foods which they had not been eating. The effect was a long-term form of sensory-specific satiety in that it was not found in refugees who had been in the camp and eaten the regular foods for two days (Rolls and de Waal 1985). It is suggested that it is important to recognize the operation of long-term sensory-specific satiety in conditions such as these, for it may enhance malnutrition if the regular foods become less acceptable and so are rejected, exchanged for other less nutritionally effective foods or goods, or are inadequately prepared. It may be advantageous in these circumstances to attempt to minimize the operation of long-term sensory-specific satiety by providing some variety, perhaps even with spices (Rolls and de Waal 1985).

2.3.2 Gastric distension

This is one of the signals that is normally necessary for satiety, as shown by the experiment in which gastric drainage of food after a meal leads to the immediate resumption of eating (Gibbs, Maddison and Rolls 1981). Gastric distension only builds up if the pyloric sphincter closes. The pyloric sphincter controls the emptying of the stomach into the next part of the gastrointestinal tract, the duodenum. The sphincter closes only when food reaches the duodenum, stimulating chemosensors and osmosensors to regulate the action of the sphincter, by both local neural circuits and by hormones, in what is called the enterogastric loop (see Gibbs *et al.* 1981; Gibbs, Fauser, Rowe, Rolls, Rolls and Maddison 1979).

2.3.3 Duodenal chemosensors

The duodenum contains receptors sensitive to the chemical composition of the food draining from the stomach. One set of receptors responds to glucose, and can contribute to satiety via the vagus nerve, which carries signals to the brain. The evidence that the vagus is the pathway is that cutting the vagus nerve (vagotomy) abolishes the satiating effects of glucose infusions into the duodenum. Fats infused into the duodenum can also produce satiety, but in this case the link to the brain may be hormonal (a hormone is a blood-borne signal), for vagotomy does not abolish the satiating effect of fat infusions into the duodenum (see Greenberg, Smith and Gibbs 1990; Mei 1993).

2.3.4 Glucostatic hypothesis

There are many lines of evidence, summarized next, that one signal that controls appetite is the concentration of glucose circulating in the plasma—we eat in order to maintain glucostasis, i.e. constancy of glucose in the internal milieu. More accurately, the actual signal appears to be the utilization of glucose by the body and brain—if the arterial minus the venous concentration is low, indicating that the body is not extracting much glucose from the bloodstream, then we feel hungry and eat; and if the utilization measured in this way is high, we feel satiated. Consistent with this correlation between glucose and eating, there is a small reduction in plasma glucose concentration just before the onset of meals in rats, suggesting that the decreasing glucose concentration initiates a meal (Campfield and Smith 1990) (see Fig. 2.5). At the end of a meal, plasma glucose concentrations (and insulin, which helps the glucose to be used by cells) increase. A second line of evidence is

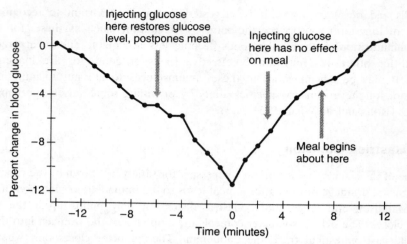

Fig. 2.5 Alterations in plasma glucose concentration that occur just before the onset of a meal in rats. (After Campfield and Smith 1990.)

that injections of insulin which reduce the concentration of glucose in the plasma (by facilitating its entry to cells and storage as fat), provoke food intake. Third, 2-Deoxyglucose, a competitive inhibitor of glucose metabolism, elicits feeding. Fourth, infusions of glucose and insulin can reduce feeding. Fifth, the brain's monitoring system for glucose availability seems to be in the area postrema in the medulla (part of the brainstem), for infusions there of a competitive inhibitor of glucose, 5-thioglucose, elicit feeding (Ritter 1986).

It is worth noting that in diabetes (that is, diabetes mellitus), the cells can become insulin-resistant, so that in this condition it is difficult to interpret whatever plasma levels of glucose are present in terms of their possible role in hunger and satiety.

2.3.5 Body fat regulation—leptin or OB protein

The signals described so far would be appropriate for regulation on the meal-to-meal timescale, but might not be adequate for the longer term regulation of body weight, and in particular of body fat. So the search has been on for another signal that might affect appetite based on, for example, the amount of fat in the body. Recent research has uncovered a candidate hormone that performs this function. Some of the evidence is as follows (see Campfield *et al.* 1995):

First, OB protein or leptin is the hormone encoded by the mouse ob gene (here ob stands for obesity).

Second, genetically obese mice that are double recessive for the ob gene, and are hence designated as obob mice, produce no leptin.

Third, leptin reduces food intake in wild type (lean) mice (who have genes which are OBOB or OBob so that they produce leptin) and in obob mice (showing that obob mice have receptors sensitive to leptin).

Fourth, the satiety effect of leptin can be produced by injections into the brain.

Fifth, leptin does not produce satiety (reduce food intake) in another type of genetically obese mouse designated dbdb. These mice may be obese because they lack the leptin receptor, or mechanisms associated with it.

Sixth, leptin has a long time-course—it fluctuates over 24 h, but not in relation to individual meals. Thus it might be appropriate for the longer-term regulation of appetite.

Seventh, leptin is found in humans.

Eighth, leptin concentration may correlate with body weight/adiposity, consistent with the possibility that it is produced by fat cells, and can signal the total amount of body fat.

A hypothesis consistent with these findings is that a hormone, leptin, is produced in proportion to the amount of body fat, and that this is normally one of the signals that controls how much food is eaten.

2.3.6   Conditioned appetite and satiety

If we eat food containing much energy (e.g. rich in fat) for a few days, we gradually eat less of it. If we eat food containing little energy, we gradually, over days, ingest more of it. This regulation involves learning, learning to associate the sight, taste, smell, texture, etc., of the food with the energy that is released from it in the hours after it is eaten. This form of learning was demonstrated by Booth (1985) who, after several days of offering sandwiches with different energy content and flavours, on a test day offered subjects medium-energy sandwiches (so that the subjects could not select by the amount of energy in the food). The subjects ate few of the sandwiches if they had the flavour of the high-energy sandwiches eaten previously, and many of the sandwiches if they had the flavour of the low-energy sandwiches eaten previously.

2.4   The brain control of eating and reward

2.4.1   The hypothalamus
2.4.1.1   Effects of damage to the hypothalamus

From clinical evidence it has been known since early this century that damage to the base of the brain can influence food intake and body weight. Later it was demonstrated that one critical region is the ventromedial hypothalamus, for bilateral lesions here in animals led to hyperphagia and obesity (see Grossman 1967, 1973; Fig. 2.6). Then Anand and Brobeck (1951) discovered that bilateral lesions of the lateral hypothalamus can produce a

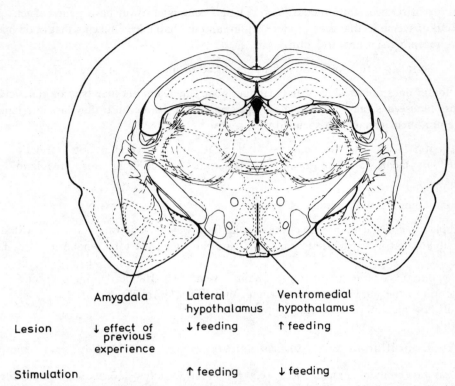

	Amygdala	Lateral hypothalamus	Ventromedial hypothalamus
Lesion	↓ effect of previous experience	↓ feeding	↑ feeding
Stimulation		↑ feeding	↓ feeding

Fig. 2.6 Coronal section through the rat hypothalamus showing the effects of lesions and stimulation of different hypothalamic regions on feeding.

reduction in feeding and body weight. Evidence of this type led in the 1950s and 1960s to the view that food intake is controlled by two interacting 'centres', a feeding centre in the lateral hypothalamus and a satiety centre in the ventromedial hypothalamus (see Stellar 1954; Grossman 1967, 1973; Fig. 2.6).

Soon, problems with this evidence for a dual-centre hypothesis of the control of food intake appeared. It appears that lesions of the ventromedial hypothalamus act indirectly to increase feeding. These lesions increase the secretion of insulin by the pancreas, this reduces plasma glucose concentration, and then feeding results. This mechanism is demonstrated by the finding that cutting the vagus nerve, which disconnects the brain from the pancreas, prevents ventromedial hypothalamic lesions from causing hypo-glycemia, and also prevents the overeating that otherwise occurs after ventromedial hypothalamic lesions (Bray *et al.* 1981). The ventromedial nucleus of the hypothalamus is thus thought of as a region which can influence the secretion of insulin and thus can indirectly influence body weight, but not as a satiety centre.

With regard to the lateral hypothalamus, a contribution to the reduced eating that follows lateral hypothalamic lesions arises from damage to fibre pathways coursing nearby, such as the dopaminergic nigro-striatal bundle. Damage to this pathway leads to motor and sensory deficits because it impairs the normal operation of the basal ganglia (striatum, globus pallidus, and substantia nigra), brain structures involved in the initiation and control of movement (Marshall *et al.* 1974). Thus by the middle 1970s it was clear that the lesion evidence for a lateral hypothalamic feeding center was not straightforward, for at least part of the effect of the lesions was due to damage to fibres of passage travelling through or near the lateral hypothalamus (Stricker and Zigmond 1976). It was thus not clear by this time what role the hypothalamus played in feeding. However, in more recent investigations it has been possible to damage the cells in the lateral hypothalamus without damaging fibres of passage, using locally injected neurotoxins such as ibotenic acid or *N*-methyl-D-aspartate (NMDA) (Winn *et al.* 1984; Dunnett *et al.* 1985; Clark *et al.* 1991). With these techniques, it has been shown that damage to lateral hypothalamic cells does produce a lasting decrease in food intake and body weight, and that this is not associated with dopamine depletion as a result of damage to dopamine pathways, or with the akinesia and sensorimotor deficits which are produced by damage to the dopamine systems (Winn *et al.* 1984; Dunnett *et al.* 1985; Clark *et al.* 1991). Moreover, the lesioned rats do not respond normally to experimental interventions which normally cause eating by reducing the availability of glucose (Clark *et al.* 1991). Thus the more recent lesion evidence does suggest that the lateral hypothalamus is involved in the control of feeding and body weight.

The evidence just described implicates the hypothalamus in the control of food intake and body weight, but does not show what functions important in feeding are being performed by the hypothalamus and by other brain areas. More direct evidence on the neural processing involved in feeding, based on recordings of the activity of single neurons in the hypothalamus and other brain regions is described next. These other brain systems include systems that perform sensory analysis involved in the control of feeding such as the taste and olfactory pathways; brain systems involved in learning about foods including the amygdala and orbitofrontal cortex; and brain systems involved in the initiation of feeding behaviour such as the striatum. Some of the brain regions and pathways described in the text are shown in Fig. 2.7 on a lateral view of the brain of the macaque monkey, and some of the connections are shown schematically in Fig. 2.8. Some of the findings described have been made in monkeys, because neuronal activity in non-human primates is especially relevant to understanding brain function and its disorders in humans.

2.4.1.2 Neuronal activity in the lateral hypothalamus during feeding

Hypothalamic neurons responsive to the sight, smell, and taste of food

It has been found that there is a population of neurons in the lateral hypothalamus and substantia innominata of the monkey with responses which are related to feeding (see Rolls 1981a,b, 1986c). These neurons, which comprised 13.6% in one sample of 764 hypothalamic neurons, respond to the taste and/or sight of food (Rolls, Burton and Mora, 1976). The neurons respond to taste in that they respond only when certain substances, such as glucose solution but not water or saline, are in the mouth, and in that their firing rates are related to the concentration of the substance to which they respond (Rolls, Burton and Mora 1980). These neurons did not respond simply in relation to mouth movements, and comprised 4.3% of the sample of 764 neurons. The responses of the

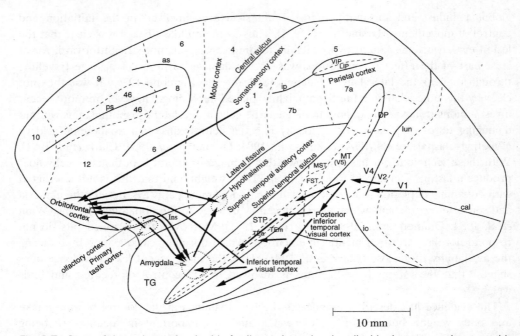

10 mm

Fig. 2.7 Some of the pathways involved in feeding and emotion described in the text are shown on this lateral view of the brain of the macaque monkey. Connections from the primary taste and olfactory cortices to the orbitofrontal cortex and amygdala are shown. Connections are also shown in the 'ventral visual system' from V1 to V2, V4, the inferior temporal visual cortex, etc., with some connections reaching the amygdala and orbitofrontal cortex. as, arcuate sulcus; cal, calcarine sulcus; cs, central sulcus; lf, lateral (or Sylvian) fissure; lun, lunate sulcus; ps, principal sulcus; io, inferior occipital sulcus; ip, intraparietal sulcus (which has been opened to reveal some of the areas it contains); sts, superior temporal sulcus (which has been opened to reveal some of the areas it contains). AIT, anterior inferior temporal cortex; FST, visual motion processing area; LIP, lateral intraparietal area; MST, visual motion processing area; MT, visual motion processing area (also called V5); PIT, posterior inferior temporal cortex; STP, superior temporal plane; TA, architectonic area including auditory association cortex; TE, architectonic area including high-order visual association cortex, and some of its sub-areas TEa and TEm; TG, architectonic area in the temporal pole; V1–V4, visual areas 1–4; VIP, ventral intraparietal area; TEO, architectonic area including posterior visual association cortex. The numerals refer to architectonic areas, and have the following approximate functional equivalence: 1,2,3, somatosensory cortex (posterior to the central sulcus); 4, motor cortex; 5, superior parietal lobule; 7a, inferior parietal lobule, visual part; 7b, inferior parietal lobule, somatosensory part; 6, lateral premotor cortex; 8, frontal eye field; 12, part of orbitofrontal cortex; 46, dorsolateral prefrontal cortex. (Modified from Rolls and Treves 1998.)

neurons associated with the sight of food occurred as soon as the monkey saw the food, before the food was in his mouth, and occurred only to foods and not to non-food objects (Rolls, Sanghera and Roper-Hall, 1979; Mora, Rolls and Burton, 1976b) (see example in Fig. 2.9). These neurons comprised 11.8% of the sample of 764 neurons (Rolls, Burton and Mora 1976, 1980). Some of these neurons (2.5% of the total sample) responded to both the sight and taste of food (Rolls *et al.* 1976, 1980). The finding that there are neurons in the lateral hypothalamus of the monkey which respond to the sight of food has been confirmed by Ono *et al.* (1980).

The discovery that there are neurons in the lateral hypothalamus that respond to the sight of food was an interesting discovery, for it emphasizes the importance in primates of vision, and not just generally but for motivational behaviour in the selection of a goal object such as food. Indeed, the sight of what we eat conveys important information that can influence not only whether we select the food but also how the food tastes to us. The hypothesis that the lateral hypothalamic neurons were involved in reward effects which the sight and taste of food might have by activating lateral hypothalamic neurons led to the next experiments which investigated whether these neurons only responded to the sight and taste of food when it was rewarding. The experiments involved reducing the reward value of the food by feeding as much of the food as was wanted, and then measuring whether the neurons still responded to the sight and taste of the food when it was no longer rewarding.

Effect of hunger

When Rolls and colleagues fed monkeys to satiety, they found that gradually the lateral hypothalamic neurons reduced the magnitude of their responses, until when the monkey was satiated the neurons did not respond at all to the sight and taste of food (Burton, Rolls and Mora 1976b; Rolls, Murzi, Yaxley, Thorpe and Simpson, 1986). An example is shown in Fig. 2.10. This finding provides evidence that these neurons have activity which is closely related to either or both autonomic responses (such as salivation to the sight of food) and behavioural responses (such as approach to a food reward) to the sight and taste of food, which only occur to food if hunger is present.

The signals which reflect the motivational state and perform this modulation probably include many of those described in Section 2.3, such as gastric distension and duodenal stimulation by food (e.g. Gibbs, Rolls and Maddison 1981) reach the nucleus of the solitary tract via the vagus as in rats (Ewart 1993; Mei 1993, 1994). The plasma glucose level may be sensed by cells in the hindbrain near the area postrema in the rat (Ritter 1986). In the monkey there is less evidence about the location of the crucial sites for glucose sensing that control food intake. It is known that there are glucose-sensitive neurons in a number of hindbrain and hypothalamic sites, as shown by micro-electro-osmotic experiments in which glucose is applied locally to a neuron being recorded by using a small current to draw out sodium ion which then drags glucose with it (Oomura and Yoshimatsu 1984; Aou et al. 1984).

The hypothalamus is not necessarily the first stage at which processing of food-related stimuli is modulated by hunger. Evidence on which is the first stage of processing where modulation by hunger occurs in primates is considered for the taste system below. To investigate whether hunger modulates neuronal responses in parts of the visual system through which visual information is likely to reach the hypothalamus (see below), the activity of neurons in the visual inferior temporal cortex was recorded in the same testing situations. It was found that the neuronal responses here to visual stimuli were not dependent on hunger (Rolls, Judge and Sanghera 1977). Nor were the responses of an initial sample of neurons in the amygdala, which connects the inferior temporal visual cortex to the hypothalamus (see below), found to depend on hunger (Sanghera, Rolls and Roper-Hall 1979; Rolls 1992b). However, in the orbitofrontal cortex, which receives inputs from the inferior temporal visual cortex, and projects into the hypothalamus (see below and Russchen et al. 1985), neurons with visual responses to food are found, and neuronal

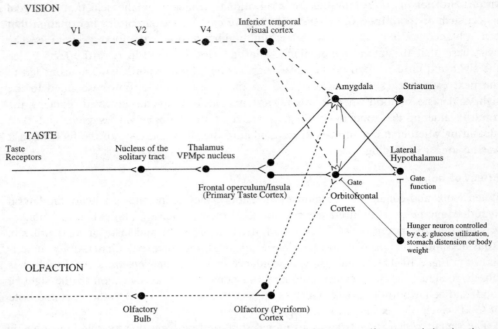

Fig. 2.8 Schematic diagram showing some of the connections of the taste, olfactory and visual pathways in the brain. V1, primary visual (striate) cortex; V2 and V4, further cortical visual areas.

responses to food in this region are modulated by hunger (Thorpe, Rolls and Maddison 1983; Critchley and Rolls, 1996b; see Sections 2.4.2.3, 2.4.4.2 and 2.4.5). Thus for visual processing, neuronal responsiveness only at late stages of sensory processing and in the hypothalamus has been found to be modulated by hunger. The adaptive value of modulation of sensory processing only at late stages of processing, which occurs also in the taste system of primates, is discussed when food-related taste processing is described below.

Sensory-specific modulation of the responsiveness of lateral hypothalamic neurons and of appetite

During these experiments on satiety it was observed that if a lateral hypothalamic neuron had ceased to respond to a food on which the monkey had been fed to satiety, then the neuron might still respond to a different food (see example in Fig. 2.10). This occurred for neurons with responses associated with the taste (Rolls 1981b; Rolls, Murzi, Yaxley, Thorpe and Simpson 1986) or sight (Rolls and Rolls 1982; Rolls *et al.* 1986) of food. Corresponding to this neuronal specificity of the effects of feeding to satiety, the monkey rejected the food on which he had been fed to satiety, but accepted other foods which he had not been fed. It was as a result of these neurophysiological discoveries that the experiments on sensory-specific satiety in humans described in Section 2.3.1 were performed.

In addition to sensory-specific satiety, it is also worth noting that the mechanism is motivation-specific, in that some hypothalamic neurons respond more to food, and others more to water, when the monkey is both hungry and thirsty (see Fig. 2.11). Feeding to satiety reduces the responses of neurons that respond to food, and drinking to satiety reduces the responses of neurons that respond to water (see Figs 2.10 and 7.7).

Effects of learning

The responses of these hypothalamic neurons in the primate become associated with the sight of food as a result of learning. This is shown by experiments in which the neurons come to respond to the sight of a previously neutral stimulus, such as a syringe, from which the monkey is fed orally; in which the neurons cease to respond to a stimulus if it is no longer associated with food (in extinction or passive avoidance); and in which the responses of these neurons remain associated with whichever visual stimulus is associated with food reward in a visual discrimination and its reversals (Mora, Rolls and Burton 1976b; Wilson and Rolls 1990). This type of learning is important for it enables organisms to respond appropriately to environmental stimuli which previous experience has shown are foods. The brain mechanisms for this type of learning are discussed below.

The responses of these neurons suggest that they are involved in responses to food. Further evidence for this is that the responses of these neurons occur with relatively short latencies of 150–200 ms, and thus precede and predict the responses of the hungry monkey to food (Rolls, Sanghera and Roper-Hall 1979) (see Fig. 2.9).

Evidence that the responses of these hypothalamic neurons are related to the reward value of food

Given that these hypothalamic neurons respond to food when it is rewarding, that is when the animal will work to obtain food, it is a possibility that their responses are related to the reward value which food has for the hungry animal. Evidence consistent with this comes from studies with electrical stimulation of the brain. It has been found that electrical stimulation of some brain regions is rewarding in that animals including humans will work to obtain electrical stimulation of some sites in the brain (see J. Olds 1977; Rolls 1975, 1976a, 1979). At some sites, including the lateral hypothalamus, the electrical stimulation appears to produce a reward which is equivalent to food for the hungry animal, in that the animal will work hard to obtain the stimulation if he is hungry, but will work much less for it if he has been satiated (see J. Olds 1977; Hoebel 1969). There is even evidence that the reward at some sites can mimic food for a hungry animal and at other sites water for a thirsty animal, in that rats chose electrical stimulation at one hypothalamic site when hungry and at a different site when thirsty (Gallistel and Beagley 1971). It was therefore a fascinating discovery when it was found that some of the neurons normally activated by food when the monkey was hungry were also activated by brain-stimulation reward (Rolls 1975, 1976a; Rolls, Burton and Mora 1980). Thus there was convergence of the effects of natural food reward and brain-stimulation reward at some brain sites (e.g. the orbitofrontal cortex and amygdala), on to single hypothalamic neurons. Further, it was shown that self-stimulation occurred through the recording electrode if it was near a region where hypothalamic neurons had been recorded which responded to food, and that this self-stimulation was attenuated by feeding the monkey to satiety (Rolls, Burton and Mora 1980).

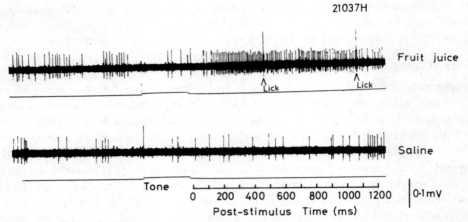

Fig. 2.9 Lateral hypothalamic neuron responding to the sight of food in a visual discrimination task. The neuron increased its firing above the spontaneous rate when a triangle was shown at time 0 which indicated that the monkey could lick a tube in front of his mouth to obtain fruit juice (top trace). The action potentials of the single neuron are the vertical spikes. The neuron did not respond when a square was shown which indicated that if the monkey licked, he would obtain aversive hypertonic saline from the lick tube (bottom trace). The latency of activation of different hypothalamic neurons by the sight of food was 150–200 ms, and compared with a latency of 250–300 ms for the earliest electrical activity associated with the motor responses of a lick made to obtain food when the food-related visual stimulus was shown. (From Rolls, Sanghera and Roper-Hall 1979b.)

The finding that these neurons were activated by brain-stimulation reward is consistent with the hypothesis that their activity is related to reward produced by food, and not to some other effect of food. *Indeed, this evidence from the convergence of brain-stimulation reward and food reward on to these hypothalamic neurons, and from the self-stimulation found through the recording electrode, suggests that animals work to obtain activation of these neurons by food, and that this is what makes food rewarding.* At the same time this accounts for self-stimulation of some brain sites, which is understood as the animal seeking to activate the neurons which he normally seeks to activate by food when he is hungry. This and other evidence (see Rolls 1975, 1982) indicates that feeding normally occurs in order to obtain the sensory input produced by food which is rewarding if the animal is hungry.

Sites in the hypothalamus and basal forebrain of neurons which respond to food

These neurons are found as a relatively small proportion of cells in a region which includes the lateral hypothalamus and substantia innominata and extends from the lateral hypothalamus posteriorly through the anterior hypothalamus and lateral preoptic area to a region ventral to and anterior to the anterior commissure (see Fig. 2.12 reproduced from Fig. 7 of Rolls, Sanghera and Roper-Hall 1979).

Useful further information about the particular populations of neurons in these regions with feeding-related activity, and about the functions of these neurons in feeding could be provided by evidence on their output connections. It is known that some hypothalamic neurons project to brainstem autonomic regions such as the dorsal motor nucleus of the vagus (Saper *et al.* 1976, 1979). If some of the hypothalamic neurons with feeding-related activity projected in this way, it would be very likely that their functions would include the generation of autonomic responses to the sight of food. Some hypothalamic neurons project to the substantia nigra (Nauta and Domesick 1978), and some neurons in the lateral hypothalamus and basal magnocellular forebrain nuclei of Meynert project directly to the cerebral cortex (Kievit and Kuypers 1975; Divac 1975; Heimer and Alheid 1990). If some of these were feeding-related neurons, then by such routes they could influence whether feeding is initiated. To determine to which regions hypothalamic neurons with feeding-related activity project, electrical stimulation is being applied to these different regions, to determine from which regions hypothalamic neurons with feeding-related activity can be antidromically activated. It has so far been found in such experiments by E. T. Rolls, E. Murzi and C. Griffiths that some of these feeding-related neurons in the lateral hypothalamus and substantia innominata project directly to the cerebral cortex, to such areas as the prefrontal cortex in the sulcus principalis and the supplementary motor cortex. This provides evidence that at least some of these neurons with feeding-related activity project this information to the cerebral cortex, where it could be used in such processes as the initiation of feeding behaviour. It also indicates that at least some of these feeding-related neurons are in the basal magnocellular forebrain nuclei of Meynert, which is quite consistent with the reconstructions of the recording sites (Fig. 2.12).

In addition to a role in food reward and thus in the control of feeding, it seems quite likely that at least some of the hypothalamic feeding-related neurons influence brainstem autonomic motor neurons. Consistent with this, it is known that there are projections from the lateral hypothalamus to the brainstem autonomic motor nuclei, and that lesions of the lateral hypothalamus disrupt conditioned autonomic responses (LeDoux *et al.* 1988).

Functions of the hypothalamus in feeding

The functions of the hypothalamus in feeding are thus related at least in part to the inputs which it receives from the forebrain, in that it contains neurons which respond to the sight of food, and which are influenced by learning. (Such pattern-specific visual responses, and their modification by learning, require forebrain areas such as the inferior temporal visual cortex and the amygdala, as described below.) This conclusion is consistent with the anatomy of the hypothalamus and substantia innominata, which receive projections from limbic structures such as the amygdala which in turn receive projections from the association cortex (Nauta 1961; Herzog and Van Hoesen 1976). The conclusion is also consistent with the evidence that decerebrate rats retain simple controls of feeding, but do not show normal learning about foods (Grill and Norgren 1978). These rats accept sweet solutions placed in their mouths when hungry and reject them when satiated, so some control of responses to gustatory stimuli which depends on hunger can occur caudal to the level of the hypothalamus. However, these rats are unable to feed themselves, and do not learn to avoid poisoned solutions. The importance of visual inputs and learning to feeding, in relation to which some hypothalamic neurons respond, is that animals, and especially primates, may eat many foods every day, and must be able to select foods from other visual stimuli, as well as produce appropriate preparative responses to them such as salivation and the release of insulin. They must also be able to initiate appropriate actions

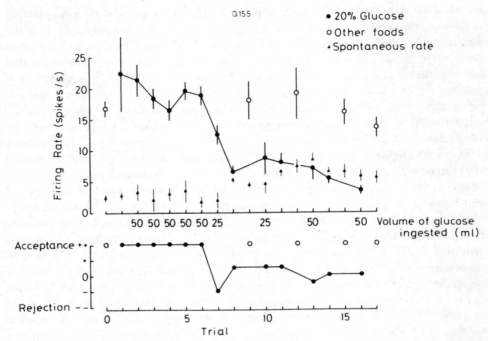

Fig. 2.10 The effect of feeding the monkey to satiety with 20% glucose solution on the responses of a lateral hypothalamic neuron to the taste of the glucose (filled circles) and to the taste of other foods (open circles). After the monkey had fed to satiety with glucose, the neuron responded much less to the taste of glucose, but still responded to the other foods. The mean responses of the neuron (±sem) are shown to the stimuli at different stages of the experiment. The satiety of the monkey, shown below, was measured by whether he accepted or rejected the glucose. (From Rolls, Murzi et al. 1986.)

in the environment to obtain food. Before any activation of motor neurons, such as those that innervate the masticatory muscles, involved in feeding, it is normally necessary to select which reinforcer in the environment should be the object of action, and then to select an appropriate (arbitrary) action to obtain the selected reinforcer. This indicates that direct connections from food reward systems or feeding control systems in the brain directly to motor neurons are likely to be involved only in the lowest level (in the sense of Hughlings Jackson, see Swash 1989) of the control of behaviour. Instead, food reward systems might be expected to project to an action-control system, and connections therefore from the lateral hypothalamus, amygdala, and orbitofrontal cortex to systems such as the basal ganglia are likely to be more important as routes for the initiation of normal feeding (see Section 2.4.8 on the striatum, below).

2.4.2 Brain mechanisms for the reward produced by the taste of food

2.4.2.1 Taste processing up to and including the primary taste cortex of primates is related to the identity of the tastant, and not to its reward value

Given that there are neurons in the hypothalamus that can respond to the taste (and/or sight) of foods but not of non-foods, and that modulation of this sensory input by motivation is seen when recordings are made from these hypothalamic neurons, it may be asked whether these are special properties of hypothalamic neurons which they show because they are specially involved in the control of motivational responses, or whether this degree of specificity and type of modulation are general properties which are evident throughout sensory systems. In one respect it would be inefficient if motivational modulation were present far peripherally, because this would imply that sensory information was being discarded without the possibility for central processing. A subjective correspondent of such a situation might be that it might not be possible to taste food, or even to see food, when satiated! It is perhaps more efficient for most of the system to function similarly whether hungry or satiated, and to have a special system (such as the hypothalamus) following sensory processing where motivational state influences responsiveness. Evidence on the actual state of affairs which exists for visual processing in primates in relation to feeding has been summarized above. In contrast, apparently there is at least some peripheral modulation of taste processing in rats (in the nucleus of the solitary tract) (see T. Scott and Giza 1992). Evidence is now being obtained for primates on the tuning of neurons in the gustatory pathways, and on whether responsiveness at different stages is influenced by motivation, as follows. These investigations on the gustatory pathways have also been able to show where flavour, that is a combination of taste and olfactory input, is computed in the primate brain. The gustatory and olfactory pathways, and some of their onward connections, are shown in Fig. 2.8.

The first central synapse of the gustatory system is in the rostral part of the nucleus of the solitary tract (Beckstead and Norgren 1979; Beckstead, Morse and Norgren 1980). The caudal half of this nucleus receives visceral afferents, and it is a possibility that such visceral information, reflecting, for example, gastric distension, is used to modulate gustatory processing even at this early stage of the gustatory system.

In order to investigate the tuning of neurons in the nucleus of the solitary tract, and whether hunger does influence processing at this first central opportunity in the gustatory system of primates, we recorded the activity of single neurons in the nucleus of the solitary tract. To ensure that our results were relevant to the normal control of feeding (and were not, for example, because of abnormally high levels of artificially administered putative satiety signals), we allowed the monkeys to feed until they were satiated, and determined whether this normal and physiological induction of satiety influenced the responsiveness of neurons in the nucleus of the solitary tract, which were recorded throughout the feeding, until satiety was reached. It was found that in the nucleus of the solitary tract, the first central relay in the gustatory system, neurons are relatively broadly tuned to the prototypical taste stimuli (sweet, salt, bitter, and sour) (T. Scott, Yaxley, Sienkiewicz and Rolls 1986a). It was also found that neuronal responses in the nucleus of the solitary tract to the taste of food are not influenced by whether the monkey is hungry or satiated (Yaxley, Rolls, Sienkiewicz and Scott 1985).

To investigate whether there are neurons in the primary gustatory cortex in the primate which are more closely tuned to respond to foods as compared to non-foods, and whether hunger modulates the responsiveness of these neurons, we have recorded the activity of single neurons in the primary gustatory cortex during feeding in the monkey. In the primary gustatory cortex in the frontal operculum and insula, neurons are more sharply

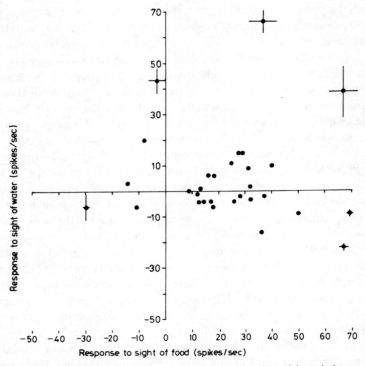

Fig. 2.11 Motivation-specific neuronal responses in the monkey lateral hypothalamus: some neurons responded more to the sight of food, and others to the sight of water, when the monkey was both hungry and thirsty. Each point represents the responses of a different single neuron to the sight of food and to the sight of water. Standard error bars are provided for some of the neurons to provide an indication that the differences in the responses of some of the neurons to the sight of food vs the sight of water were statistically significantly different. (Previously unpublished data of E. T. Rolls and E. Murzi.)

tuned to gustatory stimuli than in the nucleus of the solitary tract, with some neurons responding primarily, for example, to sweet, and much less to salt, bitter, or sour stimuli (T. Scott, Yaxley, Sienkiewicz and Rolls 1986b; Yaxley, Rolls and Sienkiewicz 1990). However, here also, hunger does not influence the magnitude of neuronal responses to gustatory stimuli (Rolls, Scott, Yaxley and Sienkiewicz 1986; Yaxley, Rolls and Sienkiewicz 1988).

2.4.2.2 Taste and taste-related processing in the secondary taste cortex, including umami taste, astringency, and fat

A secondary cortical taste area has recently been discovered in the caudolateral orbitofrontal taste cortex of the primate in which gustatory neurons can be even more sharply tuned to particular taste stimuli (Rolls, Yaxley and Sienkiewicz, 1990; Rolls and Treves 1990) (see Fig. 2.13). In addition to representations of the 'prototypical' taste stimuli sweet, salt, bitter, and sour, different neurons in this region respond to other taste and taste-related stimuli which provide information about the reward value of a potential food. One example of this additional taste information is a set of neurons that respond to umami taste, as described next.

An important food taste which appears to be different from that produced by sweet, salt, bitter, or sour is the taste of protein. At least part of this taste is captured by the Japanese word *umami*, which is a taste common to a diversity of food sources including fish, meats, mushrooms, cheese, and some vegetables such as tomatoes. Within these food sources, it is glutamates and 5′ nucleotides, sometimes in a synergistic combination, that create the umami taste (Ikeda 1909; Yamaguchi 1967; Yamaguchi and Kimizuka 1979; Kawamura and Kare 1987). Monosodium L-glutamate (MSG), guanosine 5′-monophosphate (GMP), and inosine 5′-monophosphate (IMP), are examples of umami stimuli.

These findings raise the question of whether umami taste operates through information channels in the primate taste system which are separable from those for the 'prototypical' tastes sweet, salt, bitter, and sour. (Although the concept of four prototypical tastes has been used by tradition, there is increasing discussion about the utility of the concept, and increasing evidence that the taste system is more diverse than this—see, e.g., Kawamura and Kare 1987). To investigate the neural encoding of glutamate in the primate, L. Baylis and Rolls (1991) made recordings from 190 taste-responsive neurons in the primary taste cortex and adjoining orbitofrontal cortex taste area in macaques. Single neurons were found that were tuned to respond best to monosodium glutamate (umami taste), just as other cells were found with best responses to glucose (sweet), sodium chloride (salty), HCl (sour), and quinine HCl (bitter). Across the population of neurons, the responsiveness to glutamate was poorly correlated with the responsiveness to NaCl, so that the representation of glutamate was clearly different from that of NaCl. Further, the representation of glutamate was shown to be approximately as different from each of the other four tastants as they are from each other, as shown by multidimensional scaling and cluster analysis. Moreover, it was found that glutamate is approximately as well represented in terms of mean evoked neural activity and the number of cells with best responses to it as the other four stimuli glucose, NaCl, HCl and quinine. It was concluded that in primate taste cortical areas, glutamate, which produces umami taste in humans, is approximately as well represented as are the tastes produced by: glucose (sweet), NaCl (salty), HCl (sour) and quinine HCl (bitter) (L. Baylis and Rolls 1991).

In a recent investigation, these findings have been extended beyond the sodium salt of glutamate to other umami tastants which have the glutamate ion but which do not introduce sodium ion into the experiment; and to a nucleotide umami tastant (Rolls, Critchley, Wakeman and Mason 1996d). In recordings made mainly from neurons in the orbitofrontal cortex taste area, it was shown that single neurons that had their best responses to sodium glutamate also had good responses to glutamic acid. The correlation between the responses to these two tastants was higher than between any other pair which included in addition a prototypical set including glucose (sweet), sodium chloride (salty), HCl (sour), and quinine HCl (bitter). Moreover, the responsiveness to glutamic acid clustered with the response to monosodium glutamate in a cluster analysis with this set of stimuli, and glutamic acid was close to sodium glutamate in a space created by multidimensional scaling. It was also shown that the responses of these neurons to the nucleotide

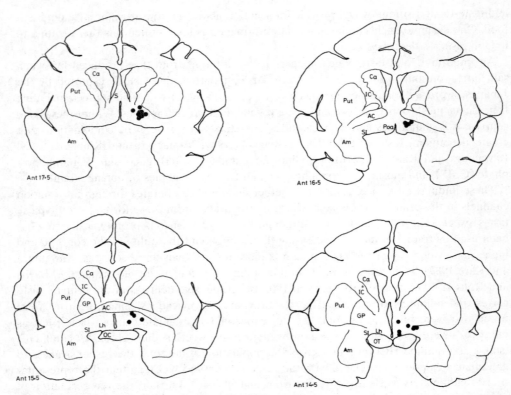

Fig. 2.12 Sites in the lateral hypothalamus and basal forebrain of the macaque at which neurons were recorded that responded to the sight of food. Abbreviations: AC, anterior commissure; Am, amygdala; Ca, caudate nucleus; GP, globus pallidus; IC, internal capsule; Lh, lateral hypothalamus; OC, optic chiasm; OT, optic tract; Poa, preoptic area; Put, putamen; S, septal region; SI, substantia innominata. (From Rolls, Sanghera and Roper-Hall 1979b.)

umami tastant inosine 5'-monophosphate were more correlated with their responses to monosodium glutamate than to any prototypical tastant.

Thus neurophysiological evidence in primates does indicate that there is a representation of umami flavour in the cortical areas which is separable from that to the prototypical tastants sweet, salt, bitter, and sour (see further Rolls, Critchley, Browning and Hernadi 1998a). This representation is probably important in the taste produced by proteins (cf. Chaudhari *et al.* 1996). These neurons are found not only in the orbitofrontal cortex taste areas, but also in the primary taste cortex (L. Baylis and Rolls 1991). Recently, evidence has started to accumulate that there may be taste receptors on the tongue specialized for umami taste (Chaudhari *et al.* 1996; Roper 1998).

Another taste-related stimulus quality which provides important information about the reward value of a potential food source is *astringency*. In humans, tannic acid elicits a characteristic astringent taste. Oral astringency is perceived as the feeling of long-lasting puckering and drying sensations on the tongue and membranes of the oral cavity. High levels of tannic acid in some potential foods makes them unpalatable without preparative techniques to reduce its presence (Johns and Duquette 1991), yet in small quantities it is commonly used to enhance the flavour of food. In this context tannic acid is a constituent of a large range of spices and condiments, such as ginger, chillies, and black pepper (Uma-Pradeep *et al.* 1993). (Tannic acid itself is not present in tea, yet a range of related polyphenol compounds are, particularly in green tea (Graham 1992)). Tannic acid is a natural antioxidant by virtue of its chemical structure (see Critchley and Rolls 1996c).

The evolutionary adaptive value of the ability to detect astringency may be related to some of the properties of tannic acid. Tannic acid is a member of the class of compounds known as polyphenols, which are present in a wide spectrum of plant matter, particularly in foliage, the skin and husks of fruit and nuts, and the bark of trees. The tannic acid in leaves is produced as a defence against insects. There is less tannic acid in young leaves than in old leaves. Large monkeys cannot obtain the whole of their protein intake from small animals, insects etc., and thus obtain some of their protein from leaves. Tannic acid binds protein (hence its use in tanning) and amino acids, and thus prevents their absorption. Thus it is adaptive for monkeys to be able to taste tannic acid, so that they can select food sources without too much tannic acid (Hladik 1978 and personal communication).

In order to investigate whether astringency is represented in the cortical taste areas concerned with taste, Critchley and Rolls (1996c) recorded from taste-responsive neurons in the orbitofrontal cortex and adjacent insula. Single neurons were found that were tuned to respond to tannic acid (0.001 M), and represented a subpopulation of neurons that was distinct from neurons responsive to the tastes of glucose (sweet), NaCl (salty), HCl (sour), quinine (bitter) and monosodium glutamate (umami). In addition, across the population of taste-responsive neurons, tannic acid was as well represented as the tastes of NaCl, HCl, quinine, or monosodium glutamate. Multidimensional scaling analysis of the neuronal responses to the tastants indicates that tannic acid lies outside the boundaries of the four conventional taste qualities (sweet, sour, bitter, and salty). Taken together these data indicate that the astringent taste of tannic acid should be considered as a distinct 'taste' quality, which receives a separate representation from sweet, salt, bitter, and sour in the primate cortical taste areas. Tannic acid may produce its 'taste' effects not through the taste nerves, but through the somatosensory inputs conveyed through the trigeminal nerve. Astringency is thus strictly not a sixth taste in the sense that umami is a fifth taste (Chaudhari *et al.* 1996). However, what has been shown in these studies is that the orosensory, probably somatosensory, sensations produced by tannic acid do converge with effects produced through taste inputs, to result in neurons in the orbitofrontal cortex responding to both taste stimuli and to astringent sensations.

Another important type of input to the same region of the orbitofrontal cortex that is concerned with detecting the reward value of a potential food is an input produced by the *texture* of food in the mouth. We have shown for example in recent recordings that single neurons influenced by taste in this region can in some cases have their responses modulated by the texture of the food. This was shown in experiments in which the texture of food was manipulated by the addition of methyl cellulose or gelatine, or by puréeing a semi-solid food (Rolls and Critchley, in preparation). The somatosensory inputs may reach this region via the rostral insula, which we have shown does project into this region, and

OFC

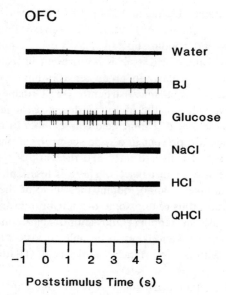

Water

BJ

Glucose

NaCl

HCl

QHCl

-1 0 1 2 3 4 5

Poststimulus Time (s)

Fig. 2.13 Examples of the responses recorded from one caudolateral orbitofrontal taste cortex neuron to the six taste stimuli, water, 20% blackcurrant juice (BJ), 1 M glucose, 1 M NaCl, 0.01 M HCl, and 0.001 M quinine HCl (QHCl). The stimuli were placed in the mouth at time 0. (From Rolls, Yaxley and Sienkiewicz 1990.)

which Mesulam and Mufson (1982a,b) and Mufson and Mesulam (1982) have shown does receive somatosensory inputs. The texture of food is an important cue about the quality of the food, for example about the ripeness of fruit. Texture in the mouth is also an important indicator of whether *fat* is present in the food, which is important not only as a high value energy source, but also as a potential source of essential fatty acids. In the orbitofrontal cortex, Rolls and Critchley have found a population of neurons that responds when fat is in the mouth. An example of such a neuron is shown in Fig. 2.14. The neuron illustrates that information about fat as well as about taste can converge onto the same neuron in this region. The neuron responded to taste in that its firing rate was significantly different within the group of tastants sweet, salt, bitter, and sour. However, its response to fat in the mouth was larger. The fat-related responses of these neurons are produced at least in part by the texture of the food rather than by chemical receptors sensitive to certain chemicals, in that such neurons typically respond not only to foods such as cream and milk containing fat, but also to paraffin oil (which is a pure hydrocarbon) and to silicone oil ($(Si(CH_3)_2O)_n$). Some of the fat-related neurons do though have convergent inputs from the chemical senses, in that in addition to taste inputs some of these neurons respond to the odour associated with a fat, such as the odour of cream (Rolls and Critchley, in preparation).

2.4.2.3 The reward value of taste is represented in the orbitofrontal cortex

In the primate orbitofrontal cortex, it is found that the responses of taste neurons to the particular food with which a monkey is fed to satiety decrease to zero (Rolls, Sienkiewicz and Yaxley 1989b). An example is shown in Fig. 2.15. This neuron reduced its responses to the taste of glucose during the course of feeding as much glucose as the monkey wanted to drink. When the monkey was fully satiated, and did not want to drink any more glucose, the neuron no longer responded to the taste of glucose. Thus the responses of these neurons decrease to zero when the reward value of the food decreases to zero. Interestingly the neuron still responded to other foods, and the monkey was willing to eat these other foods. Thus the modulation of the responses of these taste neurons occurs in a sensory-specific way. This is the first stage of the primate taste system in which this modulation of the responses of neurons to the taste of food is affected by hunger. It is of course only when hungry that the taste of food is rewarding. This is an indication that the responses of these orbitofrontal cortex taste neurons reflects the reward value of food. The firing of these orbitofrontal neurons may actually implement the reward value of a food. The hypothesis is that primates work to obtain firing of these neurons, by eating food when they are hungry. Further evidence that the firing of these neurons does actually implement the primary reward value of food is that in another experiment we showed that monkeys would work to obtain electrical stimulation of this area of the brain (Rolls, Burton and Mora 1980; Mora, Avrith, Phillips and Rolls 1979; Mora, Avrith and Rolls 1980). Moreover, the reward value of the electrical stimulation was dependent on hunger being present. If the monkey was fed to satiety, the monkey no longer found electrical stimulation at this site so rewarding, and stopped working for the electrical stimulation. Indeed, of all the brain sites tested, this orbitofrontal cortex region was the part of the brain in which the reward value of the electrical stimulation was most affected by feeding to satiety (Mora et al. 1979, 1980; Rolls, Burton and Mora 1980). Thus all this evidence indicates that the reward value of taste is decoded in the secondary taste cortex, and that primates work to obtain food in order to activate these neurons, the activation of which actually mediates reward. This is probably an innate reward system, in that taste can act as a reward in rats without prior training (Berridge et al. 1984).

The neurophysiological discoveries that feeding to satiety reduces the responses of secondary taste cortex neurons, but not neurons earlier in taste processing, are relevant to what normally produces satiety, in that in these experiments the neurons were recorded while the monkeys were fed to normal satiety. It could be that later in satiety there is some modulation of responsiveness earlier in the taste pathways, occurring perhaps as food is absorbed. But even if this does occur, such modulation would not then account for the change in acceptability of food, which of course is seen as the satiety develops, and is used to define satiety. Nor would this modulation be relevant to the decrease in the pleasantness in the taste of a food which occurs when it is eaten to satiety (Cabanac 1971; B. Rolls, Rolls, Rowe and Sweeney, 1981; B. Rolls, Rowe, Rolls, Kingston, Megson and Gunary, 1981; Rolls, Rolls B. and Rowe 1983a; Rolls and B. Rolls 1977, 1982). Thus it appears that the reduced acceptance of food as satiety develops, and the reduction in its pleasantness, are not produced by a reduction in the responses of neurons in the nucleus of the solitary tract or frontal opercular or insular gustatory cortices to gustatory stimuli. (As described above, the responses of gustatory neurons in these areas do not decrease as satiety develops.) Indeed, after feeding to satiety, humans reported that the taste of the food on which they had been satiated tasted almost as intense as when they were hungry,

Cell Be047

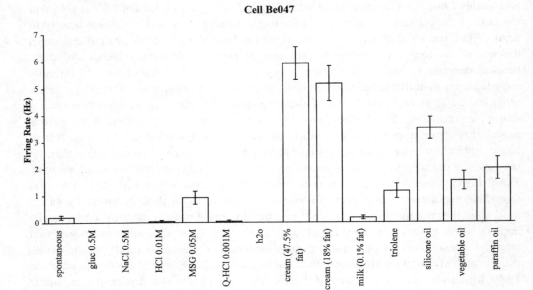

Fig. 2.14 A neuron in the primate orbitofrontal cortex responding to the texture of fat in the mouth. The cell (Be047) increased its firing rate to cream (double and single cream, with the fat proportions shown), and responded to texture rather than the chemical structure of the fat in that it also responded to 0.5 ml of silicone oil (SiO_2) or paraffin oil (hydrocarbon). The cell had a taste input too, in that it had a consistent but small response to umami taste (monosodium glutamate, MSG). Gluc, glucose; NaCl, salt; HCl, sour; QHCl, quinine, bitter. The spontaneous firing rate of the cell is also shown. (Previously unpublished data of H. Critchley, E. T. Rolls, A. D. Browning, and I. Hernadi.)

though much less pleasant (Rolls, Rolls and Rowe 1983a). This comparison is consistent with the possibility that activity in the frontal opercular and insular taste cortices as well as the nucleus of the solitary tract does not reflect the pleasantness of the taste of a food, but rather its sensory qualities independently of motivational state. On the other hand, the responses of the neurons in the orbitofrontal taste area and in the lateral hypothalamus are modulated by satiety, and it is presumably in areas such as these that neuronal activity may be related to whether a food tastes pleasant, and to whether the human or animal will work to obtain and then eat the food, that is to whether the food is rewarding. The situation is not necessarily the same in non-primates, in that in the rat some reduction in the responses of taste neurons in the nucleus of the solitary tract was produced by glucose infusions (T. Scott and Giza 1992; T. Scott, Yan and Rolls 1995).

The present results also provide evidence on the nature of the mechanisms which underlie sensory-specific satiety. Sensory-specific satiety, as noted above in Section 2.3.1, is the phenomenon in which the decrease in the palatability and acceptability of a food which has been eaten to satiety are partly specific to the particular food which has been eaten. The results just described suggest that such sensory-specific satiety for taste cannot be largely accounted for by adaptation at the receptor level, in the nucleus of the solitary tract, or in the frontal opercular or insular gustatory cortices, to the food which has been eaten to satiety, otherwise modulation of neuronal responsiveness should have been apparent in the recordings made in these regions. Indeed, the findings suggest that sensory-specific satiety is not represented in the primary gustatory cortex. It is thus of particular interest that a decrease in the response of orbitofrontal cortex neurons occurs which is partly specific to the food which has just been eaten to satiety (Rolls, Sienkiewicz and Yaxley 1989b).

These findings lead to the following proposed neuronal mechanism for sensory-specific satiety (see also Rolls and Treves 1990). The tuning of neurons becomes more specific for gustatory stimuli through the NTS, gustatory thalamus, and frontal opercular taste cortex. Satiety, habituation and adaptation are not features of the responses here. This is what is found in primates (see above). The tuning of neurons becomes even more specific in the orbitofrontal cortex, but here there is some effect of satiety by internal signals such as gastric distension and glucose utilization, and in addition habituation with a time course of several minutes which lasts for 1–2 h is a feature of the synapses which are activated. Because of the relative specificity of the tuning of orbitofrontal taste neurons, this results in a decrease in the response to that food, but different foods continue to activate other neurons. (For orbitofrontal cortex neurons that respond to two similar tastes before satiety, it is suggested that the habituation that results in a loss of the response to the taste eaten to satiety occurs because of habituation of the afferent neurons or synapses onto these orbitofrontal cortex neurons.) Then, the orbitofrontal cortex neurons have the required response properties, and it is only then necessary for other parts of the brain to use the activity of the orbitofrontal cortex neurons to reflect the reward value of that particular taste. One output of these neurons may be to the hypothalamic neurons with food-related responses, for their responses to the sight and/or taste of food show a decrease which is partly specific to a food which has just been eaten to satiety (see above). Another output may be to the ventral and adjoining striatum, which may provide an important link between reward systems and action (see below and Chapter 7).

It is suggested that the computational significance of this architecture is as follows (see also Rolls 1986c, 1989b; Rolls and Treves 1990). If satiety were to operate at an early level of sensory analysis, then because of the broadness of tuning of neurons, responses to non-foods would become attenuated as well as responses to foods (and this could well be dangerous if poisonous non-foods became undetectable). This argument becomes even more compelling when it is realized that satiety typically shows some specificity for the particular food eaten, with others not eaten in the meal remaining relatively pleasant (see above). Unless tuning were relatively fine, this mechanism could not operate, for reduction in neuronal firing after one food had been eaten would inevitably reduce behavioural responsiveness to other foods. Indeed, it is of interest to note that such a sensory-specific satiety mechanism can be built by arranging for tuning to particular foods to become relatively specific at one level of the nervous system (as a result of categorization processing in earlier stages), and then at this stage (but not at prior stages) to allow habituation to be a property of the synapses, as proposed above.

Thus information processing in the taste system illustrates an important principle of higher nervous system function in primates, namely that it is only after several or many stages of sensory information processing (which produce efficient categorization of the stimulus) that there is an interface to motivational systems, to other modalities, or to

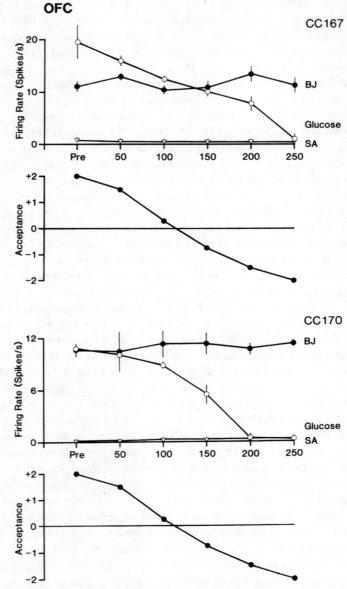

Fig. 2.15 The effect of feeding to satiety with glucose solution on the responses (rate ± sem) of two neurons in the secondary taste cortex to the taste of glucose and of blackcurrant juice (BJ). The spontaneous firing rate is also indicated (SA). Below the neuronal response data for each experiment, the behavioural measure of the acceptance or rejection of the solution on a scale from +2 (strong acceptance) to −2 (strong rejection) is shown. The solution used to feed to satiety was 20% glucose. The monkey was fed 50 ml of the solution at each stage of the experiment as indicated along the abscissa, until he was satiated as shown by whether he accepted or rejected the solution. Pre is the firing rate of the neuron before the satiety experiment started. (From Rolls, Sienkiewicz and Yaxley 1989b.)

systems involved in association memory (Rolls 1987; Rolls and Treves 1990). The rat may not be a good model for primates even for taste information processing, in that in rats there are connections from the nucleus of the solitary tract via a pontine taste area to the amygdala and hypothalamus which bypass the cortex (Norgren 1984), and in that there is some modulation by hunger of taste processing even in the nucleus of the solitary tract (T. Scott and Giza 1992; T. Scott, Yan and Rolls 1995). The fact that the connections and operation of even such a phylogenetically old system as the taste system have been reorganized in primates may be related to the importance of cortical processing in primates especially for vision, so that other sensory systems follow suit in order to build multimodal representations of objects, which are motivationally neutral and can be used for many functions, including inputs to systems for recognition, identification, object-place memory and short-term memory as well as for reward decoding in stimulus-reinforcement learning systems. One value of such organization is that objects can be recognized and learned about even when an object is not rewarding. The system is ideally suited, for example, to learning about where food is located in the environment even when hunger is not present. Modulation of visual and taste processing by hunger early on in sensory processing would mean that one would be blind and ageusic to food when not hungry.

2.4.3 Convergence between taste and olfactory processing to represent flavour

At some stage in taste processing it is likely that taste representations are brought together with inputs from different modalities, for example with olfactory inputs to form a representation of flavour. Takagi and his colleagues (Tanabe *et al.* 1975a,b) found an olfactory area in the medial orbitofrontal cortex. In a mid-mediolateral part of the caudal orbitofrontal cortex is the area investigated by Thorpe, Rolls and Maddison (1983) in which are found many neurons with visual and some with gustatory responses. During our recordings in the caudolateral orbitofrontal cortex taste area our impression was that it was different from the frontal opercular and insular primary taste cortices, in that there were neurons with responses in other modalities within or very close to the caudolateral orbitofrontal taste cortex (Rolls, Yaxley and Sienkiewicz 1990). We therefore investigated systematically whether there are neurons in the secondary taste cortex and adjoining more medial orbitofrontal cortex which respond to stimuli in other modalities, including the olfactory and visual modalities, and whether single neurons in this cortical region in some cases respond to stimuli from more than one modality.

In this investigation of the orbitofrontal cortex taste areas (Rolls and Baylis 1994), we found that of 112 single neurons which responded to any of these modalities, many were unimodal (taste 34%, olfactory 13%, visual 21%), but were found in close proximity to each other. Some single neurons showed convergence, responding, for example, to taste and visual inputs (13%), taste and olfactory inputs (13%), and olfactory and visual inputs (5%). Some of these multimodal single neurons had corresponding sensitivities in the two modalities, in that they responded best to sweet tastes (e.g. 1 M glucose), and responded more in a visual discrimination task to the visual stimulus which signified sweet fruit juice

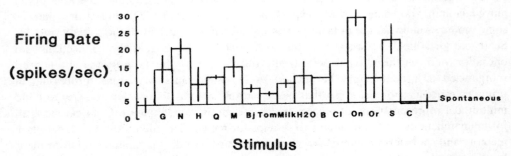

Fig. 2.16 The responses of a bimodal neuron with taste and olfactory responses recorded in the caudolateral orbitofrontal cortex. G, 1 M glucose; N, 0.1 M NaCl; H, 0.01 M HCl; Q, 0.001 M Quinine HCl; M, 0.1 M monosodium glutamate; Bj, 20% blackcurrant juice; Tom, tomato juice; B, banana odour; Cl, clove oil odour; On, onion odour; Or, orange odour; S, salmon odour; C, control no-odour presentation. The mean responses ± sem. are shown. The neuron responded best to the tastes of NaCl and monosodium glutamate and to the odours of onion and salmon. (From Rolls and Baylis 1994.)

than to that which signified saline; or responded to sweet taste, and in an olfactory discrimination task to fruit odour. An example of one such bimodal neuron is shown in Fig. 2.16. The neuron responded best among the tastants to NaCl (N), and best among the odours to onion odour (On), and well also to salmon (S). The olfactory input to these neurons was further defined by measuring their responses while the monkey performed an olfactory discrimination task. In the task, if one odour was delivered through a tube close to the nose, then the monkey could lick to obtain glucose (Reward trials). If a different odour was delivered, the monkey had to avoid licking, otherwise he obtained saline (Saline trials). The neuron shown in Fig. 2.16 responded well to the smell of onion (the discriminative stimulus on saline trials), and much less to the odour of fruit juice (the stimulus on Reward trials). The neuron had a selective and specific response to odour, and did not respond non-specifically in the discrimination task, as shown by the absence of neuronal activity while the monkey performed a visual discrimination task. The different types of neurons (unimodal in different modalities, and multimodal) were frequently found close to one another in tracks made into this region (see Fig. 2.17), consistent with the hypothesis that the multimodal representations are actually being formed from unimodal inputs to this region.

These results show that there are regions in the orbitofrontal cortex of primates where the sensory modalities of taste, vision, and olfaction converge; and that in many cases the neurons have corresponding sensitivities across modalities. It appears to be in these areas that flavour representations are built, where flavour is taken to mean a representation which is evoked best by a combination of gustatory and olfactory input. This orbitofrontal region does appear to be an important region for convergence, for there is only a low proportion of bimodal taste and olfactory neurons in the primary taste cortex (Rolls and Baylis 1994).

2.4.4 Brain mechanisms for the reward produced by the odour of food
2.4.4.1 The rules underlying the formation of olfactory representations in the primate cortex

A schematic diagram of the olfactory pathways in primates is shown in Fig. 2.8. There are direct connections from the olfactory bulb to the primary olfactory cortex, pyriform cortex, and from there a connection to a caudal part of the mid (in terms of medial and lateral) orbitofrontal cortex, area 13a, which in turn has onward projections to the lateral orbitofrontal cortex area which we have shown is secondary taste cortex, and to more rostral parts of the orbitofrontal cortex (area 11) (Price *et al.* 1991; Carmichael and Price 1994; Carmichael *et al.* 1994) (see Figs 2.18 and 2.8).

There is evidence that in the (rabbit) olfactory bulb, a coding principle is that in many cases each glomerulus (of which there are approximately 1000) is tuned to respond to its own characteristic hydrocarbon chain length of odourant (Mori *et al.* 1992; Imamura *et al.* 1992). Evidence for this is that each mitral/tufted cell in the olfactory bulb can be quite sharply tuned, responding for example best to a 5-C length aliphatic odourant (e.g. acid or aldehyde), and being inhibited by nearby hydrocarbon chain-length aliphatic odourants. An effect of this coding might appear to be to spread out the olfactory stimulus space in this early part of the olfactory system, based on the stereochemical structure of the odourant. The code would be spread out in that different parts of chemical space would be relatively evenly represented, in that each part would be represented independently of the presence of other odourants, and in that the code would be relatively sparse, leading to low correlations between the representations of different odours. (Such a coding principle might be facilitated by the presence of in the order of 1000 different genes to code for different olfactory receptor molecules, Buck and Axel 1991). Is this same coding principle, based on simple chemical properties, used later on in the (primate) olfactory system, or do other principles operate? One example of another coding principle is that representations are built that represent the co-occurrence of pairs or groups of odourants, so that particular smells in the environment, which typically are produced by combinations of chemical stimuli, are reflected in the responses of neurons. Another coding principle is that olfactory coding might represent in some sense the biological significance of an odour, for example whether it is a food odour which is normally associated with a particular taste. Another principle is that at some stage of olfactory processing the reward or hedonic value of the odourant is represented (whether the odourant smells good), rather than purely the identity of the odourant. For example, whether a food-related odour smells good depends on hunger, and this hedonic representation of odours must be represented in some part of the olfactory system. To elucidate these issues, and thus to provide principles by which the primate olfactory system may operate, the following investigations have been performed.

To investigate how olfactory information is encoded in the orbitofrontal cortex, the responses of single neurons in the orbitofrontal cortex and surrounding areas were recorded during the performance of an olfactory discrimination task (Critchley and Rolls 1996a). The task was designed to show whether there are neurons in this region that

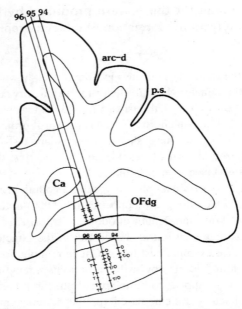

Fig. 2.17 Examples of tracks made into the orbitofrontal cortex in which taste (T) and olfactory (O) neurons were recorded close to each other in the same tracks. Some of the neurons were bimodal (T/O). arc-d, arcuate sulcus; Ca, head of Caudate nucleus; Ofdg, dysgranular part of the Orbitofrontal Cortex; p.s., principal sulcus. (From Rolls and Baylis 1994.)

categorize odours based on the taste with which the odour is associated. In the task, the delivery of one of eight different odours indicated that the monkey could lick to obtain a taste of sucrose. If one of two other odours was delivered from the olfactometer, the monkey had to refrain from licking, otherwise he received a taste of saline. It was found that 3.1% (48) of the 1580 neurons recorded had olfactory responses, and 34 (2.2%) responded differently to the different odours in the task. The neurons responded with a typical latency of 180 ms from the onset of odourant delivery. 35% of the olfactory neurons with differential responses in the task responded on the basis of the taste reward association of the odourants. Such neurons responded either to all the rewarded stimuli, and to none of the saline-associated stimuli, or vice versa. The remaining 65% of these neurons showed differential selectivity for the stimuli based on the odour quality, and not on the taste reward association of the odour. The findings show that the olfactory representation within the orbitofrontal cortex reflects for some neurons (65%) which odour is present independently of its association with taste reward, and that for other neurons (35%), the olfactory response reflects (and encodes) the taste association of the odour. The additional finding that some of the odour-responsive neurons were also responsive to taste stimuli supports the hypothesis that odour–taste association learning at the level of single neurons in the orbitofrontal cortex enables such cells to show olfactory responses which reflect the taste association of the odour.

The neurons that classify odours based on the taste with which the odour is associated are likely to respond in this way as a result of learning. Repeated pairing of an odour with a taste (especially if it is a neuron with a taste input) may by pattern-association learning lead it to respond to that odour in future. To investigate whether the responses of neurons to odours could be affected depending on the taste with which the odour was paired, we have performed a series of experiments in which the associations of odours and tastes in the olfactory discrimination task have been reversed. For example, the monkey might learn that when amyl acetate was delivered, a lick response would result in the delivery of a drop of glucose, and that when cineole was delivered, a lick would result in the delivery of a drop of saline. After this had been learned, the contingency was then reversed, so that cineole might after the reversal be associated with the taste of glucose. Rolls, Critchley, Mason and Wakeman (1996b) found that 68% of the odour-responsive neurons analysed modified their responses following the changes in the taste reward associations of the odourants. Full reversal of the neuronal responses was seen in 25% of the neurons analysed. (In full reversal, the odour to which the neuron responded reversed when the taste with which it was associated reversed.) Extinction of the differential neuronal responses after task reversal was seen in 43% of these neurons. (These neurons simply stopped discriminating between the two odours after the reversal.) These findings demonstrate directly a coding principle in primate olfaction whereby the responses of some orbitofrontal cortex olfactory neurons are modified by and depend upon the taste with which the odour is associated. This modification is likely to be important for setting the motivational or reward value of olfactory stimuli for feeding and other rewarded behaviour. It was of interest however that this modification was less complete, and much slower, than the modifications found for orbitofrontal visual neurons during visual–taste reversal (Rolls, Critchley, Mason and Wakeman, 1996b). This relative inflexibility of olfactory responses is consistent with the need for some stability in odour–taste associations to facilitate the formation and perception of flavours.

2.4.4.2 The effects of hunger on olfactory processing in the orbitofrontal cortex: evidence that the reward value of odour is represented

It has also been possible to investigate whether the olfactory representation in the orbitofrontal cortex is affected by hunger. In satiety experiments, Critchley and Rolls (1996b) have been able to show that the responses of some olfactory neurons to a food odour are reduced when the monkey is fed to satiety with a food (e.g. fruit juice) with that odour. In particular, seven of nine olfactory neurons that were responsive to the odours of foods, such as blackcurrant juice, were found to reduce their responses to the odour of the satiating food. The decrease was typically at least partly specific to the odour of the food that had been eaten to satiety, potentially providing part of the basis for sensory-specific satiety. (It was also found for eight of nine neurons that had selective responses to the sight of food that they demonstrated a sensory-specific reduction in their visual responses to foods following satiation.) These findings show that the olfactory and visual representations of food, as well as the taste representation of food, in the primate orbitofrontal cortex are modulated by hunger. Usually a component related to sensory-specific satiety can be demonstrated. The findings link at least part of the processing of olfactory and

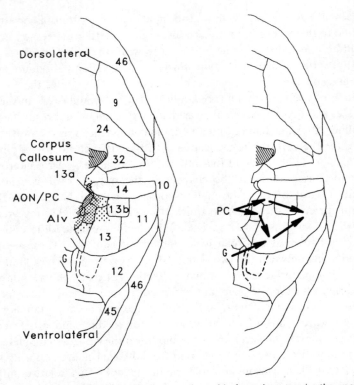

Fig. 2.18 The progression of olfactory inputs to the orbitofrontal cortex in the monkey, drawn on unfolded maps of the frontal lobe. The cortex was unfolded by splitting it along the principal sulcus, which is therefore located at the top and bottom of each map. (Reference to Figs 2.7 and 4.16 may help to show how the map was constructed.) Left: inputs from the primary olfactory (pyriform) cortex (PC) terminate in the shaded region, that is in the caudal medial part of area 13, i.e. 13a, and in the ventral agranular insular cortex (AIv), which could therefore be termed secondary olfactory cortex. Right: the secondary olfactory cortices then project into the caudolateral orbitofrontal cortex, that is into the secondary taste cortex in that it receives from the primary taste cortex (G); and there are further projections into more anterior and medial parts of the orbitofrontal cortex. (After Price et al. 1991, with permission.)

visual information in this brain region to the control of feeding-related behaviour. This is further evidence that part of the olfactory representation in this region is related to the hedonic value of the olfactory stimulus, and in particular that at this level of the olfactory system in primates, the pleasure elicited by the food odour is at least part of what is represented.

To investigate whether the sensory-specific reduction in the responsiveness of the orbitofrontal olfactory neurons might be related to a sensory-specific reduction in the pleasure produced by the odour of a food when it is eaten to satiety, Rolls and Rolls (1997) measured humans' responses to the smell of a food which was eaten to satiety. It was found that the pleasantness of the odour of a food, but much less significantly its intensity, was reduced when the subjects ate it to satiety. It was also found that the pleasantness of the smell of other foods (i.e. not foods eaten in the meal) showed much less decrease. This finding has clear implications for the control of food intake; for ways to keep foods presented in a meal appetitive; and for effects on odour pleasantness ratings that could occur following meals. In an investigation of the mechanisms of this odour-specific sensory-specific satiety, Rolls and Rolls (1997) allowed humans to chew a food without swallowing, for approximately as long as the food is normally in the mouth during eating. They demonstrated a sensory-specific satiety with this procedure, showing that the sensory-specific satiety does not depend on food reaching the stomach. Thus at least part of the mechanism is likely to be produced by a change in processing in the olfactory pathways. It is not yet known which is the earliest stage of olfactory processing at which this modulation occurs. It is unlikely to be in the receptors, because the change in pleasantness found was much more significant than the change in the intensity (Rolls and Rolls 1997).

In addition to this modulation of neuronal responses to the taste and smell of foods eaten, there will be effects of the energy ingested on taste and smell responses to food. These are likely to depend on factors such as gastric distension, and the concentration of glucose and other indicators of hunger/satiety in the systemic circulation (see Karadi *et al.* 1990, 1992; Oomura *et al.* 1991; LeMagnen 1992; Rolls 1993, 1994c; Campfield *et al.* 1995).

2.4.4.3 The representation of information about odours by populations of neurons in the orbitofrontal cortex

To investigate how information about odours is represented by the responses of neurons in the orbitofrontal cortex, Rolls, Critchley and Treves (1996c) applied information theoretic analyses to the responses of these neurons recorded to 7–9 odours in an olfactory discrimination task. The information reflected by the firing rate of the response accounted for the majority of the information present (86%) when compared with that which was decodable if temporal encoding in the spike train was taken into account. This indicated that temporal encoding had a very minor role in the encoding of olfactory information by single orbitofrontal olfactory cells. The average information about which odourant was presented, averaged across the 38 neurons, was 0.09 bits, a figure that is low when compared with the information values previously published for the responses of temporal lobe face-selective neurons. However, it was shown that the information available from the population as a whole of these neurons increased approximately linearly with the number of neurons in the population (Rolls, Treves and Critchley, in preparation). Given that information is a log measure, the number of stimuli that can be encoded increases exponentially with the number of neurons in the sample. Thus the principle of encoding by the populations of neurons is that the combinatorial potential of distributed encoding is used. The significance of this is that with relatively limited numbers of neurons, information about a large number of stimuli can be represented. This means that receiving neurons need only receive from limited numbers of neurons of the type described here, and can nevertheless reflect the information about many stimuli. This type of combinatorial encoding makes brain connectivity possible. The fact that the information can largely be read out from the firing rates of a population of these neurons also makes the decoding of this information (by other neurons) relatively simple (see Rolls and Treves 1998).

2.4.5   The responses of orbitofrontal cortex taste and olfactory neurons to the sight of food

Many of the neurons with visual responses in this region also show olfactory or taste responses (Rolls and Baylis 1994), reverse rapidly in visual discrimination reversal (Rolls, Critchley, Mason and Wakeman, 1996b, see above), and only respond to the sight of food if hunger is present (Critchley and Rolls 1996b). This part of the orbitofrontal cortex thus seems to implement a mechanism which can flexibly alter the responses to visual stimuli depending on the reinforcement (e.g. the taste) associated with the visual stimulus (see Thorpe, Rolls and Maddison 1983; Rolls 1996a). This enables prediction of the taste associated with ingestion of what is seen, and thus in the visual selection of foods (see Rolls 1986c, 1993, 1994c). This cortical region is implicated more generally in a certain type of learning, namely in extinction and in the reversal of visual discriminations. It is suggested that the taste neurons in this region are important for these functions, for they provide information about whether a reward has been obtained (see Thorpe, Rolls and Maddison 1983; Rolls 1986c, 1990b, 1992a). These taste neurons represent a number of important primary reinforcers. The ability of this part of the cortex to perform rapid learning of associations between visual stimuli and primary reinforcers such as taste provides the basis for the importance of this part of the brain in food-related and emotion-related learning (see Rolls 1990b, 1992a, 1994c, 1996a) (see Chapter 3). Consistent with this function, parts of the orbitofrontal cortex receive direct projections from the inferior temporal visual cortex (Barbas 1988; Seltzer and Pandya 1989), a region important in high-order visual information processing (Rolls 1992b, 1994c).

The convergence of visual information onto neurons in this region not only enables associations to be learned between the sight of a food and its taste and smell, but also may provide the neural basis for the well-known effect which the sight of a food has on its perceived taste.

2.4.6   Functions of the amygdala and temporal cortex in feeding
2.4.6.1   Effects of lesions

Bilateral damage to the temporal lobes of primates leads to the Kluver–Bucy syndrome, in which lesioned monkeys, for example, select and place in their mouths non-food as well as food items shown to them, and repeatedly fail to avoid noxious stimuli (Kluver and Bucy 1939; Jones and Mishkin 1972; Aggleton and Passingham 1982; L. Baylis and Gaffan 1991). Rats with lesions in the basolateral amygdala also display altered food selection, in that they ingest relatively novel foods (Rolls and Rolls 1973; Borsini and Rolls 1984), and do not normally learn to avoid to ingest a solution which has previously resulted in sickness (B. Rolls and Rolls 1973). (The deficit in learned taste avoidance in rats may be because of damage to the insular taste cortex, which has projections through and to the amygdala, see Dunn and Everitt 1988.) The basis for these alterations in food selection and in food-related learning are considered next (see also Rolls 1990b, 1992b and Section 4.4).

The monkeys with temporal lobe damage have a visual discrimination deficit, in that they are impaired in learning to select one of two objects under which food is found, and thus fail to form correctly an association between the visual stimulus and reinforcement (Jones and Mishkin 1972; D. Gaffan 1992). D. Gaffan and Harrison (1987) and E. Gaffan, Gaffan and Harrison (1988) have shown that the tasks which are impaired by amygdala lesions in monkeys typically involve a cross-modal association from a previously neutral stimulus to a primary reinforcing stimulus (such as the taste of food), consistent with the hypothesis that the amygdala is involved in learning associations between stimuli and primary reinforcers (see also D. Gaffan 1992; D. Gaffan, Gaffan and Harrison 1989; Section 4.4). Further evidence linking the amygdala to reinforcement mechanisms is that monkeys will work in order to obtain electrical stimulation of the amygdala, and that single neurons in the amygdala are activated by brain-stimulation reward of a number of different sites (Rolls 1975; Rolls, Burton and Mora 1980; Chapter 4).

The Kluver–Bucy syndrome is produced by lesions which damage the cortical areas in the anterior part of the temporal lobe and the underlying amygdala (Jones and Mishkin 1972), or by lesions of the amygdala (Weiskrantz 1956; Aggleton and Passingham 1981; D. Gaffan 1992), or of the temporal lobe neocortex (Akert et al. 1961). Lesions to part of the temporal lobe neocortex, damaging the inferior temporal visual cortex and extending into the cortex in the ventral bank of the superior temporal sulcus, produce visual aspects of the syndrome, seen for example as a tendency to select non-food as well as food items (Weiskrantz and Saunders 1984). Anatomically, there are connections from the inferior temporal visual cortex to the amygdala (Herzog and Van Hoesen 1976), which in turn projects to the hypothalamus (Nauta 1961), thus providing a route for visual information to reach the hypothalamus (see Rolls 1981b, 1990b, 1992b; Amaral et al. 1992). This evidence, together with the evidence that damage to the hypothalamus can disrupt feeding (see Winn et al. 1984, 1990; Clark et al. 1991; LeMagnen 1992), thus indicates that there is a system which includes visual cortex in the temporal lobe, projections to the amygdala, and further connections to structures such as the lateral hypothalamus, which is involved in behavioural responses made on the basis of learned associations between visual stimuli and primary (unlearned) reinforcers such as the taste of food (see Fig. 2.8). Given this evidence from lesion and anatomical studies, the contribution of each of these regions to the visual analysis and learning required for these functions in food selection will be considered using evidence from the activity of single neurons in these regions.

2.4.6.2 Inferior Temporal Visual Cortex

Recordings were made from single neurons in the inferior temporal visual cortex while rhesus monkeys performed visual discriminations, and while they were shown visual stimuli associated with positive reinforcement such as food, with negative reinforcement such as aversive hypertonic saline, and neutral visual stimuli (Rolls, Judge and Sanghera 1977). It was found that during visual discrimination inferior temporal neurons often had sustained visual responses with latencies of 100–140 ms to the discriminanda, but that

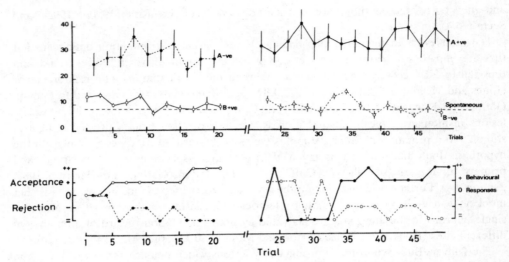

Fig. 2.19 Examples of the responses of a neuron in the inferior temporal visual cortex, showing that its responses (firing rate in spikes s^{-1}, upper panel) do not reverse when the reward association of the visual stimuli reverses. For the first 21 trials of the visual discrimination task, visual stimulus A was aversive (−ve, because if the monkey licked he obtained saline), and visual stimulus B was associated with reward (+ve, because if the monkey licked when he saw this stimulus, he obtained fruit juice). The neuron responded more to stimulus A than to stimulus B. After trial 21, the contingencies reversed (so that A was now +ve, and B −ve). The monkey learned the reversal correctly by about trial 35 (lower panel). However, the inferior temporal cortex neuron did not reverse when the reinforcement contingency reversed—it continued to respond to stimulus A after the reversal, even though the stimulus was now +ve. Thus this, and other inferior temporal cortex neurons, respond to the physical aspects of visual stimuli, and not to the stimuli based on their reinforcement association or the reinforcement contingency. (From Rolls, Judge and Sanghera 1977a.)

these responses did not depend on whether the visual stimuli were associated with reward or punishment. This was shown in a visual discrimination learning paradigm in which one visual stimulus is associated with reward (for example glucose taste, or fruit-juice taste), and another visual stimulus is associated with an aversive taste, such as saline, and then the reinforcement contingency was reversed. (That is, the visual stimulus, for example a triangle, to which the monkey had to lick in order to obtain a taste of fruit juice, was after the reversal associated with saline: if the monkey licked to the triangle after the reversal, he obtained mildly aversive salt solution.) An example of such an experiment is shown in Fig. 2.19. The neuron responded more to the triangle, both before reversal when it was associated with fruit juice, and after reversal, when the triangle was associated with saline. Thus the reinforcement association of the visual stimuli did not alter the response to the visual stimuli, which was based on the physical properties of the stimuli (for example their shape, colour, or texture). The same was true for the other neurons recorded in this study. This independence from reward association seems to be characteristic of neurons right through the temporal visual cortical areas, and must be true in earlier cortical areas too, in that they provide the inputs to the inferior temporal visual cortex.

This conclusion, that the responses of inferior temporal neurons during visual discriminations do not code for whether a visual stimulus is associated with reward or punishment, is also consistent with the findings of Ridley *et al.* (1977), Jarvis and Mishkin (1977), Gross *et al.* (1979), and Sato *et al.* (1980). Further it was found that inferior temporal neurons did not respond only to food-related visual stimuli, or only to aversive stimuli, and were not dependent on hunger, but rather that in many cases their responses depended on physical aspects of the stimuli such as shape, size, orientation, colour, or texture (Rolls, Judge and Sanghera 1977).

2.4.6.3 Why reward and punishment associations of stimuli are not represented early in information processing in the primate brain

The processing stream that has just been considered is that concerned with objects, that is with *what* is being looked at. Two fundamental points about pattern association networks for stimulus-reinforcement association learning can be made from what we have considered. The first point is that sensory processing in the primate brain proceeds as far as the invariant representation of objects (invariant with respect to, for example, size, position on the retina, and even view), independently of reward vs punishment association. Why should this be, in terms of systems-level brain organization? The suggestion that is made is that the visual properties of the world about which reward associations must be learned are generally objects (for example the sight of a banana, or of an orange), and are not just raw pixels or edges, with no invariant properties, which is what is represented in the retina and V1. The implication is that the sensory processing must proceed to the stage of the invariant representation of objects before it is appropriate to learn reinforcement associations. The invariance aspect is important too, for if we had different representations for an object at different places in our visual field, then if we learned when an object was at one point on the retina that it was rewarding, we would not generalize correctly to it when presented at another position on the retina. If it had previously been punishing at that retinal position, we might find the same object rewarding when at one point on the retina, and punishing when at another. This is inappropriate given the world in which we live, and in which our brain evolved, in that the most appropriate assumption is that objects have the same reinforcement association wherever they are on the retina.

These findings thus indicate that the responses of neurons in the inferior temporal visual cortex do not reflect the association of visual stimuli with reinforcers such as food. Given these findings and the lesion evidence described above, it is thus likely that the inferior temporal cortex is an input stage for this process. The next structure on the basis of anatomical connections (see Fig. 2.8) is the amygdala, and this is considered next.

2.4.6.4 Amygdala

In recordings made from 1754 amygdaloid neurons, it was found that 113 (6.4%), of which many were in a dorsolateral region of the amygdala known to receive directly from the inferior temporal visual cortex (Herzog and Van Hoesen 1976), had visual responses which in most cases were sustained while the monkey looked at effective visual stimuli (Sanghera, Rolls and Roper-Hall 1979). The latency of the responses was 100–140 ms or more. The majority (85%) of these visual neurons responded more strongly to some stimuli than to others, but physical factors which accounted for the responses such as orientation, colour, and texture could not usually be identified. It was found that 22 (19.5%) of these visual neurons responded primarily to foods and to objects associated with food (see e.g. Fig. 4.13a), but for none of these neurons did the responses occur uniquely to food-related stimuli, in that they all responded to one or more aversive or neutral stimuli. Further, although some neurons responded in a visual discrimination to the visual stimulus which indicated food reward, but not to the visual stimulus associated with aversive saline, only minor modifications of the neuronal responses were obtained when the association of the stimuli with reinforcement was reversed in the reversal of the visual discrimination. Thus even the responses of these neurons were not invariably associated with whichever stimulus was associated with food reward (see further Rolls 1992b; Section 4.4). A comparable population of neurons with responses apparently partly but not uniquely related to aversive visual stimuli was also found (Sanghera, Rolls and Roper-Hall 1979).

Amygdala neurons with responses which are probably similar to these have also been described by Ono *et al.* (1980, 1989), Nishijo *et al.* (1988), and Ono and Nishijo (1992). When Nishijo *et al.* (1988) tested four amygdala neurons in a simpler relearning situation than reversal in which salt was added to a piece of food such as a water melon, the neurons' responses to the sight of the water-melon appeared to diminish. However, in this task it was not clear whether the monkeys continued to look at the stimuli during extinction. It will be of interest in further studies to investigate whether in extinction evidence can be found for a rapid decrease in the neuronal responses to visual stimuli formerly associated with reward, even when fixation of the stimuli is adequate (see Rolls 1992b).

Wilson and Rolls (1999; see also Rolls 1992b) extended the analysis of the responses of these amygdala neurons by showing that while they do respond to (some) stimuli associated with primary reinforcement such as food, they do not respond if the reinforcement must be determined on the basis of a rule (such as stimuli when novel are negatively reinforced, and when familiar are positively reinforced). This is consistent with the evidence that the amygdala is involved when reward must be determined, as normally occurs during feeding, by association of a stimulus with a primary reinforcer such as the taste of food, but is not involved when reinforcement must be determined in some other ways (see D. Gaffan 1992; Rolls 1992b). In the same study (Wilson and Rolls 1999), it was shown that these amygdala neurons that respond to food can also respond to some other stimuli while they are relatively novel. It is suggested that it is by this mechanism that when relatively novel stimuli are encountered, they are investigated, e.g. by being smelled and then placed in the mouth, to assess whether the new stimuli are foods (see Rolls 1992b).

The failure of this population of amygdala neurons to respond only to reinforcing stimuli, and the difficulty in reversing their responses, are in contrast with the responses of certain populations of neurons in the caudal orbitofrontal cortex and in a region to which it projects, the basal forebrain, which do show very rapid (in one or two trials) reversals of their responses in visual discrimination reversal tasks (Thorpe, Rolls and Maddison 1983; Wilson and Rolls 1990; see Section 4.5). On the basis of these findings, it is suggested that the orbitofrontal cortex is more involved than the amygdala in the rapid readjustments of behavioural responses made to stimuli such as food when their reinforcement value is repeatedly changing, as in discrimination reversal tasks (Thorpe, Rolls and Maddison 1983; Rolls 1986b, 1990b). The ability to flexibly alter responses to stimuli based on their changing reinforcement associations is important in motivated behaviour (such as feeding) and in emotional behaviour, and it is this flexibility which it is suggested the orbitofrontal cortex adds to a more basic capacity which the amygdala implements for stimulus-reinforcement learning (Rolls 1990b).

These findings thus suggest that the amygdala could be involved at an early but rather inflexible stage of the processing by which visual stimuli are associated with reinforcement. Neuronal responses here do not code uniquely for whether a visual stimulus is associated with reinforcement, partly because the neurons do not reverse rapidly, and partly because the neurons can respond to relatively novel stimuli, which monkeys frequently pick up and place in their mouths for further exploration. Neurons with responses more closely related to reinforcement are found in areas to which the amygdala projects, such as the lateral hypothalamus, substantia innominata, and ventral striatum, and this may be because of the inputs these structures receive from the orbitofrontal cortex. The amygdala may thus be a somewhat slow and inflexible system, compared with the orbitofrontal cortex which has developed greatly in primates, in learning about which visual stimuli have the taste and smell of food. Consistent with the hypothesis that the amygdala can play some role in learning associations of visual stimuli to the taste and smell of food (see Fig. 2.8), some neurons with taste and olfactory responses are found in the primate amygdala (Sanghera, Rolls and Roper-Hall 1979; Ono *et al.* 1980, 1989; Nishijo *et al.* 1988; Ono and Nishijo 1992).

2.4.7 Functions of the orbitofrontal cortex in feeding

Damage to the orbitofrontal cortex alters food preferences, in that monkeys with damage to the orbitofrontal cortex select and eat foods which are normally rejected (Butter, McDonald and Snyder 1969; L. Baylis and Gaffan 1991) (Fig. 2.20). Their food choice behaviour is very similar to that of monkeys with amygdala lesions (L. Baylis and Gaffan 1991). Lesions of the orbitofrontal cortex also lead to a failure to correct feeding responses when these become inappropriate. Examples of the situations in which these abnormalities in feeding responses are found include: (a) extinction, in that feeding responses continue to be made to the previously reinforced stimulus; (b) reversals of visual discriminations, in that the monkeys make responses to the previously reinforced stimulus or object; (c) Go/Nogo tasks, in that responses are made to the stimulus which is not associated with food reward; and (d) passive avoidance, in that feeding responses are made even when they are punished (Butter 1969; Iversen and Mishkin 1970; Jones and Mishkin 1972; Tanaka 1973; see also Rosenkilde 1979; Fuster 1996). (It may be noted that in contrast, the formation of associations between visual stimuli and reinforcement is less affected by these lesions than by temporal lobe lesions, as tested during visual discrimination learning and reversals—Jones and Mishkin 1972).

To investigate how the orbitofrontal cortex may be involved in feeding and in the correction of feeding responses when these become inappropriate, recordings were made

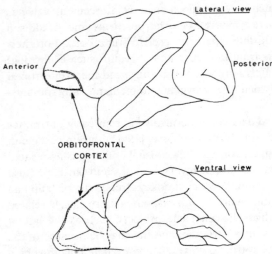

Lateral view

Anterior

Posterior

ORBITOFRONTAL
CORTEX

Ventral view

Effects of Orbitofrontal lesions:

(a) Changes in emotional behavior
(b) Changes in food-selection behavior
(c) Impaired extinction
(d) Difficulty in reversing responses
    during visual discrimination reversal

Fig. 2.20 The orbitofrontal cortex of the monkey. The effects of orbitofrontal lesions include: (a) changes in emotional behaviour; (b) changes in food-selection behaviour; (c) impaired extinction; (d) difficulty in reversing responses during visual discrimination reversal.

of the activity of 494 orbitofrontal neurons during the performance of a Go/Nogo task, reversals of a visual discrimination task, extinction, and passive avoidance (Thorpe, Rolls and Maddison 1983). First, neurons were found which responded in relation to the preparatory auditory or visual signal used before each trial (15.1%), or non-discriminatively during the period in which the discriminative visual stimuli were shown (37.8%). These neurons are not considered further here. Second, 8.6% of neurons had responses which occurred discriminatively during the period in which the visual stimuli were shown. The majority of these neurons responded to whichever visual stimulus was associated with reward, in that the stimulus to which they responded changed during reversal. However, six of these neurons required a combination of a particular visual stimulus in the discrimination *and* reward in order to respond. Further, none of this second group of neurons responded to all the reward-related stimuli including different foods which were shown, so that in general this group of neurons coded for a combination of one or several visual stimuli *and* reward. Thus information that particular visual stimuli had previously been associated with reinforcement was represented in the responses of orbitofrontal neurons. Third, 9.7% of neurons had responses which occurred after the lick response was made in the task to obtain reward. Some of these responded independently of whether fruit juice reward was obtained, or aversive hypertonic saline was obtained on trials on which the monkey licked in error or was given saline in the first trials of a reversal. Through these neurons information that a lick had been made was represented in the orbitofrontal cortex. Other neurons in this third group responded only when fruit juice was obtained, and thus through these neurons information that food reward had been given on that trial was represented in the orbitofrontal cortex. Such neurons reflect the taste of the liquid received, and are in a part of the orbitofrontal cortex which is close to, and probably receives inputs from, the secondary taste cortex (Rolls 1989b; Rolls, Yaxley and Sienkiewicz

1990). Other neurons in this group responded when saline was obtained when a response was made in error, or when saline was obtained on the first few trials of a reversal (but not in either case when saline was simply placed in the mouth), or when reward was not given in extinction, or when food was taken away instead of being given to the monkey, but did not respond in all these situations in which reinforcement was omitted or punishment was given. Thus through these neurons task-selective information that reward had been omitted or punishment given was represented in the responses of these neurons.

These three groups of neurons found in the orbitofrontal cortex could together provide for computation of whether the reinforcement previously associated with a particular stimulus was still being obtained, and generation of a signal if a match was not obtained. This signal could be partly reflected in the responses of the last subset of neurons with task-selective responses to non-reward or to unexpected punishment. This signal could be used to alter the monkey's behaviour, leading for example to reversal to one particular stimulus but not to other stimuli, to extinction to one stimulus but not to others, etc. It could also lead to the altered responses of the orbitofrontal differential neurons found as a result of learning in reversal, so that their responses indicate appropriately whether a particular stimulus is now associated with food reinforcement.

Thus the orbitofrontal cortex contains neurons which appear to be involved in altering behavioural responses when these are no longer associated with reward or become associated with punishment. In the context of feeding it appears that without these neurons the primate is unable to suppress his behaviour correctly to non-food objects, in that altered food preferences are produced by orbitofrontal damage (Butter *et al.* 1969). It also appears that without these neurons the primate is unable to correct his behaviour when it becomes appropriate to break a learned association between a stimulus and a reward such as food (Jones and Mishkin 1972). The orbitofrontal neurons could be involved in the actual breaking of the association, or in the alteration of behaviour when other neurons signal that the connection is no longer appropriate. As shown here, the orbitofrontal cortex contains neurons with responses which could provide the information necessary for, and the basis for, the unlearning. This type of unlearning is important in enabling animals to alter the environmental stimuli to which motivational responses such as feeding have previously been made, when experience shows that such responses have become inappropriate. In this way they can ensure that their feeding and other motivational responses remain continually adapted to a changing environment.

This evidence on how the primate orbitofrontal cortex is involved in feeding has been greatly extended by the discoveries described in Sections 2.4.2–2.4.4 that the secondary and tertiary taste and olfactory cortices are present in the orbitofrontal regions, that it is the reward value of food that is represented here as shown by the finding that satiety reduces the responsiveness of these neurons, and that the representation of the flavour of food is formed here in the brain. These findings show that the primary reward value of food produced by its taste and smell is represented in the primate orbitofrontal cortex. Consistent with this, in humans a representation of the taste and smell of food has been demonstrated in the orbitofrontal cortex (Rolls, Francis *et al.* 1997b) (Fig. 2.21 (see plate section) and Fig. 2.22). The findings described in Section 2.4.5 also confirm the very rapid visual-to-taste learning and reversal that take place in the primate orbitofrontal cortex.

Taste fMRI

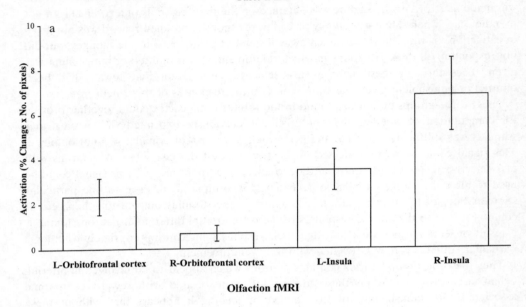

Olfaction fMRI

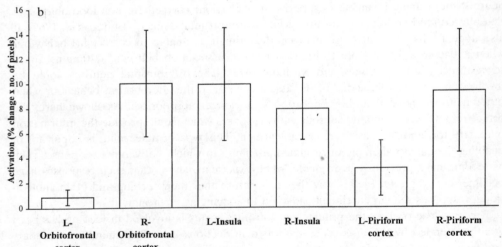

Fig. 2.22 Histograms showing the mean ($\pm$ s.e.m., across seven experiments) of the change in activation of different brain regions during the taste (a) and olfactory (b) stimulation. L, left; OFC, orbitofrontal cortex; PIR, pyriform (primary olfactory) cortex; R, right. (After Rolls, Francis et al. 1997b.)

The fact that the texture of food in the mouth, and the mouth feel of fat, an important factor in the palatability of food, are also represented in the primate orbitofrontal cortex, also implicates this region as a crucial region for indicating the reward value of food, as well as for learning which stimuli are associated with food reward.

The more rapid reversal of neuronal responses in the orbitofrontal cortex, and in a region to which it projects, the basal forebrain (Thorpe, Rolls and Maddison 1983; Wilson and Rolls 1990), than in the amygdala suggest that the orbitofrontal cortex is more involved than the amygdala in the rapid readjustments of behavioural responses made to stimuli when their reinforcement value is repeatedly changing, as in discrimination reversal tasks (Thorpe, Rolls and Maddison 1983; Rolls 1986c, 1990b). The ability to flexibly alter responses to stimuli based on their changing reinforcement associations is important in motivated behaviour (such as feeding) and in emotional behaviour, and it is this flexibility which it is suggested the orbitofrontal cortex adds to a more basic capacity which the amygdala implements for stimulus-reinforcement learning (Rolls 1986c, 1990b). The great development of the orbitofrontal cortex in primates, yet the similarity of its connections to those of the amygdala (see Fig 4.11), and its connections with the amygdala, lead to the suggestion that in evolution, and as part of continuing corticalization of functions, the orbitofrontal cortex has come to be placed hierarchically above the amygdala, and is especially important when rapid readjustment of stimulus-reinforcement associations is required (see Rolls 1990b). This suggestion is also consistent with the indication that whereas in rodents subcortical structures such as the amygdala and hypothalamus have access to taste information from the precortical taste system, the same does not occur in primates; and that some precortical processing of taste in relation to the control of feeding occurs in rodents (see above and T. Scott and Giza 1992). In contrast, there is great development and importance of cortical processing of taste in primates, and it is very appropriate that the orbitofrontal cortex area just described is found just medial to the secondary taste cortex, which is in primates in the caudolateral orbitofrontal cortex. It appears that close to this orbitofrontal taste cortex the orbitofrontal cortical area just described develops, and receives inputs from the visual association cortex (inferior temporal cortex), the olfactory (pyriform) cortex, and probably from the somatosensory cortex, so that reward associations between these different modalities can be determined rapidly. An interesting topic for the future is whether the satiety signals summarized in Sections 2.2 and 2.3 also gain access to the orbitofrontal cortex, and how they modulate there the taste, olfactory and visual neuronal responses to food.

2.4.8 Functions of the striatum in feeding

Parts of the striatum receive inputs from many of the structures involved in the control of feeding, and have connections on through other parts of the basal ganglia which may influence behavioural output. Moreover, damage to different parts of the striatum can affect feeding in a number of ways. We therefore discuss here its role as one of the behavioural output systems for feeding which enable the structures such as the orbitofrontal cortex and amygdala which decode the reward value of sensory stimuli including food to connect to behaviour. Further aspects of basal ganglia function in terms of an output system for emotional stimuli to produce behavioural responses will be described in Chapter 4, and a more complete description (with figures) including its implication in the pharmacology of reward is provided in Chapter 6. Figure 6.5 shows where the striatum (which includes the caudate nucleus, the putamen, and the ventral striatum consisting of the nucleus accumbens and olfactory tubercle) is in the primate brain. Figure 6.6 shows some of the connections of the different parts of the striatum. These figures will be useful for the whole of Section 2.4.8, and for Chapters 4–6. Hypotheses on how the basal ganglia actually operate as neural networks are described in Chapter 6 and by Rolls and Treves (1998, Chapter 9). In this section, we focus on the role of the striatum in feeding.

2.4.8.1 Effects of lesions of the striatum on feeding, and connections of the striatum.

Damage to the nigrostriatal bundle, which depletes the striatum of dopamine, produces aphagia (lack of eating) and adipsia (lack of drinking) associated with a sensori-motor disturbance in the rat (Ungerstedt 1971; Marshall *et al*. 1974; Stricker and Zigmond 1976; Stricker 1984). Many of the brain systems implicated in the control of feeding, such as the amygdala and orbitofrontal cortex, have projections to the striatum, which could provide a route for these brain systems to lead to feeding responses (see Rolls 1979, 1984b, 1986c; Mogenson *et al*. 1980; Rolls and Williams 1987a; Rolls and Johnstone 1992; Williams, Rolls, Leonard and Stern 1993; see Figs 6.5 and 6.6 and Section 6.4). We now consider how each part of the striatum is involved in the control of feeding, using evidence from the connections of each part, the effects of lesions to each part, and especially the type of neuronal activity in each part of the primate striatum during feeding. A more general discussion of basal ganglia function is provided in Section 6.4, and only aspects especially relevant to feeding are considered here.

2.4.8.2 The ventral striatum

The ventral striatum, which includes the nucleus accumbens, the olfactory tubercle (or anterior perforated substance of primates), and the islands of Calleja, receives inputs from limbic structures such as the amygdala and hippocampus, and from the orbitofrontal cortex, and projects to the ventral pallidum (see further Groenewegen *et al*. 1991; Rolls and Treves 1998; Figs 6.5 and 6.6). The ventral pallidum may then influence output regions by the subthalamic nucleus/globus pallidus/ventral thalamus/premotor cortex route, or via the mediodorsal nucleus of the thalamus/prefrontal cortex route (Heimer *et al*. 1982). The ventral striatum may thus be for limbic structures what the neostriatum is for neocortical structures, that is a route for limbic structures to influence output regions. There is evidence linking the ventral striatum and its dopamine input to reward, for manipulations of this system alter the incentive effects which learned rewarding stimuli (e.g. a light associated with food) have on behaviour (Everitt and Robbins 1992; Robbins and Everitt 1992). For example, depletion of dopamine in the ventral striatum of rats using the neurotoxin 6-hydroxydopamine abolished the effect that a light previously associated with the delivery of food normally has in prolonging responding when food is no longer being delivered (Everitt and Robbins 1992; Robbins and Everitt 1992). Eating and body weight, were not impaired. Thus it is the effects on feeding that result from stimulus-rein-forcement association learning, in which the amygdala and orbitofrontal cortex are implicated, that the ventral striatum appears to link to behavioural output.

Glucose

Olfaction

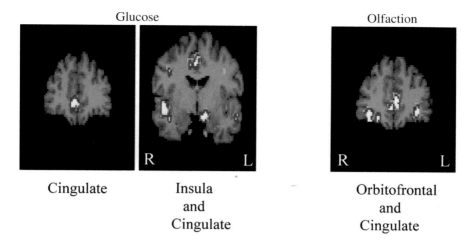

Cingulate   Insula   Orbitofrontal
                  and   and
                Cingulate   Cingulate

Fig. 2.21 Coronal MRI sections of the brain of one subject showing the areas activated by the taste of glucose and by the smell of vanilla. The areas of significant activation are shown coloured on isotropic, grey matter nulled images, for all pixels with a probability of $P < 0.005$, corrected for the multiple comparisons problem using the method of Gaussian random fields (Friston *et al.* 1995). The activations shown were calculated from the difference in pixel intensity over the 6-s period during which the activation for each brain region was maximal, from that measured during the control period with no stimulation. Activation was produced in the orbitofrontal cortex, insula, and some other brain regions (After Rolls, Francis *et al.* 1997b.)

Pleasant Touch

Neutral Touch

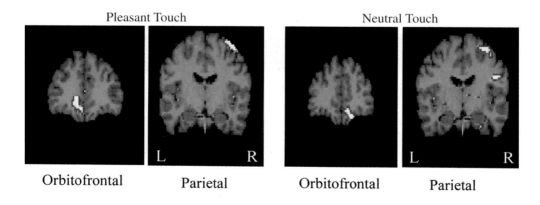

Orbitofrontal   Parietal   Orbitofrontal   Parietal

Fig. 4.5 Coronal MRI sections of the brain of one of the subjects showing the areas activated by the pleasant touch. The activations which exceeded a *t* value of 3.25 for the somatosensory cortex and 2.0 for the other regions are shown. These activations were averaged over 32 16-s repetitions of the somatosensory stimuli. The activations shown were calculated over the 6-s period during which the activation for each brain region was at its maximum, and the values shown are those during the pleasant touch minus those during the control period with no somatosensory stimulation. Activation was produced in the somatosensory cortex, in the lateral orbitofrontal cortex, and in some other brain regions. (After Rolls, Francis *et al.* 1997a.)

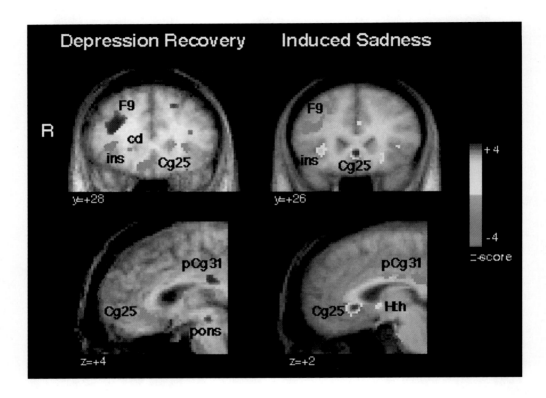

Fig. 4.25 Changes in the subgenual cingulate area (Cg25) associated with the recovery from depression (left), and with the induction of a mood state of sadness (right). Left images: Z-score maps demonstrating changes in regional glucose metabolism (fluorodeoxyglucose PET) in depressed patients following 6 weeks of treatment with the antidepressant fluoxetine. Upper: coronal view; lower, saggital view). Green indicates that the change is a decrease, and red or yellow an increase (see calibration bar on far right). Right images: changes in regional cerebral blood flow (oxygen-15 water PET) in healthy volunteers 10 min after induction of acute sadness. The recovery from depression and the induction of sadness produce opposite changes in Cg25. Reciprocal changes were seen in the dorsal part of the prefrontal cortex, labelled F9. F, frontal; cd, caudate nucleus; ins, anterior insula; Cg25, subgenual cingulate; Hth, hypothalamus; pCG31, posterior cingulate; R, right. (Reproduced with permission from Mayberg 1997.)

Because of its possible role as an output structure for the amygdala and orbitofrontal cortex to enable learned associations between previously neutral stimuli and rewards such as food to influence behaviour, the activity of neurons in the ventral striatum has been analysed in macaques during feeding and during tasks which require stimulus-reinforcement association learning, such as visual discrimination tasks in which one visual stimulus predicts (is a discriminative stimulus for) the taste of food, and the other visual stimulus is a discriminative stimulus for the taste of saline (Rolls and Williams 1987a,b; Williams, Rolls, Leonard and Stern 1993). A number of different types of neuronal response were found. One population of neurons was found to respond differently to visual stimuli which indicate that if a lick response is made, the taste of glucose will be obtained, and to other visual stimuli which indicate that if a lick response will be made, the taste of aversive saline will be obtained (Rolls 1990b). Responses of an example of a neuron of this type are shown in Fig. 6.7. The neuron increased its firing rate to the visual stimulus which indicated that saline would be obtained if a lick was made (the S−), and decreased its firing rate to the visual stimulus which indicated that a response could be made to obtain a taste of glucose (the S+). The differential response latency of this neuron to the reward-related and to the saline-related visual stimulus was approximately 150 ms (see Fig. 6.7), and this value was typical.

Of the neurons which responded to visual stimuli that were rewarding, relatively few responded to all the rewarding stimuli used. That is, only few (1.8%) ventral striatal neurons responded both when food was shown and to the positive discriminative visual stimulus, the S+ (e.g. a triangle shown on a video monitor), in a visual discrimination task. Instead, the reward-related neuronal responses were typically more context- or stimulus-dependent, responding, for example, to the sight of food but not to the S+ which signified food (4.3%), differentially to the S+ or S− but not to food (4.0%), or to food if shown in one context but not in another context. Some neurons were classified as having taste or olfactory responses to food (see Table 6.1; Williams, Rolls, Leonard and Stern 1993). Some other neurons (1.4%) responded to aversive stimuli. These neurons did not respond simply in relation to arousal, which was produced in control tests by inputs from different modalities, for example by touch of the leg.

These neurons with reinforcement-related responses represented 13.9% of the neurons recorded in the ventral striatum, and may receive their inputs from structures such as the amygdala and orbitofrontal cortex, in which some neurons with similar responses are found (see above).

In that the majority of the neurons recorded in the ventral striatum did not have unconditional sensory responses, but instead the response typically depended on memory, for whether the stimulus was recognized, or for whether it was associated with reinforcement, the function of this part of the striatum does not appear to be purely sensory. Rather, it may provide one route for such memory-related and emotional and motivational stimuli to influence motor output. This is consistent with the hypothesis that the ventral striatum is a link for learned incentive (e.g. rewarding) stimuli (see, e.g., Everitt and Robbins 1992), and also for other limbic-processed stimuli such as faces and novel stimuli, to influence behaviour (Mogenson et al. 1980; Rolls 1984b, 1989a, 1990a; Rolls and Williams 1987a,b; Rolls and Johnstone 1992; Williams, Rolls, Leonard and Stern 1993;

Rolls and Treves 1998). The role of the ventral striatum in feeding may thus be to provide a route for learned incentive stimuli such as the sight of food to influence behavioural responses such as approach to food.

2.4.8.3 The caudate nucleus

In the **head of the caudate nucleus** (Rolls, Thorpe and Maddison 1983b), which receives inputs particularly from the prefrontal cortex (see Figs 6.5 and 6.6), many neurons responded to environmental stimuli which were cues to the monkey to prepare for the possible initiation of a feeding response. Thus, 22.4% of neurons recorded responded during a cue given by the experimenter that a food or non-food object was about to be shown, and fed if food, to the monkey. Comparably, in a visual discrimination task made to obtain food, 14.5% of the neurons (including some of the above) responded during a 0.5-s tone/light cue which preceded and signalled the start of each trial. It is suggested that these neurons are involved in the utilization of environmental cues for the preparation for movement, and that disruption of the function of these neurons contributes to the akinesia or failure to initiate movements (including those required for feeding) found after depletion of dopamine in the striatum (Rolls, Thorpe and Maddison 1983b). Some other neurons (25.8%) responded if food was shown to the monkey immediately prior to feeding by the experimenter, but the responses of these neurons typically did not occur in other situations in which food-related visual stimuli were shown, such as during the visual discrimination task. Comparably, some other neurons (24.3%) responded differentially in the visual discrimination task, for example to the visual stimulus which indicated that the monkey could initiate a lick response to obtain food, yet typically did not respond when food was simply shown to the monkey prior to feeding. The responses of these neurons thus occur to particular stimuli which indicate that particular motor responses should be made, and are thus situation-specific, so that it is suggested that these neurons are involved in stimulus-motor response connections. In that their responses are situation-specific, they are different from the responses of the orbitofrontal cortex and hypothalamic neurons described above with visual responses to the sight of food (Rolls, Thorpe and Maddison 1983b). It is thus suggested that these neurons in the head of the caudate nucleus could be involved in relatively fixed feeding responses made in particular, probably well-learned, situations to food, but do not provide a signal which reflects whether a visual stimulus is associated with food, and on the basis of which any response required to obtain the food could be initiated. Rather, it is likely that the systems described above in the temporal lobe, hypothalamus and orbitofrontal cortex are involved in this more flexible decoding of the food value of visual stimuli.

In the **tail of the caudate nucleus**, which receives inputs from the inferior temporal visual cortex (see Figs 6.5 and 6.6), neurons were found which responded to visual stimuli such as gratings and edges, but which showed habituation which was rapid and pattern-specific (Caan, Perrett and Rolls 1984). It was suggested that these neurons are involved in orientation to patterned visual stimuli, and in pattern-specific habituation to these stimuli (Caan, Perrett and Rolls 1984). These neurons would thus appear not to be involved directly in the control of feeding, although a disturbance in the ability to orient normally to a changed visual stimulus could indirectly have an effect on the ability to react normally.

2.4.8.4 The putamen

In the putamen, which receives from the sensori-motor cortex, neurons were found with activity which occurred just before mouth or arm movements made by the monkey (Rolls, Thorpe *et al.* 1984). Disturbances in the normal function of these neurons might be expected to affect the ability to initiate and execute movements, and thus might indirectly affect the ability to feed normally.

2.4.8.5 Synthesis: the functions of the striatum in feeding and reward

These neurophysiological studies show that in different regions of the striatum neurons are found which may be involved in orientation to environmental stimuli, in the use of such stimuli in the preparation for and initiation of movements, in the execution of movements, in stimulus-response connections appropriate for particular responses made in particular situations to particular stimuli, and in allowing learned reinforcers, including food, to influence behaviour. Because of its many inputs from brain systems involved in feeding and from other brain systems involved in action, it may provide a crucial route for signals which have been decoded through sensory pathways and limbic structures, and which code for the current reward value of visual, olfactory, and taste stimuli, to be interfaced in an arbitration mechanism, to produce behavioural output. The issue then arises of how the striatum, and more generally the basal ganglia, might operate to perform such functions.

We can start by commenting on what functions must be performed in order to link the signals that control feeding to action. It has been shown above that through sensory pathways representations of objects in the environment are produced. These are motivation-independent, and are in, for example, the primary taste cortex and the inferior temporal visual cortex in primates (see Fig. 2.8). After this stage, the sensory signals are interfaced to motivational state, so that the signals in, for example, the orbitofrontal cortex reflect not only the taste of the food, but also whether the monkey is hungry. The sensory signals are also passed in these structures (e.g. the orbitofrontal cortex and amygdala) through association memories, so that the outputs reflect whether a particular stimulus has been previously, and is still, associated with a primary reward. (This process will include conditioned effects from previous ingestion which reflect the energy obtained from the food, sickness produced by it, etc.) These neurons thus reflect the reward value of food, and neurons in this system can be driven by visual, olfactory, and/or taste stimuli. Now, it is of fundamental importance that these reward-related signals should not be interfaced directly to feeding movements, such as chewing. (Brainstem systems which perform such functions might, in a limited way, assist in the execution of feeding movements later in the feeding sequence.) Instead, what is required is that the food-related reward signals should enter an arbitration mechanism, which takes into account not only the other rewards (with their magnitude) that are currently available, but also the cost of obtaining each reward (see further Sections 10.3 and 6.4).

The proposal is developed at the conceptual level elsewhere that the basal ganglia perform this function (Section 6.4; Rolls 1984b, 1994a; Rolls and Williams 1987a; Rolls and Johnstone 1992; Rolls and Treves 1998, Chapter 9). The striatum receives the appropriate signals for this function, including not only information from limbic structures and the orbitofrontal cortex about rewards available; and cognitive information from the association areas of the cerebral cortex; but also information from the motor, premotor, somatosensory, and parietal cortical areas which provides information about action and movements. The hypothesis is that the striatum, followed by the globus pallidus and substantia nigra, provide a two-stage system for bringing these signals together. Such convergence is implied and provided for by the dendritic organization of the basal ganglia (Percheron *et al.* 1984a,b; Rolls 1984b; Rolls and Williams 1987a; Rolls and Johnstone 1992; see Section 6.4). By virtue of such anatomy, the basal ganglia would allow in its output stages signals indicating that food was available, was currently rewarding, and that the costs of obtaining it were not too high as indicated perhaps by frontal cortical inputs, to be combined with, for example, signals from parietal and premotor areas reflecting what position in space is being visually fixated, and actions or movements being made to approach that position in space. These signals might well lead to the activation of individual neurons as a result of previous repeated co-occurrence, and associated synaptic modification in the basal ganglia. The output of such neurons would then indicate that actions should be made to approach and obtain rewarding targets in the environment. If a signal arrived in the basal ganglia from another cortical or limbic area (indicating for example that a novel visual stimulus had appeared), then lateral inhibitory connections and the competitive interactions it makes possible within the striatum would lead to interruption of feeding, and would implement an arbitration system (see further Rolls 1984b; Rolls and Williams 1987a; Rolls and Johnstone 1992). It is suggested that part of what is implemented in this way is a relatively simple interface between sensory and action systems, in that the signals reaching the striatum about reward need only to signify that reward is available, with the details about where it is being implied, for example, by which position in space is being visually fixated, and is the current subject of attention. Limiting sensory analysis in this way allows the reward signal, reflecting the output of the 'what' system in perception, to be linked unambiguously with the output of the 'where' system in perception (cf. Rolls 1991; Rolls 1992a, page 18), and this is part of what simplifies the interface between systems that specify what targets in the environment should be the targets for action, and the systems which lead to action. The action system in this case can be general-purpose, in that it can be organized to perform general-purpose operations (which are not different for each type of goal object or reward), to approach and acquire the objects in space which are currently the focus of attention. (Of course, if the object that is the object of attention is associated with punishment, as shown by inputs carried by other neurons from limbic structures, then the basal ganglia should access or 'look up' operations learned previously that will lead to withdrawal from the current focus of attention.) The ways in which reward systems provide for an interface to action systems, and in which the basal ganglia may operate to map signals into actions, are discussed more fully elsewhere (Rolls 1984b, 1990b, 1994a; Rolls and Williams 1987a; Rolls and Johnstone 1992; Rolls and Treves 1998).

These ideas address some of the crucial current questions in understanding how brain systems involved in decoding rewards, including food reward, are interfaced to action systems to produce, for example, feeding. It is likely that understanding the functions of the basal ganglia will be crucial in understanding these issues.

3 The nature of emotion

In this chapter the nature of emotion, and its functions, are considered, to provide a foundation for exploring the brain mechanisms involved in emotion in Chapter 4. It is important when considering the neural bases of emotion to know what types of stimuli elicit emotions. This is considered here, and helps to focus analysis on certain types of brain processing in Chapter 4. It is also important to know what the functions of emotion are, for they provides a guide to the neural output systems which may be expected to receive inputs from the brain regions involved in emotions.

Certain more general issues about emotion are left until later in the book, after the brain mechanisms involved in emotion and in related behaviours have been described. One such issue is that of emotional feelings, which is part of the much larger issue of consciousness. This issue is left until Chapter 9. Another issue is the interesting one of emotion and brain design. Why do we have emotions? Are emotions crucial to brain design and evolution? This issue, which deals with the adaptive value of emotion in relation to evolution by natural selection, is left until Chapter 10, where it is suggested that emotion is fundamental to the design of any adaptive brain with flexible behaviour. That will conclude our exploration of reward, punishment, emotion, motivation, their brain mechanisms, and why we have these processes.

3.1 A theory of emotion

3.1.1 Introduction

What are emotions? This is a question that almost everyone is interested in. There have been many answers, many of them surprisingly unclear and ill-defined (see Strongman 1996; Oatley and Jenkins 1996). William James (1884) was at least clear about what he thought. He believed that emotional experiences were produced by sensing bodily changes, such as changes in heart rate or in skeletal muscles. His view was that "We feel frightened because we are running away". But he left unanswered the crucial question even for his theory, which is: Why do some events make us run away (and then feel emotional), whereas others do not?

A more modern theory is that of Frijda (1986), who argues that a change in action readiness is the central core of an emotion. Oatley and Jenkins (1996, p. 96) make this part of their definition too, stating that the core of an emotion is readiness to act and the prompting of plans. But surely subjects in reaction time experiments in psychology who are continually for thousands of trials altering their action readiness are very far indeed from having normal or strong emotional experiences? Similarly, we can perform an action in response to a verbal request (e.g. open a door), yet may not experience great emotion when performing this action. Another example might be the actions that are performed in driving a car on a routine trip—we get ready, and many actions are performed, often quite automatically, and little emotion occurs. So it appears that there is no necessary link between performing actions and emotion. This may not be a clear way to define emotion.

Because it is useful to be able to specify what emotions are, in this chapter we consider a systematic approach to this question. Part of the route is to ask what causes emotions. Can clear conditions be specified for the circumstances in which emotions occur? This is considered in Section 3.1.2. Continuing with this theme, when we have come to understand the conditions under which emotions occur, does this help us to classify and describe different emotions systematically, in terms of differences between the different conditions that cause emotions to occur? A way in which a systematic account of different emotions can be provided is described in Section 3.1.3. A major help in understanding emotions would be provided by understanding what the functions of emotion are. It turns out that emotions have quite a number of different functions, each of which helps us to understand emotions a little more clearly. These different functions of emotion are described in Section 3.1.5. Understanding the different functions of emotion helps us to understand also the brain mechanisms of emotion, for it helps us to see that emotion can operate to affect several different output systems of the brain. With this background of the factors that cause emotion, and what emotion in turn does, we are in a good position to understand the brain systems that determine whether emotion is produced and that implement behavioural, autonomic, and endocrine responses to emotion-provoking stimuli. These analyses leave open though a major related question, which is why emotional states feel like something to us. This it transpires is part of the much larger, though more speculative, issue of consciousness, and why anything should feel like something to us. This aspect of emotional feelings, because it is part of the much larger issue of consciousness, is deferred until Chapter 9. In this chapter, in considering the function of emotions, the idea is presented that emotions are part of a system which helps to map certain classes of stimuli, broadly identified as rewarding and punishing stimuli, to action systems. Part of the idea is that this enables a simple interface between such stimuli and actions. This is an important area in its own right, which goes to the heart of why animals are built to respond to rewards and punishments. This issue is taken up in a comprehensive way in Chapter 10.

The suggestion is that we now have a way of systematically approaching the nature of emotion, their functions, and their brain mechanisms. Doubtless in time there will be changes and additions to the overall picture. But the suggestion is that the ideas presented here do provide a firm and systematic foundation for understanding emotions, their functions, and their brain mechanisms.

3.1.2 Definitions

I will first introduce the definition of emotion that I propose (Rolls 1986a,b, 1990b, 1995c). The essence of the proposal is that emotions are states elicited by rewards and punishers, including changes in rewards and punishments. A reward is anything for which an animal will work. A punisher is anything that an animal will work to escape or avoid. An example of an emotion might thus be happiness produced by being given a reward, such as a hug, a pleasant touch, praise, winning a large sum of money, or being with someone whom one loves. All these things are rewards, in that we will work to obtain them. Another example of an emotion might be fear produced by the sound of a rapidly approaching bus when we are cycling, or the sight of an angry expression on someone's face. We will work to avoid such stimuli, which are punishers. Another example might be frustration, anger, or sadness produced by the omission of an expected reward such as a prize, or the termination of a reward such as the death of a loved one. Another example might be relief, produced by the omission or termination of a punishing stimulus, for example the removal of a painful stimulus, or sailing out of danger. These examples indicate how emotions can be produced by the delivery, omission, or termination of rewarding or punishing stimuli, and go some way to indicate how different emotions could be produced and classified in terms of the rewards and punishers received, omitted, or terminated.

Before accepting this proposal, we should consider whether there are any exceptions to the proposed rule. Are any emotions caused by stimuli, events, or remembered events that are not rewarding or punishing? Do any rewarding or punishing stimuli not cause emotions? We will consider these questions in more detail in the next few pages. The point is that if there are no major exceptions, or if any exceptions can be clearly encapsulated, then we may have a good working definition at least of what causes emotions. Moreover, it is worth pointing out that many approaches to or theories of emotion have in common that part of the process involves 'appraisal' (e.g. Frijda 1986; Oatley and Johnson-Laird 1987; Lazarus 1991; Izard 1993; Stein, Trabasso and Liwag 1994). This is part, for example, of the suggestion made by Oatley and Jenkins (1996), who on p. 96 write that "an emotion is usually caused by a person consciously or unconsciously evaluating an event as relevant to a concern (a goal) that is important; the emotion is felt as positive when a concern is advanced and negative when a concern is impeded". The concept of appraisal presumably involves in all these theories assessment of whether something is rewarding or punishing, that is whether it will be worked for or avoided. The description in terms of reward or punishment adopted here simply seems much more precisely and operationally specified. In the remainder of this section, we will also consider a slightly more formal definition than rewards or punishers, in which the concept of reinforcers is used, and show how there has been a considerable history in the development of ideas along this line.

Emotions can usefully be defined as states produced by instrumental reinforcing stimuli (Millenson 1967; Weiskrantz 1968; J. Gray 1975, Chapter 7; J. Gray 1981). (Earlier views, to which these more recent theories are related, include those of Watson 1929, 1930; Harlow and Stagner 1933; and Amsel 1958, 1962.) This definition is extended below. (Instrumental reinforcers are stimuli which if their occurrence, termination, or omission is made contingent upon the making of a response, alter the probability of the future emission of that response. Part of the point of introducing reinforcers into the definition of emotion-provoking stimuli, events, or remembered events, is that this provides an operational definition of what causes an emotion. Another reason for introducing reinforcers into the definition is that different emotions can then be partly classified in terms of different reinforcement contingencies. I note that the definition provided above should be taken to include the formulation 'emotions can be defined as states produced by stimuli which can be shown to be instrumental reinforcers', for the formal conditions for demonstrating that a stimulus is a reinforcer may not always be present when such a stimulus is delivered, omitted, or terminated.) Some stimuli are unlearned (or 'primary') reinforcers (e.g. the taste of food if the animal is hungry, or pain); while others may become reinforcing by learning, because of their association with such primary reinforcers, thereby becoming 'secondary reinforcers'. This type of learning may thus be called 'stimulus–reinforcement association', and probably occurs via a process like that of classical conditioning. It is a form of pattern association between two stimuli, one of which is a primary reinforcer, and the other of which becomes a secondary reinforcer (see Rolls and Treves 1998). (It is not stimulus–response or habit learning, in which the association is to a response, and in which other brain systems are implicated—see Rolls and Treves 1998, Chapter 9.) If a reinforcer increases the probability of emission of a response on which it is contingent, it is said to be a 'positive reinforcer' or 'reward'; if it reduces the probability of such a response it is a 'negative reinforcer' or 'punisher'. For example, fear is an emotional state which might be produced by a sound that has previously been associated with an electrical shock. Shock in this example is the primary negative reinforcer, and fear is the emotional state which occurs to the tone stimulus as a result of the learning of the stimulus (i.e. tone)–reinforcement (i.e. shock) association. The tone in this example is a conditioned stimulus because of classical conditioning, and has secondary reinforcing properties in that responses will be made to escape from it and thus avoid the primary reinforcer, shock.

The converse reinforcement contingencies produce the opposite effects on behaviour. The omission or termination of a positive reinforcer ('extinction' and 'time out' respectively, sometimes described as 'punishing'), reduce the probability of responses. Responses followed by the omission or termination of a negative reinforcer increase in probability, this pair of reinforcement operations being termed 'active avoidance' and 'escape', respectively (see J. Gray 1975, Chapter 4; Mackintosh 1983, pp. 19–21; Dickinson 1980; and Pearce 1996, for further discussions of this terminology).

A useful convention to distinguish between emotion and a mood state is as follows. An emotion consists of cognitive processing which results in a decoded signal that an environmental event (or remembered event) is reinforcing, together with the mood state produced as a result. If the mood state is produced in the absence of the external sensory input and the cognitive decoding (for example by direct electrical stimulation of the amygdala, see Section 5.2), then this is described only as a mood state, and is different from an emotion in that there is no object in the environment towards which the mood state is directed. (In that emotions are produced by stimuli or objects, and thus emotions "take or have an object", emotional states are examples of what philosophers call intentional states.) It is useful to point out that there is great opportunity for cognitive processing (whether conscious or not) in emotions, for cognitive processes will very often be required to determine whether an environmental stimulus or event is reinforcing (see further Section 3.1.4).

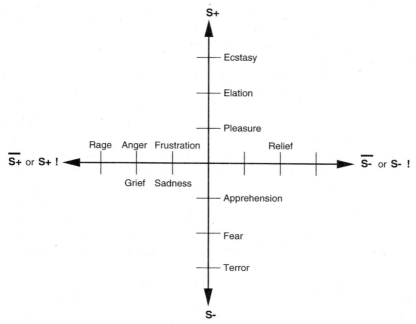

Fig. 3.1 Some of the emotions associated with different reinforcement contingencies are indicated. Intensity increases away from the centre of the diagram, on a continuous scale. The classification scheme created by the different reinforcement contingencies consists of: (1) the presentation of a positive reinforcer (S+); (2) the presentation of a negative reinforcer (S−); (3) the omission of a positive reinforcer ($\overline{S+}$) or the termination of a positive reinforcer (S+!); and (4) the omission of a negative reinforcer ($\overline{S−}$) or the termination of a negative reinforcer (S−!).

3.1.3 Different emotions

The different emotions can be described and classified according to whether the reinforcer is positive or negative, and by the reinforcement contingency. An outline of the classification scheme thus created is shown in Fig. 3.1. Movement away from the centre of the diagram represents increasing intensity of emotion, on a continuous scale. The diagram shows that emotions associated with the presentation of a positive reinforcer (S+) include pleasure, elation and ecstasy. Of course, other emotional labels can be included along the same axis. Emotions associated with the presentation of a negative reinforcer (S−) include apprehension, fear, and terror (see Fig. 3.1). Emotions associated with the omission of a positive reinforcer ($\overline{S+}$) or the termination of a positive reinforcer (S+!) include frustration, anger and rage. Emotions associated with the omission of a negative reinforcer ($\overline{S−}$) or the termination of a negative reinforcer (S−!) include relief. Although the classification of emotion presented here differs from earlier theories, the approach adopted here of defining and classifying emotions by reinforcing effects is one that has been developed in a number of earlier analyses (Millenson 1967; J. Gray 1975, 1981; Rolls 1986a,b, 1990b; see Strongman 1996).

The mechanisms described here would not be limited in the range of emotions for which they could account. First, different classes of emotion could arise because of different reinforcement contingencies, as described above and indicated in Fig. 3.1.

Second, different intensities within these classes can produce different degrees of emotion (see above and Millenson 1967). For example, as the strength of a positive reinforcer being presented increases, emotions might be labelled as pleasure, elation, and ecstasy. Similarly, as the strength of a negative reinforcer being presented increases, emotions might be labelled as apprehension, fear, and terror (see Fig. 3.1). It may be noted here that anxiety can refer to the state produced by stimuli associated with non-reward or punishment (J. Gray 1987).

Third, any environmental stimulus might have a number of different reinforcement associations. For example, a stimulus might be associated both with the presentation of a reward and of a punishment, allowing states such as conflict and guilt to arise. The different possible combinations greatly increase the number of possible emotions.

Fourth, emotions elicited by stimuli associated with different primary reinforcers will be different even within a reinforcement category (i.e. with the same reinforcement contingency), because the original reinforcers are different. Thus, for example, the state elicited by a stimulus associated with a positive reinforcer such as the taste of food will be different from that elicited by a positive reinforcer such as grooming. Indeed, it is an important feature of the association memory mechanisms described here that when a stimulus is applied, it acts as a key which 'looks up' or recalls the original primary reinforcer with which it was associated. Thus emotional stimuli will differ from each other in terms of the original primary reinforcers with which they were associated. A summary of many different primary reinforcers is provided in Table 10.1, and inspection of this will show how quite a number of emotions are produced typically by certain primary reinforcers. For example, from Table 10.1 it might be surmised that one of the biological origins of the emotion of jealousy might be the state elicited in a male when his partner is courted by another male, because this threatens his parental investment.

A fifth way in which emotions can be different from each other is in terms of the particular (conditioned) stimulus which elicits the emotion. Thus, even though the reinforcement contingency and even the unconditioned reinforcer may be identical, emotions will still be different cognitively, if the stimuli which give rise to the emotions are different (that is, if the objects of the emotion are different). For example, the emotional state elicited by the sight of one person may be different from that elicited by the sight of another person because the people, and thus the cognitive evaluation associated with the perception of the stimuli, are different.

A sixth possible way in which emotions can vary arises when the environment constrains the types of behavioural response which can be made. For example, if an active behavioural response can occur to the omission of an S+, then anger might be produced, but if only passive behaviour is possible, then sadness, depression or grief might occur.

By realizing that these six possibilities can occur in different combinations, it can be seen that it is possible to account for a very wide range of emotions, and this is believed to be one of the strengths of the approach described here. It is also the case that the extent to which a stimulus is reinforcing on a particular occasion (and thus the emotion produced) depends on the prior history of reinforcements (both recently and in the longer term), and that mood state can affect the degree to which a stimulus is reinforcing (see Section 4.8).

3.1.4   Refinements of the theory of emotion

The definition of emotions given above, that they are states produced by reinforcing stimuli, is refined now (see further Rolls 1990b).

First, when positively reinforcing stimuli (such as the taste of food or water) are relevant to a drive state produced by a change in the internal milieu (such as hunger and thirst), then we do not normally classify these stimuli as emotional, though they do produce pleasure (see Chapters 2 and 7). In contrast, emotional states are normally initiated by reinforcing stimuli that have their origin in the external environment, such as an (external) noise associated with pain (delivered by an external stimulus). We may then have identified a class of reinforcers (in our example, food) which we do not want to say cause emotions. This then is a refinement of the definition of emotions given above. Fortunately, we can encapsulate the set of reinforcing stimuli that we wish to exclude from our definition of stimuli which produce emotion. They are the set of external reinforcers (such as the sight of food) which are relevant to internal homeostatic drives such as hunger and thirst, which are controlled by internal need-related signals such as the concentration of glucose in the plasma (see Chapters 2 and 7). However, there is room for plenty of further discussion and refinement here. Perhaps some people (especially French people?) might say that they do experience emotion when they savour a wonderful food. There may well be cultural differences here in the semantics of whether such reinforcing stimuli should be included within the category that produce emotions. Another area for discussion is how we wish to categorize the reinforcers associated with sexual behaviour. Such stimuli may be made to be rewarding, and to feel pleasurable, partly because of the internal hormonal state. Does this mean that we wish to exclude such stimuli from the class that we call emotion-provoking, in the same way that we might exclude food reward from the class of stimuli that are said to cause emotion, because the reward value of food depends on an internal controlling signal? I am not sure that there is a perfectly clear answer to this. But this may not matter, as long as we understand that there are some rewarding stimuli that some may wish to exclude from those that cause emotional states.

Second, emotional states can be produced by remembered external reinforcing stimuli. (Indeed, the remembered neuronal states are, it is thought, very similar to those produced by a real sensory input, in all but the early stages of sensory processing; see Rolls 1989a; Rolls and Treves 1998).

Third, the stimulus which produces the emotional state does not have to be shown to be a reinforcer when producing the emotional state—it simply has to be capable of being shown to have reinforcing properties. The emotion-provoking stimulus has rewarding or punishing properties, and is a goal for action.

Fourth, the definition given provides great opportunity for cognitive processing (whether conscious or not) in emotions, for cognitive processes will very often be required to determine whether an environmental stimulus or event is reinforcing. Normally an emotion consists of this cognitive processing which results in a decoded signal that the environmental event is reinforcing, together with the mood state produced as a result. If the mood state is produced in the absence of the external sensory input and the cognitive decoding (for example by direct electrical stimulation of the amygdala, see Rolls 1975), then this is described only as a mood state, and is different from an emotion in that there is no object in the environment towards which the mood state is directed. It is suggested that, in order to produce some stability of mood, the firing rates of the neurons that are activated by external reinforcing stimuli to produce mood states must therefore have their spontaneous firing rates carefully controlled by the brain. (Many brain systems use lateral inhibition in order to maintain sensitivity to contrast constant, but this is not possible in the emotion system in which absolute levels of reinforcer must be represented over moderately long time spans.) The difficulty of maintaining a constant absolute level of firing in neurons such as these may contribute to 'spontaneous' mood swings, depression which occurs without a clear external cause, and the multiplicity of hormonal and transmitter systems which seem to be involved in the control of mood (see Chapter 6).

Having said this, it also seems to be the case that there is some 'regression to a constant value' for emotional stimuli. What I mean by this is that we are sensitive to some extent not just to the absolute level of reinforcement being received, but also to the change in the rate or magnitude of reinforcers being received. This is well shown by the phenomena of positive and negative contrast effects with rewards. Positive contrast occurs when the magnitude of a reward is increased. An animal will work very much harder for a period (perhaps lasting for minutes or longer) in this situation, before gradually reverting to a rate close to that at which the animal was working for the small reinforcement. A comparable contrast effect is seen when the reward magnitude (or rate at which rewards are obtained) is reduced—there is a negative overshoot in the rate of working for a time. This phenomenon is adaptive. It is evidence that animals are in part sensitive to a change in reinforcement, and this helps them to climb gradients to obtain better rewards. In effect, regardless of the absolute level of reinforcement being achieved, it is adaptive to be sensitive to a change in reinforcement. If this were not true, an animal receiving very little reinforcement but then obtaining a small increase in positive reinforcement might still be working very little for the reward. But it is much more adaptive to work hard in this situation, as the extra little bit of reward might make the difference between survival or not. A similar phenomenon may be evident in humans. People who have very little in the way of rewards, who may be poor, have a poor diet, and may suffer from disease, may nevertheless not have a baseline level of happiness that is necessarily very different from that of a person in an affluent society who in absolute terms apparently has many more rewards. This may be due in part to resetting of the baseline of expected rewards to a constant value, so that we are especially sensitive to changes in rewards (or punishers) (cf. Solomon and Corbit 1974; Solomon 1980).

The approach described above shows that the learning of stimulus–reinforcer associations is the learning involved when emotional responses are learned. In so far as the majority of stimuli which produce our emotional responses do so as a result of learning, this type of learning, and the brain mechanisms which underlie it, are crucial to the majority of our emotions. This, then, provides a theoretical basis for understanding the functions of some brain systems such as the amygdala in emotion. Ways in which this approach can be applied are given below.

It also follows from this approach towards a theory of emotion that brain systems involved in disconnecting stimulus–reinforcer associations which are no longer appropriate will also be very important in emotion. Failure of this function would be expected to lead, for example, in frustrating situations to inappropriate perseveration of behaviour to stimuli no longer associated with positive reinforcement. The inability to correct behaviour when reinforcement contingencies change would be evident in a number of emotion-provoking situations, such as frustration (i.e. non-reward), and the punishment of previously rewarded behaviour. It will be shown in Chapter 4 that this approach, which emphasizes the necessity, in, for example, social situations, to update and correct the decoded reinforcement value of stimuli continually, provides a basis for understanding the functions of some other brain regions such as the orbitofrontal cortex in emotion.

3.1.5 The functions of emotion

Understanding the functions of emotion is also important for understanding the nature of emotions, and for understanding the brain systems involved in the different types of response that are produced by emotional states. Emotion appears to have many functions, which are not necessarily mutually exclusive. Some of these functions are described next, and in more detail by Rolls (1990b).

The first function proposed for emotion is the elicitation of autonomic responses (e.g. a change in heart rate) and endocrine responses (e.g. the release of adrenaline). It is of clear survival value to prepare the body, for example by increasing the heart rate, so that actions which may be performed as a consequence of the reinforcing stimulus, such as running, can be performed more efficiently. The projections from the amygdala and orbitofrontal cortex via the hypothalamus as well as directly towards the brainstem autonomic motor nuclei may be particularly involved in this function. The James–Lange theory (see Schachter and Singer 1962; Grossman 1967; Reisenzein 1983), and theories which are closely related to it in supposing that feedback from parts of the periphery, such as the face (see Adelmann and Zajonc 1989) or body (Damasio 1994), leads to emotional feelings, have the major weakness that they do not give an adequate account of how the peripheral change is produced only by stimuli which happen to be emotion-provoking. Perhaps the most important issue in emotion is why only some stimuli give rise to emotions. We have prepared the way for answering this by identifying the stimuli which produce emotions as reinforcing stimuli. It is then possible to answer the question of *how* emotions are produced by investigating which parts of the brain decode whether stimuli are reinforcing. Such investigations are described in Chapter 4.

The second function proposed is flexibility of behavioural responses to reinforcing stimuli. The thesis here is that when a stimulus in the environment elicits an emotional state, we can perform any appropriate response to obtain the reward, or avoid the punishment. This is more flexible than simply learning a fixed behavioural response to a stimulus. More formally, the first stage in learning, for example, avoidance would be classical conditioning of an emotional response such as fear to a tone associated with shock. The amygdala and orbitofrontal cortex appear to be especially involved in this first stage of this type of learning, by virtue of their function in forming and correcting stimulus-reinforcement associations (see below). The second stage would be instrumental learning of an operant response, motivated by and performed in order to terminate the fear-inducing stimulus (see J. Gray 1975; Rolls 1990b). This two-stage learning process was suggested as being important for avoidance learning by N. E. Miller and O. H. Mowrer (see J. Gray 1975). The suggestion made here is that this general type of two-stage learning process is closely related to the design of animals for many types of behaviour, including emotional behaviour. It simplifies the interface of sensory systems to motor systems. Instead of having to learn a particular response to a particular stimulus by slow, habit, trial and error, learning, two-stage learning allows very fast (often one trial) learning of an emotional state to a rewarding or punishing stimulus. Then the motor system can operate in quite a general way, using many previously learned strategies, to approach the reward or avoid the punisher, which act as goals. This not only gives great flexibility to the interface, but also makes it relatively simple. It means that the reward value of a number of different stimuli can be decoded at roughly the same time. A behavioural decision system can then compare the different rewards available, in that they have a form of 'common currency'. (The value of each type of reward in this 'common currency' will be affected by many different factors, such as need state, e.g. hunger; how recently that reward has been obtained (see Chapter 10); the necessity in evolution to set each type of reward so that it sometimes is chosen if it is important for survival; etc.) The decision system can then choose between the rewards, based on their value, but also on the cost of obtaining each reward (see Chapter 10). After the choice has been made, the action or motor system can then switch on any behavioural responses possible, whether learned or not, in order to maximize the reward signal being obtained. The magnitude of the reward signal being obtained would be indicated just by the firing of the neurons which reflect the value of reward being obtained (e.g. the taste of a food if hungry, the pleasantness of touch, etc.), as described in Chapters 2 and 4. The actual way in which the appropriate response or action is learned may depend on response–reinforcer association learning, or on some more general type of purposive behaviour that can be learned to obtain goals (see Mackintosh and Dickinson 1979; Pearce 1996 Chapter 6).

A third function of emotion is that it is motivating. For example, fear learned by stimulus–reinforcer association formation provides the motivation for actions performed to avoid noxious stimuli. Similarly, positive reinforcers elicit motivation, so that we will work to obtain the rewards. Another example where emotion affects motivation is when a reward becomes no longer available, that is frustrative non-reward (see Fig. 3.1). If an action is possible, then increased motivation facilitates behaviour to work harder to obtain that reinforcer again or another reinforcer. If no action is possible to obtain again that positive reinforcer (e.g. after a death in the family), then as described in Section 3.1.3, grief or sadness may result. This may be adaptive, by preventing continuing attempts to regain the positive reinforcer which is no longer available, and helping the animal in due course to therefore be sensitive to other potential reinforcers to which it might be adaptive to switch. As described in Chapter 9, if such frustrative non-reward occurs in humans when no action is possible, depression may occur. A depressed state which lasts for a short time may be seen as being adaptive for the reason just given. However, the depression may last for a very long time perhaps because long-term explicit (conscious) knowledge in humans enables the long-term consequences of loss of the positive reinforcer to be evaluated and repeatedly brought to mind as described in Chapter 9 and in Section 10.6, and this may make long-term (psychological) depression maladaptive.

A fourth function of emotion is in communication. For example, monkeys may communicate their emotional state to others, by making an open-mouth threat to indicate the extent to which they are willing to compete for resources, and this may influence the behaviour of other animals. Communicating emotional states may have survival value, for example by reducing fighting. There are neural systems in the amygdala and overlying temporal cortical visual areas which are specialized for the face-related aspects of this processing, that is for decoding for example facial expression or gesture (see Chapter 4).

A fifth function of emotion is in social bonding. Examples of this are the emotions associated with the attachment of the parents to their young, with the attachment of the young to their parents, and with the attachment of the parents to each other. In the theory of the ways in which the genes affect behaviour ('selfish gene' theory, see R. Dawkins 1989), it is held that (because, e.g., of the advantages of parental care) all these forms of emotional attachment have the effect that genes for such attachment are more likely to survive into the next generation. Kin-altruism can also be considered in these terms (see e.g. R. Dawkins 1989; Chapter 10, Footnote 1).

A sixth function of emotion may be generalized from the above. It may be suggested that anything that feels pleasant to the organism, and is positively reinforcing, so that actions made to obtain it are performed, has survival value. (Stimuli which act as implicit or unconscious rewards should also act to produce pleasant feelings in the explicit or conscious processing system, so that both the implicit and explicit routes to action operate largely consistently—see Chapter 9.) One example of this is slight novelty, which may feel good and be positively reinforcing because it may lead to the discovery of better opportunities for survival in the environment (e.g. a new food). It is crucial that animals that succeed in the genetic competition which drives evolution have genes which encourage them to explore new environments, for then it is possible for the genes which happen to be present in an individual to explore the large multidimensional space of the environment in which they might succeed. Another example is gregariousness, which may assist the identification of new social partners, which could provide advantage. Probably related to the effects of novelty is sensory-specific satiety, the phenomenon whereby pleasant tastes during a meal gradually become less pleasant as satiety approaches (see Rolls 1986c, 1989b, 1993a). This may be an aspect of a more general adaptation to ensure that behaviour does eventually switch from one reinforcer to another. Comparably, it is likely that natural selection acting on genes will lead to unpleasant feelings, and negative reinforcement, being associated with behaviour which does not have survival value, at least in cases where genes can influence matters. (Of course the genes may be misled sometimes and lead to behaviour which does not have survival value, as when for example the non-nutritive sweetener saccharin is eaten by animals. This does not disprove the theory, but only points out that the genes cannot specify correctly for every possible stimulus or event in the environment, but must only on average lead to behaviour feeling pleasant that increases fitness, i.e. is appropriate for gene survival.)

A seventh effect of emotion is that the current mood state can affect the cognitive evaluation of events or memories (see Blaney 1986), and this may have the function of facilitating continuity in the interpretation of the reinforcing value of events in the environment. A theory of how this occurs is presented in Section 4.8 'Effects of emotions on cognitive processing'.

An eighth function of emotion is that it may facilitate the storage of memories. One way in which this occurs is that episodic memory (i.e. one's memory of particular episodes) is facilitated by emotional states. This may be advantageous in that storage of as many details as possible of the prevailing situation when a strong reinforcer is delivered may be useful in generating appropriate behaviour in situations with some similarities in the future. This function may be implemented by the relatively non-specific projecting systems to the cerebral cortex and hippocampus, including the cholinergic pathways in the basal forebrain and medial septum, and the ascending noradrenergic pathways (see Section 4.7; Rolls and Treves 1998; Wilson and Rolls 1990a,b). A second way in which emotion may affect the storage of memories is that the current emotional state may be stored with episodic memories, providing a mechanism for the current emotional state to affect which memories are recalled. In this sense, emotion acts as a contextual retrieval cue, that as with other contextual effects influences the retrieval of episodic memories (see Rolls and Treves 1998). A third way in which emotion may affect the storage of memories is by guiding the cerebral cortex in the representations of the world which are set up. For example, in the visual system, it may be useful to build perceptual representations or analysers which are different from each other if they are associated with different reinforcers, and to be less likely to build them if they have no association with reinforcement. Ways in which backprojections from parts of the brain important in emotion (such as the amygdala) to parts of the cerebral cortex could perform this function are discussed in Section 4.8, 'Effects of emotions on cognitive processing'; by Rolls (1989a, 1990b, 1992b); and by Rolls and Treves (1998).

A ninth function of emotion is that by enduring for minutes or longer after a reinforcing stimulus has occurred, it may help to produce persistent motivation and direction of behaviour.

A tenth function of emotion is that it may trigger recall of memories stored in neocortical representations. Amygdala backprojections to the cortex could perform this for emotion in a way analogous to that in which the hippocampus could implement the retrieval in the neocortex of recent (episodic) memories (see Rolls and Treves 1998).

It is useful to have these functions of emotion in mind when considering the neural basis of emotion, for each function is likely to have particular output pathways from emotional systems associated with it.

3.1.6 The James–Lange and other bodily theories of emotion

James (1884) believed that emotional experiences were produced by sensing bodily changes, such as changes in heart rate or in skeletal muscles. Lange (1885) had a similar

James-Lange theory of emotion

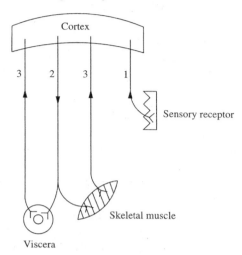

Fig. 3.2 The James–Lange theory of emotion proposes that there are three steps in producing emotional feelings. The first step is elicitation by the emotion-provoking stimulus (received by the cortex via pathway 1 in the Figure) of peripheral changes, such as skeleto-muscular activity to run away, and autonomic changes, such as alteration of heart rate (via pathways labelled 2 in the Figure). The second step is the sensing of the peripheral responses (e.g. altered heart rate, and somatosensory effects produced by running away) (via pathways labelled 3 in the Figure). The third step is elicitation of the emotional feeling in response to the sensed feedback from the periphery.

view, although he emphasized the role of autonomic feedback (for example from the heart) in producing the experience of emotion. The theory, which became known as the James–Lange theory, suggested that there are three steps in producing emotional feelings (see Fig. 3.2). The first step is elicitation by the emotion-provoking stimulus of peripheral changes, such as skeleto–muscular activity to produce running away, and autonomic changes, such as alteration of heart rate. But, as pointed out above, the theory leaves unanswered perhaps the most important issue in any theory of emotion: Why do some events make us run away (and then feel emotional), whereas others do not? This is a major weakness of this type of theory. The second step is the sensing of the peripheral responses (e.g. running away, and altered heart rate). The third step is elicitation of the emotional feeling in response to the sensed feedback from the periphery.

The history of research into peripheral theories of emotion starts with the fatal flaw that step one (the question of which stimuli elicit emotion-related responses in the first place) leaves unanswered this most important question. The history continues with the accumulation of empirical evidence which has gradually weakened more and more the hypothesis that peripheral responses made during emotional behaviour have anything to do with producing the emotional behaviour (which has largely already been produced anyway according to the James–Lange theory), or the emotional feeling. Some of the landmarks in this history are as follows. First, the peripheral changes produced during emotion are not sufficiently distinct to be able to carry the information which would enable one to have subtly different emotional feelings to the vast range of different stimuli that can produce different emotions. The evidence suggests that by measuring many peripheral changes in emotion, such as heart rate, skin conductance, breathing rate, and hormones such as adrenaline and noradrenaline (known in the United States by their Greek names epinephrine and norepinephrine), it may be possible to make coarse distinctions between, for example, anger and fear, but not much finer distinctions (Wagner 1989; Cacioppo *et al.* 1993; Oatley and Jenkins 1996). Second, when emotions are evoked by imagery, then the peripheral responses are much less marked and distinctive than during emotions produced by external stimuli (Ekman *et al.* 1983; Stemmler 1989; Levenson *et al.* 1990). This makes sense in that although an emotion evoked by imagery may be strong, there is no need to produce strong peripheral responses, because no behavioural responses are required. Third, disruption of peripheral responses and feedback from them surgically (for example in dogs, Cannon 1927, 1929, 1931), or as a result of spinal cord injury in humans (Hohmann 1966; Bermond *et al.* 1991) does not abolish emotional responses. What was found was that in some patients there was apparently some reduction in emotions in some situations (Hohmann 1966), but this could be related to the fact that some of the patients were severely disabled which could have produced its own consequences for emotionality, and that in many cases the patients were considerably older than before the spinal cord damage, which could itself have been a factor. What was common to both studies was that emotions could be felt by all the patients; and that in some cases, emotions resulting from mental events were even reported as being stronger (Hohmann 1966; Bermond *et al.* 1991). Fourth, when autonomic changes are elicited by injections of, for example, adrenaline or noradrenaline, particular emotions are not produced. Instead, the emotion that is produced depends on the cognitive decoding of the reinforcers present in the situation, for example an actor who insults your parents to make you angry, or an actor who plays a game of hula hoop to make you feel happy (Schachter and Singer 1962). In this situation, the hormone adrenaline or noradrenaline can alter the magnitude of the emotion, but not which emotion is felt. This is further evidence that it is the decoded reinforcement value of the input stimulus or events which determines which emotion is felt. The fact that the hormone injections produced some change in the magnitude of an emotion is not very surprising. If you felt your heart pounding for no explicable reason, you might wonder what was happening, and therefore react more or abnormally. Fifth, if the peripheral changes associated with emotion are blocked with drugs, then this does not block the perception of emotion (Reisenzein 1983). Sixth, it is found that in normal life, behavioural expressions of emotion (for example smiling at a bowling alley) do not usually occur when one might be expected to feel happy because of a success, but instead occur when one is looking at one's friends (Kraut and Johnson 1979). These body responses, which can be very brief, thus often serve the needs of communication, or of action, not of producing emotional feelings.

3.1.6.1 The somatic marker hypothesis

Despite this rather overwhelming evidence against an important role for body responses in producing emotions or emotional feelings, Damasio (1994) has effectively tried to resurrect a weakened version of the James–Lange theory of emotion from the last century, by arguing with his somatic marker hypothesis that after reinforcers have been evaluated, a bodily response ('somatic marker') normally occurs, then this leads to a bodily feeling, which in turn is appreciated by the organism to then make a contribution to the decision-making process. (In the James–Lange theory, it was emotional feelings that depend on peripheral feedback; for Damasio, it is the decision of which behavioural response to make that is normally influenced by the peripheral feedback. A quotation from Damasio (1994, p190) follows: 'The squirrel did not really think about his various options and calculate the costs and benefits of each. He saw the cat, was jolted by the body state, and ran.' Here it is clear that the pathway to action uses the body state as part of the route. Damasio would also like decisions to be implemented using the peripheral changes elicited by emotional stimuli. Given all the different reinforcers which may influence behaviour, Damasio (1994) even suggests that the net result of them all is reflected in the net peripheral outcome, and then the brain can sense this net peripheral result, and thus know what decision to take.) The James–Lange theory has a number of major weaknesses just outlined which apply also to the somatic marker hypothesis. Another major weakness, which applies to both the James–Lange and to Damasio's somatic marker hypothesis, is that they do not take account of the fact that once an information processor has determined that a response should be made or inhibited based on reinforcement associa-tion, a function attributed in the theory proposed in this chapter and by Rolls (1986a,b, 1990b) to the orbitofrontal cortex, it would be very inefficient and noisy to place in the execution route a peripheral response, and transducers to attempt to measure that peripheral response, itself a notoriously difficult procedure (see, e.g., Grossman 1967). Even for the cases when Damasio (1994) might argue that the peripheral somatic marker and its feedback can be by-passed using conditioning of a representation in, e.g., the somatosensory cortex to a command signal (which might originate in the orbitofrontal cortex), he apparently would still wish to argue that the activity in the somatosensory cortex is important for the emotion to be appreciated or to influence behaviour. (Without this, the somatic marker hypothesis would vanish.) The prediction would apparently be that if an emotional response were produced to a visual stimulus, then this would necessarily involve activity in the somatosensory cortex or other brain region in which the 'somatic marker' would be represented. This prediction could be tested (for example in patients with somatosensory cortex damage), but it seems most unlikely that an emotion produced by a visual reinforcer would *require* activity in the somatosensory cortex to feel emotional or to elicit emotional decisions. The alternative view proposed here (and by Rolls 1986a,b, 1990b) is that where the reinforcement value of the visual stimulus is decoded, namely in the orbitofrontal cortex and the amygdala, is the appropriate part of the brain for outputs to influence behaviour (via, e.g., the orbitofrontal-to-striatal connec-tions), and that the orbitofrontal cortex and amygdala, and brain structures that receive connections from them, are the likely places where neuronal activity is directly related to the felt emotion (see further Rolls 1997a,d and Chapter 9).

3.1.7 Individual differences in emotion, and personality

H. J. Eysenck developed the theory that personality might be related to different aspects of conditioning. He analysed the factors that accounted for the variance in the differences between the personality of different humans (using, for example, questionnaires), and suggested that the first two factors in personality (those which accounted for most of the variance) were introversion vs extraversion, and neuroticism (related to a tendency to be anxious). He performed studies of classical conditioning on groups of subjects, and also obtained measures of what he termed arousal. Based on the correlations of these measures with the dimensions identified in the factor analysis, he suggested that introverts showed greater conditionability than extraverts; and that neuroticism raises the general intensity of emotional reactions (see Eysenck and Eysenck 1968).

J. Gray (1970) reinterpreted the findings, suggesting that introverts are more sensitive to punishment and frustrative non-reward than are extraverts; and that neuroticism reflects the extent of sensitivity to both reward and punishment.

I do not wish to consider this research area in detail. However, I do point out that insofar as sensitivity to reward and punishment, and the ability to learn and be influenced by reward and punishment, may be important in personality, and are closely involved in emotion according to the theory developed here, there may be close links between the neural bases of emotion, to be described in Chapter 4, and personality.

4   The neural bases of emotion

In this chapter the neural bases of emotion are considered. Particular attention is paid to research in non-human primates as well as in humans, partly because the developments in primates in the structure and connections of neural systems involved in emotion such as the amygdala and orbitofrontal cortex make studies in primates particularly important for understanding emotion in humans.

4.1   Introduction

Some of the main brain regions implicated in emotion will now be considered in the light of the introduction given in Chapter 3 on the nature and functions of emotion. These brain regions include the amygdala, orbitofrontal cortex, and basal forebrain areas including the hypothalamus. Some of these brain regions are indicated in Figs 4.1 and 4.2. Particular attention is paid to the functions of these regions in primates, for in primates the neocortex undergoes great development and provides major inputs to these regions, in some cases to parts of these structures thought not to be present in non-primates. An example of this is the projection from the primate neocortex in the anterior part of the temporal lobe to the basal accessory nucleus of the amygdala (see below). Studies in primates are thus particularly relevant to understanding the neural basis of emotion in the human.

    The way in which recent studies in primates indicate that the neural processing of emotion is organized is as follows (see Fig. 4.3). First, there are brain mechanisms that are involved in computing the reward value of primary (unlearned) reinforcers. The primary reinforcers include taste, touch (both pleasant touch and pain), and to some extent smell, and perhaps certain visual stimuli, such as face expression. Then some brain regions are concerned with learning associations between previously neutral stimuli, such as the sight of objects or of individuals' faces, with primary reinforcers. These brain regions include the amygdala and orbitofrontal cortex. For the processing of primary reinforcers, and especially for secondary reinforcers, the brain is organized to process the stimulus first to the object level (so that if the input is visual, the object can be recognized independently of its position on the retina, or size, or view), and then to determine whether the stimulus is rewarding or punishing. Once the relevant brain regions have determined whether the input is reinforcing, whether primary or secondary, the signal is passed directly to output regions of the brain, with no need to produce peripheral body or autonomic responses. The brain regions in which the reinforcing, and hence emotional, value of stimuli are represented interface to three main types of output system. The first is the autonomic and endocrine system, for producing such changes as increased heart rate and release of

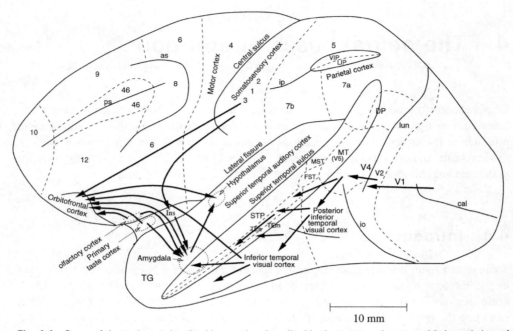

Fig. 4.1 Some of the pathways involved in emotion described in the text are shown on this lateral view of the brain of the macaque monkey. Connections from the primary taste and olfactory cortices to the orbitofrontal cortex and amygdala are shown. Connections are also shown in the 'ventral visual system' from V1 to V2, V4, the inferior temporal visual cortex, etc., with some connections reaching the amygdala and orbitofrontal cortex. In addition, connections from the somatosensory cortical areas 1, 2, and 3 that reach the orbitofrontal cortex directly and via the insular cortex, and that reach the amygdala via the insular cortex, are shown. as, arcuate sulcus; cal, calcarine sulcus; cs, central sulcus; lf, lateral (or Sylvian) fissure; lun, lunate sulcus; ps, principal sulcus; io, inferior occipital sulcus; ip, intraparietal sulcus (which has been opened to reveal some of the areas it contains); sts, superior temporal sulcus (which has been opened to reveal some of the areas it contains). AIT, anterior inferior temporal cortex; FST, visual motion processing area; LIP, lateral intraparietal area; MST, visual motion processing area; MT, visual motion processing area (also called V5); PIT, posterior inferior temporal cortex; STP, superior temporal plane; TA, architectonic area including auditory association cortex; TE, architectonic area including high order visual association cortex, and some of its subareas TEa and TEm; TG, architectonic area in the temporal pole; V1–V4, visual areas 1–4; VIP, ventral intraparietal area; TEO, architectonic area including posterior visual association cortex. The numerals refer to architectonic areas, and have the following approximate functional equivalence: 1,2,3, somatosensory cortex (posterior to the central sulcus); 4, motor cortex; 5, superior parietal lobule; 7a, inferior parietal lobule, visual part; 7b, inferior parietal lobule, somatosensory part; 6, lateral premotor cortex; 8, frontal eye field; 12, part of orbitofrontal cortex; 46, dorsolateral prefrontal cortex. (Modified from Rolls and Treves 1998.)

adrenaline, which prepare the body for action. The second type of output is to brain systems concerned with performing actions unconsciously or implicitly, in order to obtain rewards or avoid punishers. These brain systems include the basal ganglia. The third type of output is to a system capable of planning many steps ahead, and for example deferring short-term rewards in order to execute a long-term plan. This system may use syntactic processing in order to perform the planning, and is therefore part of a linguistic system which performs explicit (conscious) processing, as described more fully in Chapter 9.

4.2   Decoding[1] primary reinforcers

Emotions can be produced by primary reinforcers. (Primary reinforcers are unlearned reinforcers, that is they are innately reinforcing.) Other, previously neutral, stimuli, such as the sight of an object, can by association learning with a primary reinforcer come to be a secondary (or learned) reinforcer, which can also produce an emotional response. For these reasons, in order to understand the neural basis of emotion it is necessary to know where in the processing systems in the brain a sensory input comes to be decoded as and treated by the rest of the brain (which may try to maximize or minimize its activity) as a primary reinforcer.

In primates, the evidence that the representation of taste is independent of its rewarding properties as far as the primary taste cortex is described in Chapter 2. In the secondary taste cortex, the representation is of the food reward value of the taste, in that the taste responses of neurons are modulated by hunger, and decrease to zero when the animal is satiated, and the taste is no longer rewarding.

For olfaction, it is known that some orbitofrontal cortex olfactory neurons respond to the smell of food only when a monkey has an appetite for that food (Critchley and Rolls 1996b). The responses of these neurons thus reflect the reward value of these food-related olfactory stimuli. It is not yet known in primates whether this modulation of olfactory neuronal responses occurs at earlier processing stages. In rats, there is some evidence that signals about hunger can influence olfactory processing as far peripherally as the olfactory bulb (Pager *et al.* 1972; Pager 1974). Although some of these orbitofrontal cortex olfactory neurons may respond because they are secondary reinforcers as a result of olfactory-to-taste association learning (Rolls, Critchley. Mason and Wakeman 1996b), it is known that some olfactory neurons in the orbitofrontal cortex do not alter their responses during olfactory-to-taste association learning (Critchley and Rolls 1996a). The responses of these olfactory neurons *could* thus reflect information about whether the odour is a primary reinforcer. However, the neurons could also simply be representing the identity of the odour. This issue has not yet been settled. In humans there is some evidence that there is a vomero–nasal olfactory system, which is sensitive to pheromones. In particular, there may be a system in women that is especially sensitive to the pheromones PH56 and PH94B, and in men to the pheromone pregna-diene-dione (see Chapter 8). These signals in the

---

[1] By decoding, I mean what is made explicit in the representation. If the firing of neurons (in for example the inferior temporal visual cortex) reflects which object has been seen invariantly with respect to size, position, reward association, etc., then it can be said that representations of objects have been decoded from the sensory information reaching the retina. Although information about which object has been seen is of course present in the retinal neuronal firing, it is not made explicit at this stage of processing. Instead, local contrast over small regions of the retina is made explicit at the retinal level. If the firing of neurons in, for example, the orbitofrontal cortex reflects whether an object is currently associated with reward, then we can say that the reward value of objects has been decoded by this stage of processing. The most common way for information to be made explicit in the firing is by altering the firing rate of neurons, though it has been hypothesized that some additional information might be available in the relative time of firing of different neurons. This issue of the representation of information by populations of neurons is considered more comprehensively by Rolls and Treves (1998).

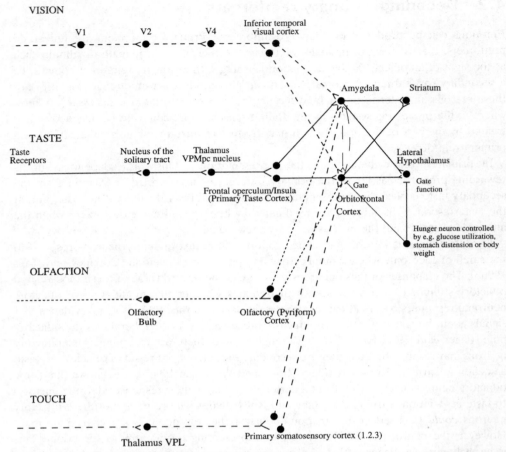

Fig. 4.2 Schematic diagram showing some of the connections of the taste, olfactory, somatosensory, and visual pathways in the brain. V1, primary visual (striate) cortex; V2 and V4, further cortical visual areas. VPL, ventro-postero-lateral nucleus of the thalamus, which conveys somatosensory information to the primary somatosensory cortex (areas 1, 2 and 3).

accessory olfactory system could act as primary reinforcers which affect attractiveness. There may also be a system in which attractiveness can be influenced by other body odours, perhaps as a means for producing genetic diversity (see Chapters 8 and 10).

Experiments have recently been performed to investigate where in the human touch-processing system (see Figs 4.1 and 4.2) tactile stimuli are decoded and represented in terms of their rewarding value or the pleasure they produce. In order to investigate this, Rolls, Francis *et al.* (1997a) performed functional magnetic resonance imaging (fMRI) of humans who were receiving pleasant and neutral tactile stimuli. They found that a weak but very pleasant touch of the hand with velvet produced much stronger activation of the orbitofrontal cortex than a more intense but affectively neutral touch of the hand with wood. In contrast, the pleasant stimuli produced approximately the same activation as the neutral stimuli of the primary somatosensory cortex (see Fig. 4.4, and Fig. 4.5 in the plates section). It was concluded that part of the orbitofrontal cortex is concerned with representing the positively affective aspects of somatosensory stimuli. Nearby, but separate, parts of the human orbitofrontal cortex were shown in the same series of experiments to be activated by taste and olfactory stimuli. Thus the pleasantness of tactile stimuli, which can be powerful primary reinforcers (Taira and Rolls 1996), is correlated with the activity of a part of the orbitofrontal cortex. This part of the orbitofrontal cortex probably receives its somatosensory inputs via the somatosensory cortex both via direct projections and via the insula (see Mesulam and Mufson 1982a, b; Rolls and Treves 1998). In contrast, the pleasantness of a tactile stimulus does not appear to be represented explicitly in the somatosensory cortex. The indication thus is that only certain parts of the somatosensory input, which reflect its pleasantness, are passed on (perhaps after appropriate processing) to the orbitofrontal cortex by the somatosensory cortical areas.

The issue of where the reinforcing properties of activation of the pain pathways is decoded is complex (see Melzack 1973; Melzack and Wall 1996; Perl and Kruger 1996). There are clearly specialized peripheral nerves (including C fibres) that convey painful stimulation to the central nervous system. At the spinal cord level, there are reflexes that enable a limb to be withdrawn from painful stimulation. But the essence of a reinforcer is that it should enable the probability of an arbitrary (that is any) instrumental response or action to be altered in probability. For this learning to occur, it is probably necessary that the activity should proceed past the central gray in the brainstem, which is an important region for pain processing, to at least the diencephalic (hypothalamus/thalamus) level. This level may be sufficient for at least simple operant responses, such as lifting the tail, to be learned to avoid footshock (Huston and Borbely 1973). For more complex operant responses, it is likely that the basal ganglia must be intact (see Section 4.6.2 and Chapter 6). There appears to be a focus for pain inputs in part of area 3 of the primary somatosensory cortex, as shown by loss of pain sensation after a lesion to this region (Marshall 1951), and by activation measured in PET studies of regions in the primary and the secondary somatosensory cortex (Coghill *et al.* 1994), although a more recent PET study from the same Centre implicates the cingulate cortex rather than the somatosensory cortex in the affective aspects of pain (Rainville *et al.* 1997). However, there is evidence that structures as recently developed as the orbitofrontal cortex of primates are important in the subjective aspects of pain, for patients with lesions or disconnection of the orbitofrontal cortex may say that they can identify the input as painful, but that it does not produce the same affective feeling as previously (Freeman and Watts 1950; Melzack 1973; see also Price *et al.* 1996).

Although most visual stimuli are not primary reinforcers, but may become secondary reinforcers as a result of stimulus−reinforcement association learning, it is possible that some visual stimuli, such as the sight of a smiling face or of an angry face, could be primary reinforcers. It has been shown that there is a population of neurons in the cortex in the anterior part of the macaque superior temporal sulcus that categorize face stimuli based on the expression on the face, not based on the identity of the face (Hasselmo, Rolls and Baylis 1989a; Section 4.3.5). Thus it is possible that the reinforcing value of face expression could be being decoded by this stage of cortical processing (which is at the same stage approximately as the inferior temporal visual cortex; see Rolls and Treves

Brain Mechanisms of Emotion

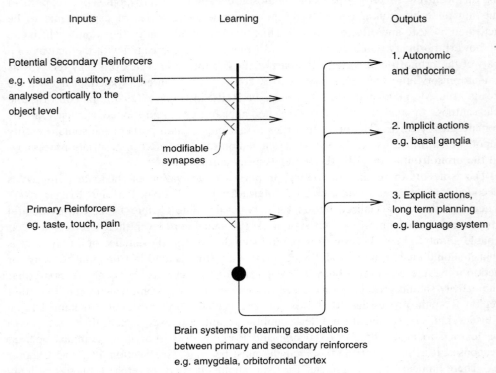

Inputs   Learning   Outputs

Potential Secondary Reinforcers
e.g. visual and auditory stimuli,
analysed cortically to the
object level

modifiable
synapses

Primary Reinforcers
eg. taste, touch, pain

1. Autonomic
and endocrine

2. Implicit actions
e.g. basal ganglia

3. Explicit actions,
long term planning
e.g. language system

Brain systems for learning associations
between primary and secondary reinforcers
e.g. amygdala, orbitofrontal cortex

Fig. 4.3 Schematic diagram showing the organization of some of the brain mechanisms underlying emotion, including those involved in learning the reinforcement associations of visual stimuli.

1998; G. Baylis, Rolls and Leonard 1987). This cortical region projects into the amygdala, in which face-selective neurons are also found (Leonard, Rolls, Wilson and Baylis 1985). Although it is not yet known whether amygdala face-selective neurons can code for expression or reward as well as identity (Leonard *et al.* 1985), this does seem likely given that these amygdala neurons receive some of their inputs from the neurons in the cortex in the superior temporal sulcus. Another population of face-selective neurons is also found in the orbitofrontal cortex (observations of Critchley and Rolls; see Rolls 1996d), and some of these neurons could also represent the primary reinforcing value of a face. However, it seems likely that, in addition, at least some of the face-selective neurons in the amygdala and orbitofrontal cortex reflect the secondary reinforcing value of a face, given the role these brain regions play in stimulus–reinforcement association learning (see below).

It is possible that some auditory stimuli can be primary reinforcers. Where the reinforcement value may be decoded is not yet known.

As discussed in Sections 10.2.1 and 4.4.4, novel stimuli are somewhat rewarding and in this sense act as primary reinforcers. The value of this type of reinforcer is that it encourages animals to explore new environments in which their genes might produce a fitness advantage (see Section 10.2.1).

Further examples of primary reinforcers are given in Section 10.2.2 and Table 10.1.

4.3 Representing potential secondary reinforcers

Many stimuli, such as the sight of an object, have no intrinsic emotional effect. They are not primary reinforcers. Yet they can come as a result of learning to have emotional significance. This type of learning is called stimulus–reinforcement association, and the association is between the sight of the neutral visual stimulus (the potential secondary reinforcer) and the primary reward or punisher (the taste of food, or a painful stimulus). How are the representations of objects built in the brain, and what is the form of the representation appropriate for it to provide the input stimulus in stimulus–reinforcement association learning? These issues are addressed in detail by Rolls and Treves (1998), but some of the relevant issues in the present context of how stimuli should be represented if they are to be appropriate for subsequent evaluation by stimulus–reinforcement association learning brain mechanisms are described here.

4.3.1 The requirements of the representation

From an abstract, formal point of view we would want the representation of the to-be-associated stimulus, neutral before stimulus–reinforcement association learning, to have some of the following properties.

4.3.1.1 Invariance

The representation of the object should be invariant with respect to physical transforms of the object such as size (which varies with distance), position on the retina (translation invariance), and view. The reason that invariance is such an important property is that if we learned, for example, an association between one view of an object and a reward or punisher, it would be extremely unadaptive if when we saw the object again from a different view we did not have the same emotional response to it, or recognize it as a food with a good taste. We need to learn about the reward and punishment associations of objects, not of particular images with a fixed size and position on the retina. This is the fundamental reason why perceptual processing in sensory systems should proceed to the level at which objects are represented invariantly before the representation is used for emotional and motivation-related learning by stimulus–reinforcement association. There are only exceptional circumstances in which we wish to learn, or it would be adaptive to learn, associations to stimuli represented early on in sensory processing streams, before invariant representations are computed. There are exceptional cases though, such as it being appropriate to learn an emotional response to a loud sound represented only as tones, as has been studied by LeDoux (1994) in his model system. We should realise that

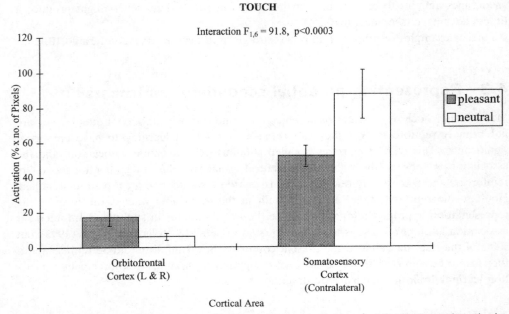

Fig. 4.4 Histograms showing the mean (±s.e.m., across seven subjects) of the % change in activation (×number of significant pixels) of different brain regions (left and right orbitofrontal cortex, and left and right somatosensory cortex) during touch to the left hand which was pleasant (velvet) or neutral (wood). (After Rolls, Francis *et al.* 1997a.)

such cases are exceptions, and that the fundamental design principle is very different, with representations normally being at the object level before there is an interface to emotion learning systems, as described in the work considered below and elsewhere (e.g. Rolls 1986a,b, 1990b). While the example taken has been from vision, the same is true for other modalities. For example, in audition, we would want to make the same emotional decoding to the word 'Fire' independently of whether we hear it spoken (with extremely different pitches) by a child, by a woman, or by a man. This could not be decoded without high-level cortical processing, emphasizing the point that normally we need to have emotional responses to stimuli decoded correctly to the level where an object has been made explicit in the representation.

The capacity for view-invariant representation of objects may be especially well developed in primates, as implied, for example, by the great development in primates of the parts of the temporal lobe concerned with vision (inferior temporal visual cortex, cortex in the superior temporal sulcus, etc., see Section 4.3.4). The issue then arises of the organization of vision in non-primates, and whether their view-invariant representations are formed when there is a much less well-developed temporal lobe. It may be that for many objects, a sufficiently good representation of objects which is effectively view-invariant can be formed without explicitly computing a view-invariant representation. Take for example the representation of a small fruit such as a raspberry. The nature of this object is that it can be recognized from almost any viewing angle based on the presence of three simple features, (two-dimensional) shape, surface texture, and colour. (Moreover, once one has been identified by, for example, taste, there are likely to be others present locally, and serial feeding (concentrating on one type of food, then switching to another) may take advantage of this.) Thus much behaviour towards objects may take place based on the presence of a simple list of identifying features, rather than by computing true view-invariant representations of objects that look different from different angles (see also Rolls and Treves 1998, Section 8.8). The sophisticated mechanism present in the primate temporal lobe for computing invariant representations of objects may be associated with the evolution of hands, tool use, and stereoscopic vision, and the necessity to recognize and manipulate objects from different angles to make artefacts. At a slightly simpler level, primates often eat more than 100 different types of food in a day, and the ability to perform view-invariant representations of large numbers of small objects is clearly adaptive in this situation too.

It is certainly of interest that apparently quite complex behaviour, including food selection in birds and insects, may be based on quite simple computational processes, such as in this case object identification based on a list of simple features. We should always be cautious about inferring more complex substrates for behaviour than is really necessary given the capacities. Part of the value of neurophysiological investigation of the primate temporal cortex is that it shows that view-invariant representations are actually computed, even for objects that look very different from different viewing angles (see Booth and Rolls, 1998; Rolls and Treves, 1998).

4.3.1.2 Generalization

If we learn an emotional response to an object, we usually want to generalize the emotional response to other similar objects. An example might be the sight of a pin, which, after stimulus–reinforcement association learning, would generalize to the shape of other similar sharp-pointed objects such as a pencil, a pen, etc. Generalization occurs most easily if each object is represented by a population of neurons firing, each perhaps reflecting different properties of the object. Then if the object alters a little, in that some of its features change, there will still be sufficient similarity of the representation for it to be reasonably correlated with the original representation.

The way in which this occurs in the types of neuronal network found in the brain, and the nature of the representation needed, have been fully described by Rolls and Treves (1998). A synopsis of some of the key ideas as they apply most directly to pattern associators, which are types of network involved in learning about which environmental stimuli are associated with reward or with punishment, is provided in the Appendix. The approach is introduced in Fig. 4.6. The unconditioned or primary reinforcer activates the neuron shown (one of many) by unmodifiable synaptic connections (only one of which is drawn in Fig. 4.6). The to-be-conditioned stimulus activates the neuron through a population of modifiable synapses. The association is learned by strengthening those synapses from active conditioned stimulus input axons when the postsynaptic neuron is activated by the primary reinforcer. This is known as the Hebb learning rule (after D. O. Hebb, who in 1949 envisaged a synaptic learning rule of this general form). Later, when only the conditioned stimulus is presented, it activates the postsynaptic neuron through

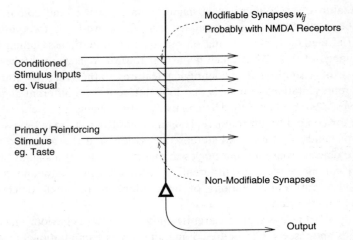

Fig. 4.6 Pattern association between a primary reinforcer, such as the taste of food, which activates neurons through non-modifiable synapses, and a potential secondary reinforcer, such as the sight of food, which has modifiable synapses on to the same neurons. Such a mechanism appears to be implemented in the amygdala and orbitofrontal cortex. (Homosynaptic) long-term depression (see Appendix) in a pattern associator in the amygdala could account for the habituating responses to novel visual stimuli which are not associated with primary reinforcers.

the modified synapses, producing the same firing as that originally produced by the unconditioned stimulus. If the conditioned stimulus is represented by the firing of a set of axons, then we can think of this as a vector. In the same way, we can think of the synaptic weights as another vector. If the input vector matches the weight vector, then the maximal activation of the neuron is produced. If the input vector uses distributed encoding (with perhaps each axon reflecting the presence of one or several features of the object), then a similar vector of firing will represent a similar object. Because many of the strengthened synapses activated by the original stimulus will also be activated by the similar stimulus, the similar stimulus will produce activation of the neuron that is similar to that produced by the original conditioned stimulus. The neuron can thus be thought of as computing the similarity of input patterns of firing, and it is this which results in good generalization (see the Appendix). This consideration leads to the suggestion that in order to enable good generalization to occur, the to-be-conditioned stimulus, i.e. the potential secondary reinforcer, should be represented with a distributed representation. If, in contrast to a distributed representation, there was a local representation (in which a single neuron would be so specifically tuned that it carried all the information about which stimulus was present), then generalization would be much more difficult. If one learned an association to a single neuron firing that represented the object, then any small alteration of the stimulus would lead to another neuron firing (so that small perceptual differences between stimuli could be represented), and there would be no generalization.

4.3.1.3 Graceful degradation

If there is minor damage to the nervous system, for example if some neurons die or some synapses are lost, there is no catastrophic change in performance. Instead, as the damage becomes more and more major, there is generally a gradual decline in the performance of the function affected. This is known as graceful degradation (and is a form of fault tolerance). Graceful degradation is a simple property of neural networks that use distributed representations. It arises in a very similar way to generalization. Because each object is represented by an ensemble (or vector) of neuronal activity, if a few of the input axons or the synapses are damaged, then the remainder of the input axons and synapses can still produce activation of the neuron that approximates the correct activation. (As explained in the Appendix and by Rolls and Treves 1998, the operation performed by a neuron may be thought of as computing the inner or dot product of the input firing vector of neuronal activity and the synaptic weight vector. The result is a scalar value, the activation of the neuron. The dot product effectively measures the similarity of the input firing-rate vector and the stored synaptic-weight vector. Provided that the two vectors use distributed representations, then graceful degradation will occur.) Given that the output of the network is produced in practice not by a single neuron but by a population of neurons, loss of a few output neurons (which of course provide the input to the next stage) does not produce catastrophic degradation either (see further Rolls and Treves 1998; and the Appendix).

4.3.1.4 High capacity

We would like the object representation to convey much information, that is to be capable of representing separately (discriminating between) many different objects. At the same time, we would like this high capacity representation to be readable by a pattern associator of the type just described, which reads out the information from the representation using a dot product operation. It turns out that this can be achieved by a distributed representation of the type found in the brain. One property of the representation is that each neuron should convey essentially independent information. The implication of this is that the number of stimuli that can be represented increases exponentially with the number of neurons in the population (because information is a log measure). Another property of the representation is that it should be readable by a simple operation such as a dot product, with each input neuron conveying an approximately similar amount of information. (This is described further in the Appendix. The point is that a binary code would be too compact for the properties required). It turns out that exactly the type of representation required is built for objects in the visual system, and is found elsewhere in the brain too (see Rolls and Treves 1998; and the Appendix). Another advantage of this type of representation is that a great deal of information about which object was shown can be read by taking the activity of any reasonably large subset of the population. This means that neurons in the brain do not need to have an input connection from every neuron in the sending population; and this makes the whole issue of brain wiring during development tractable (see Rolls and Treves 1998).

It turns out that not only does the inferior temporal visual cortex have a representation of both faces and non-face objects with the properties described above, but also it transpires that the inferior temporal visual cortex does not contaminate its representation of objects (which must be used for many different functions in the brain) by having reward representations associated on to the neurons there. Instead, because its outputs are used for many functions, the reward value of objects is not what determines the response of inferior temporal cortex neurons. (If it did, then we might go blind to objects if they changed from being rewarding to being neutral. Exactly this change of reward value does occur if we eat a food to satiety, yet we can still see the food.) This issue, that the inferior temporal visual cortex is the stage in the object processing stream at which objects become represented, and from which there are major inputs to other parts of the brain which do learn reward and punishment associations of objects, the orbitofrontal cortex and amygdala, is considered next. The reasons for this architectural design are also considered.

4.3.2 Objects, and not their reward and punishment associations, are represented in the inferior temporal visual cortex

We now consider whether associations between visual stimuli and reinforcement are learned, and stored, in the visual cortical areas which proceed from the primary visual cortex, V1, through V2, V4, and the inferior temporal visual cortex (see Figs. 4.1 and 4.2). Is the emotional or motivational valence of visual stimuli represented in these regions? A schematic diagram summarizing some of the conclusions that will be reached is shown in Fig. 4.3.

One way to answer the issue just raised is to test monkeys in a learning paradigm in which one visual stimulus is associated with reward (for example glucose taste, or fruit juice taste), and another visual stimulus is associated with an aversive taste, such as strong saline. Rolls, Judge and Sanghera (1977) performed just such an experiment and found that single neurons in the inferior temporal visual cortex did not respond differently to objects based on their reward association. To test whether a neuron might be influenced by the reward association, the monkey performed a visual discrimination task in which the reinforcement contingency could be reversed during the experiment. (That is, the visual stimulus, for example a triangle, to which the monkey had to lick to obtain a taste of fruit juice, was after the reversal associated with saline—if the monkey licked to the triangle after the reversal, he obtained mildly aversive salt solution.) An example of such an experiment is shown in Fig. 2.19. The neuron responded more to the triangle, both before reversal when it was associated with fruit juice, and after reversal, when the triangle was associated with saline. Thus the reinforcement association of the visual stimuli did not alter the response to the visual stimuli, which was based on the physical properties of the stimuli (for example their shape, colour, or texture). The same was true for the other neurons recorded in this study. This independence from reward association seems to be characteristic of neurons right through the temporal visual cortical areas, and must be true in earlier cortical areas too, in that they provide the inputs to the inferior temporal visual cortex.

4.3.3 Why reward and punishment associations of stimuli are not represented early in information processing in the primate brain

The processing stream that has just been considered is that concerned with objects, that is with *what* is being looked at. Two fundamental points about pattern association networks for stimulus–reinforcement association learning can be made from what we have considered. The first point is that sensory processing in the primate brain proceeds as far as the invariant representation of objects (invariant with respect to, for example, size, position on the retina, and even view), independently of reward vs punishment association. Why should this be, in terms of systems level brain organization? The suggestion that is made is that the visual properties of the world about which reward associations must be learned are generally objects (for example the sight of a banana, or of an orange), and are not just raw pixels or edges, with no invariant properties, which is what is represented in the retina and V1. The implication is that the sensory processing must proceed to the stage of the invariant representation of objects before it is appropriate to learn reinforcement associations. The invariance aspect is important too, for if we had different representations for an object at different places in our visual field, then if we learned when an object was at one point on the retina that it was rewarding, we would not generalize correctly to it when presented at another position on the retina. If it had previously been punishing at that retinal position, we might find the same object rewarding when at one point on the retina, and punishing when at another. This is inappropriate given the world in which we live, and in which our brain evolved, in that the most appropriate assumption is that objects have the same reinforcement association wherever they are on the retina.

The same systems-level principle of brain organization is also likely to be true in other sensory systems, such as those for touch and hearing. For example, we do not generally want to learn that a particular pure tone is associated with reward or punishment. Instead, it might be a particular complex pattern of sounds such as a vocalization that carries a reinforcement signal, and this may be independent of the exact pitch at which it is uttered. Thus, cases in which some modulation of neuronal responses to pure tones in parts of the brain such as the medial geniculate (the thalamic relay for hearing) (LeDoux 1994) where tonotopic tuning is found may be rather special *model* systems (that is simplified systems on which to perform experiments), and not reflect the way in which auditory-to-reinforcement pattern associations are normally learned. The same may be true for touch in so far as one considers associations between objects identified by somatosensory input, and primary reinforcers. An example might be selecting a food object from a whole collection of objects in the dark.

The second point, which complements the first, is that the visual system is not provided with the appropriate primary reinforcers for such pattern-association learning, in that visual processing in the primate brain is mainly unimodal to and through the inferior temporal visual cortex (see Fig. 4.2). It is only after the inferior temporal visual cortex, when it projects to structures such as the amygdala and orbitofrontal cortex, that the appropriate convergence between visual processing pathways and pathways conveying information about primary reinforcers such as taste and touch/pain occurs (Fig. 4.2). We now, therefore, turn our attention to the amygdala and orbitofrontal cortex, to consider whether they might be the brain regions that contain the neuronal networks for pattern associations involving primary reinforcers. We note at this stage that in order to make the results as relevant as possible to brain function and its disorders in humans, the system being described is that present in primates such as monkeys. In rats, although the

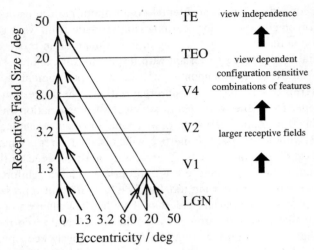

Fig. 4.7 Schematic diagram showing convergence achieved by the forward projections in the visual system, and the types of representation that may be built by competitive networks operating at each stage of the system from the primary visual cortex (V1) to the inferior temporal visual cortex (area TE) (see text). LGN, lateral geniculate nucleus. Area TEO forms the posterior inferior temporal cortex. The receptive fields in the inferior temporal visual cortex (for example in the TE areas) cross the vertical midline (not shown).

organization of the amygdala may be similar, the areas which may correspond to the primate inferior temporal visual cortex and orbitofrontal cortex are hardly developed.

4.3.4 Invariant representations of faces and objects in the inferior temporal visual cortex
4.3.4.1 Processing to the inferior temporal cortex in the primate visual system

A schematic diagram to indicate some aspects of the processing involved in object identification from the primary visual cortex, V1, through V2 and V4 to the posterior inferior temporal cortex (TEO) and the anterior inferior temporal cortex (TE) is shown in Fig. 4.7. Their approximate location on the brain of a macaque monkey is shown in Fig. 4.8, which also shows that TE has a number of different subdivisions. The different TE areas all contain visually responsive neurons, as do many of the areas within the cortex in the superior temporal sulcus (G. Baylis, Rolls and Leonard 1987). For the purposes of this summary, these areas will be grouped together as the anterior inferior temporal cortex (IT), except where otherwise stated. Some of the information processing that takes place through these pathways that must be addressed by computational models is as follows. A fuller account is provided by Rolls (1994a, 1995b, 1997d; Wallis and Rolls 1997; Rolls and Treves 1998, Chapter 8). Many of the studies on neurons in the inferior temporal cortex and cortex in the superior temporal cortex have been performed with neurons which respond particularly to faces, because such neurons can be found regularly in recordings in this region, and therefore provide a good population for systematic studies (see Rolls 1994a, 1997d).

4.3.4.2   Receptive field size and translation invariance

There is convergence from each small part of a region to the succeeding region (or layer in the hierarchy) in such a way that the receptive field sizes of neurons (for example 1° near the fovea in V1) become larger by a factor of approximately 2.5 with each succeeding stage (and the typical parafoveal receptive field sizes found would not be inconsistent with the calculated approximations of, for example, 8° in V4, 20° in TEO, and 50° in inferior temporal cortex, Boussaoud et al. 1991) (see Fig. 4.7). Such zones of convergence would overlap continuously with each other (see Fig. 4.7). This connectivity provides part of the basis for the fact that many neurons in the temporal cortical visual areas respond to a stimulus relatively independently of where it is in their receptive field, and moreover maintain their stimulus selectivity when the stimulus appears in different parts of the visual field (Gross et al. 1985; Tovee, Rolls and Azzopardi 1994). This is called translation or shift invariance. In addition to having topologically appropriate connections, it is necessary for the connections to have the appropriate synaptic weights to perform the mapping of each set of features, or object, to the same set of neurons in IT. How this could be achieved is addressed in the neural network model described by Wallis and Rolls (1997) and Rolls and Treves (1998).

4.3.4.3   Size and spatial frequency invariance

Some neurons in IT/STS respond relatively independently of the size of an effective face stimulus, with a mean size invariance (to a half maximal response) of 12 times (3.5 octaves) (Rolls and Baylis 1986). This is not a property of a simple single-layer network (see Fig. 8.1 of Rolls and Treves 1998), nor of neurons in V1, which respond best to small stimuli, with a typical size-invariance of 1.5 octaves. (Some neurons in IT/STS also respond to face stimuli which are blurred, or which are line drawn, showing that they can also map the different spatial frequencies with which objects can be represented to the same represen-tation in IT/STS, see Rolls, Baylis and Leonard 1985.)

Some neurons in the temporal cortical visual areas actually represent the absolute size of objects such as faces independently of viewing distance (Rolls and Baylis 1986). This could be called neurophysiological size constancy. The utility of this representation by a small population of neurons is that the absolute size of an object is a useful feature to use as an input to neurons which perform object recognition. Faces only come in certain sizes.

4.3.4.4   Combinations of features in the correct spatial configuration

Many cells in this processing stream respond to combinations of features (including objects), but not to single features presented alone, and the features must have the correct spatial arrangement. This has been shown, for example, with faces, for which it has been shown by masking out or presenting parts of the face (for example eyes, mouth, or hair) in isolation, or by jumbling the features in faces, that some cells in the cortex in IT/STS respond only if two or more features are present, and are in the correct spatial arrange-ment (Perrett, Rolls and Caan 1982; Rolls, Tovee, Purcell et al. 1994b). Corresponding evidence has been found for non-face cells. For example, Tanaka et al. (1990) showed that

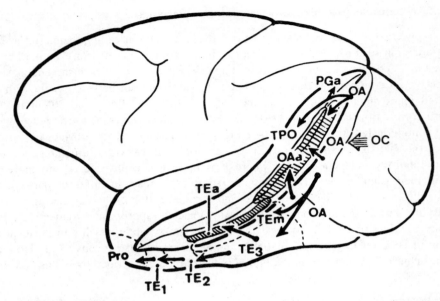

Fig. 4.8 Lateral view of the macaque brain showing the different architectonic areas (for example TEm, TPO) in and bordering the anterior part of the superior temporal sulcus (STS) of the macaque (see text). The borders of the opened superior temporal sulcus are indicated by bold outline. Terminology of Seltzer and Pandya (1978).

some posterior inferior temporal cortex neurons might only respond to the combination of an edge and a small circle if they were in the correct spatial relation to each other. Evidence consistent with the suggestion that neurons are responding to combinations of a few variables represented at the preceding stage of cortical processing is that some neurons in V2 and V4 respond to end-stopped lines, to tongues flanked by inhibitory subregions, or to combinations of colours (see references cited by Rolls 1991c). Neurons that respond to combinations of features but not to single features indicate that the system is non-linear.

4.3.4.5 A view-independent representation

For recognizing and learning about objects (including faces), it is important that an output of the visual system should be not only translation- and size-invariant, but also relatively view-invariant. In an investigation of whether there are such neurons, we found that some temporal cortical neurons reliably responded differently to the faces of two different individuals independently of viewing angle (Hasselmo, Rolls, Baylis and Nalwa 1989b), although in most cases (16/18 neurons) the response was not perfectly view-independent. Mixed together in the same cortical regions there are neurons with view-dependent responses (for example Hasselmo, Rolls, Baylis and Nalwa 1989b; Rolls and Tovee 1995a). Such neurons might respond, for example, to a view of a profile of a monkey but not to a full-face view of the same monkey (Perrett *et al.* 1985). These findings, of view-dependent, partially view-independent, and view-independent representations in the same cortical regions are consistent with the hypothesis discussed below that view-independent representations are being built in these regions by associating together the outputs of neurons that respond to different views of the same individual. These findings also provide evidence that one output of the visual system includes representations of what is being seen, in a view-independent way that would be useful for object recognition and for learning associations about objects; and that another output is a view-based representation that would be useful in social interactions to determine whether another individual is looking at one, and for selecting details of motor responses, for which the orientation of the object with respect to the viewer is required. Further evidence that some neurons in the temporal cortical visual areas have object-based responses comes from a population of neurons that responds to moving faces, for example to a head undergoing ventral flexion, irrespective of whether the view of the head was full face, of either profile, or even of the back of the head (Hasselmo, Rolls, Baylis and Nalwa 1989b).

4.3.4.6 Distributed encoding

An important question for understanding brain function is whether a particular object (or face) is represented in the brain by the firing of one or a few gnostic (or 'grandmother') cells (Barlow 1972), or whether instead the firing of a group or ensemble of cells each with somewhat different responsiveness provides the representation. Advantages of distributed codes (see the Appendix and Rolls and Treves 1998) include generalization and graceful degradation (fault tolerance), and a potentially very high capacity in the number of stimuli that can be represented (that is exponential growth of capacity with the number of neurons in the representation). If the ensemble encoding is sparse, this provides a good input to an associative memory, for then large numbers of stimuli can be stored (see Chapters 2 and 3 of Rolls and Treves 1998). We have shown that in the IT/STS, responses of a group of neurons, but not of a single neuron, provide evidence on which face was shown. We showed, for example, that these neurons typically respond with a graded set of firing to different faces, with firing rates from 120 spikes s^{-1} to the most effective face, to no response at all to a number of the least effective faces (G. Baylis, Rolls and Leonard 1985; Rolls and Tovee 1995a). The sparseness a of the activity of the neurons was 0.65 over a set of 68 stimuli including 23 faces and 45 non-face natural scenes, and a measure called the response sparseness a_r of the representation, in which the spontaneous rate was subtracted from the firing rate to each stimulus so that the responses of the neuron were being assessed, was 0.38 across the same set of stimuli (Rolls and Tovee 1995a). (For the definition of sparseness see the Appendix. For binary neurons firing, e.g. either at a high rate or not at all, the sparseness is the proportion of neurons that are active during the presentation of any one stimulus.)

It has been possible to apply information theory to show that each neuron conveys on average approximately 0.4 bits of information about which face in a set of 20 faces has been seen (Tovee and Rolls 1995; cf. Tovee, Rolls, Treves and Bellis 1993, Rolls, Treves, Tovee and Panzeri 1997d). If a neuron responded to only one of the faces in the set of 20, then it could convey (if noiseless) 4.6 bits of information about one of the faces (when that face was shown). If, at the other extreme, it responded to half the faces in the set, it would convey 1 bit of information about which face had been seen on any one trial. In fact, the average maximum information about the best stimulus was 1.8 bits of information. This provides good evidence not only that the representation is distributed, but also that it is a sufficiently reliable representation that useful information can be obtained from it.

The most impressive result obtained so far is that when the information available from a population of neurons about which of 20 faces has been seen is considered, the information increases approximately linearly as the number of cells in the population increases from 1 to 14 (Abbott, Rolls and Tovee 1996; Rolls, Treves and Tovee 1997c; see Fig. 4.9). Remembering that the information in bits is a logarithmic measure, this shows that the representational capacity of this population of cells increases exponentially. This is the case both when an optimal, probability estimation, form of decoding of the activity of the neuronal population is used, and also when the neurally plausible dot product type of decoding is used (Fig. 4.9a). (The dot product decoding assumes that what reads out the information from the population activity vector is a neuron or a set of neurons which operates just by forming the dot product of the input population vector and its synaptic weight vector—see Rolls, Treves and Tovee 1997c.) By simulation of further neurons and further stimuli, we have shown that the capacity grows very impressively, approximately as shown in Fig. 4.9c (Abbott, Rolls and Tovee 1996). This result is exactly what would be hoped for from a distributed representation. This result is not what would be expected for local encoding, for which the number of stimuli that could be encoded would increase linearly with the number of cells. (Even if the grandmother cells were noisy, adding more replicates to increase reliability would not lead to more than a linear increase in the number of stimuli that can be encoded as a function of the number of cells.) These findings provide very firm evidence that the encoding built at the end of the visual system *is* distributed, and that part of the power of this representation is that by receiving inputs from relatively small numbers of such neurons, neurons at the next stage of processing (for example in memory structures such as the hippocampus, amygdala, and orbitofrontal cortex) would obtain information about which of a very great number of stimuli had been shown. This representational capacity of neuronal populations has fundamental implications for the connectivity of the brain, for it shows that neurons need not have hundreds of thousands or millions of inputs to have available to them information about what is represented in another population of cells, but that instead the real numbers of perhaps 8000–10000 synapses per neuron would be adequate for them to receive considerable information from the several different sources between which this set of synapses is allocated. Similar results have been found for objects (Booth and Rolls 1998).

It may be noted that it is unlikely that there are further processing areas beyond those described where ensemble coding changes into grandmother cell encoding. Anatomically, there does not appear to be a whole further set of visual processing areas present in the brain; and outputs from the temporal lobe visual areas such as those described are taken to limbic and related regions such as the amygdala and via the entorhinal cortex to the hippocampus (see Rolls 1994a, 1997d; Rolls and Treves 1998). Indeed, tracing this pathway onwards, we have found a population of neurons with face-selective responses in the amygdala, and in the majority of these neurons, different responses occur to different faces, with ensemble (not local) coding still being present (Leonard, Rolls, Wilson and

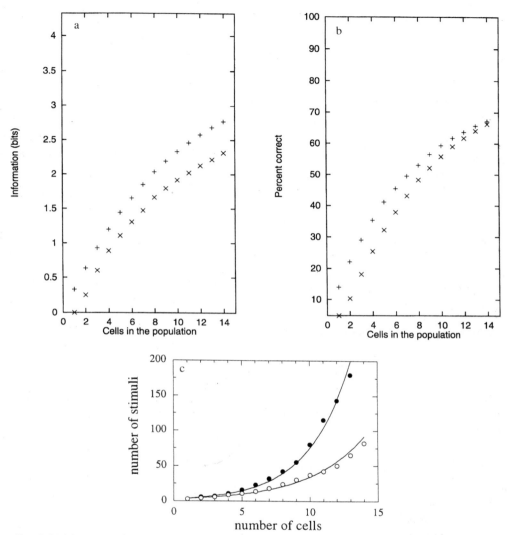

Fig. 4.9 (a) The values for the average information available in the responses of different numbers of neurons in the temporal cortical visual areas on each trial in a 500-ms period, about which of a set of 20 face stimuli has been shown. The decoding method was Dot Product (×) or Probability Estimation (+). (b) The percentage correct for which one of 20 faces was shown based on the firing rate responses of different numbers of neurons on a single trial (i.e. the corresponding data to those shown in Fig. 4.9a). (Fig. 4 of Rolls, Treves and Tovee 1997c.). (c) The number of stimuli (in this case from a set of 20 faces) that are encoded in the responses of different numbers of neurons in the temporal lobe visual cortex. (After Abbott, Rolls and Tovee 1996; Rolls, Treves and Tovee 1997c; see Rolls and Treves 1998, Section 10.4.3 and Appendix A2.)

Baylis 1985; Rolls 1992a). The amygdala, in turn, projects to another structure which may be important in other behavioural responses to faces, the ventral striatum, and compara-ble neurons have also been found in the ventral striatum (Williams, Rolls, Leonard and

Stern 1993). We have also recorded from face-responding neurons in the part of the orbitofrontal cortex that receives from the IT/STS cortex, and have found that the encoding there is also not local (Rolls and Critchley, in preparation; Rolls 1996d).

4.3.5 Face expression, gesture and view represented in a population of neurons in the cortex in the superior temporal sulcus

In addition to the population of neurons that code for face identity, which tend to have object-based representations and are in areas TEa and TEm on the ventral bank of the superior temporal sulcus, there is a separate population in the cortex in the superior temporal sulcus (e.g. area TPO) which conveys information about facial expression (Hasselmo, Rolls and Baylis 1989a) (see e.g. Fig. 4.10). Some of the neurons in this region tend to have view-based representations (so that information is conveyed, for example, about whether the face is looking at one, or is looking away), and might respond to moving faces, and to facial gesture (Hasselmo, Rolls and Baylis 1989b; Rolls 1992a,c).

Thus information in cortical areas which project to the amygdala is about face identity, and about face expression and gesture. Both types of information are important in social and emotional responses to other primates, which must be based on who the individual is as well as on the face expression or gesture being made. One output from the amygdala for this information is probably via the ventral striatum, for a small population of neurons has been found in the ventral striatum with responses selective for faces (Rolls and Williams 1987b; Williams, Rolls, Leonard and Stern 1993).

4.3.6 The brain mechanisms that build the appropriate view-invariant representations of objects required for learning emotional responses to objects, including faces

This book has a main goal of advancing understanding of the function of many systems of the brain, taking mainly a systems-level approach, and an approach related to biological adaptation. The main goal of the book by Rolls and Treves (1998) was to provide some of the foundations for understanding at the computational and neuronal network level *how* the brain performs its functions. Some of the ways in which the visual system may produce the distributed invariant representations of objects needed for inputs to emotion-learning systems have been described by Rolls and Treves 1998, Chapter 8 (see also Rolls 1992a, 1994d, 1997e; Wallis and Rolls 1997; Parga and Rolls, 1998), and include a hierarchical feed-forward series of competitive networks using convergence from stage to stage; and the use of a modified Hebb synaptic learning rule which incorporates a short-term memory trace of previous neuronal activity to help learn the invariant properties of objects from the temporo-spatial statistics produced by the normal viewing of objects.

4.4 The amygdala

Bilateral damage to the amygdala produces a deficit in learning to associate visual and

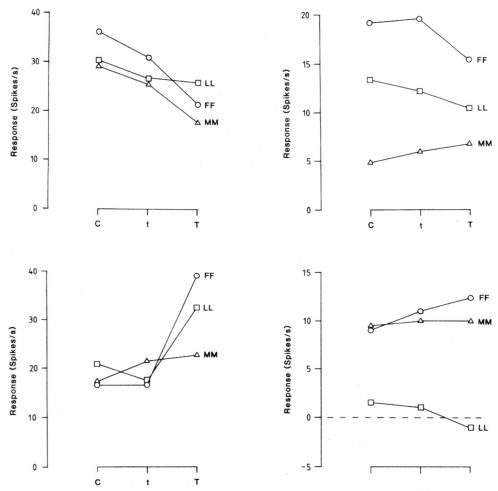

Fig. 4.10 There is a population of neurons in the cortex in the superior temporal sulcus with responses tuned to respond differently to different face expressions. The cells in the two left panels did not discriminate between individuals (faces MM, FF, and LL), but did discriminate between different expressions on the faces of those individuals (C, calm expression; t, mild threat; T, strong threat). In contrast, the cells in the right two panels responded differently to different individuals, and did not discriminate between different expressions. The neurons that discriminated between expressions were found mainly in the cortex in the fundus of the superior temporal sulcus; the neurons that discriminated between identity were in contrast found mainly in the cortex in lateral part of the ventral lip of the superior temporal sulcus (areas Tea and Tem). (From Hasselmo, Rolls and Baylis 1989a.)

other stimuli with a primary (i.e. unlearned) reward or punisher. For example, monkeys with damage to the amygdala when shown foods and non-foods pick up both and place them in their mouths. When such visual or auditory discrimination learning and learned emotional responses to stimuli are tested more formally, it is found that animals have difficulty in associating the sight or sound of a stimulus with whether it produces a reward, or is noxious and should be avoided (see Rolls 1990c, 1992a). Similar changes in behaviour have been seen in humans with extensive damage to the temporal lobe. The primate amygdala also contains a population of neurons specialized to respond to faces, and damage to the human amygdala can alter the ability to discriminate between different facial expressions.

4.4.1 Connections of the amygdala

The amygdala is a subcortical region in the anterior part of the temporal lobe. It receives massive projections in the primate from the overlying temporal lobe cortex (see Amaral *et al*. 1992; Van Hoesen 1981) (see Fig. 4.11). These come in the monkey to overlapping but partly separate regions of the lateral and basal amygdala from the inferior temporal visual

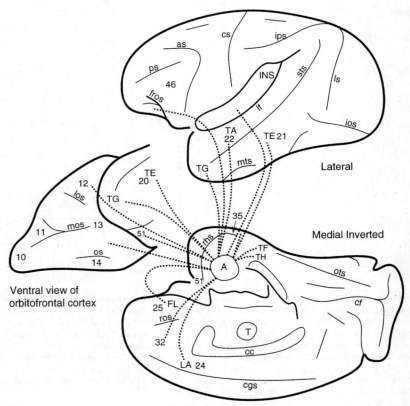

Fig. 4.11 Connections of the amygdala shown on lateral, ventral, and medial views of the monkey brain (after Van Hoesen 1981). Abbreviations: as, arcuate sulcus; cc, corpus callosum; cf., calcarine fissure; cgs, cingulate sulcus; cs, central sulcus; ls, lunate sulcus; ios, inferior occipital sulcus; mos, medial orbital sulcus; os, orbital sulcus; ots, occipito-temporal sulcus; ps, principal sulcus; rhs, rhinal sulcus; sts, superior temporal sulcus; lf, Lateral (or Sylvian) fissure (which has been opened to reveal the insula); A, amygdala; INS, insula; T, thalamus; TE (21), inferior temporal visual cortex; TA (22), superior temporal auditory association cortex; TF and TH, parahippocampal cortex; TG, temporal pole cortex; 12, 13, 11, orbitofrontal cortex; 24, part of the cingulate cortex; 35, perirhinal cortex; 51, olfactory (prepyriform and periamygdaloid) cortex. The cortical connections shown provide afferents to the amygdala, but are reciprocated.

cortex, the superior temporal auditory cortex, the cortex of the temporal pole, and the cortex in the superior temporal sulcus. These inputs thus come from the higher stages of sensory processing in the visual and auditory modalities, and not from early cortical processing areas. Via these inputs, the amygdala receives inputs about objects that could become secondary reinforcers, as a result of pattern association in the amygdala with primary reinforcers. The amygdala also receives inputs that are potentially about primary reinforcers, e.g. taste inputs (from the secondary taste cortex, via connections from the orbitofrontal cortex to the amygdala), and somatosensory inputs, potentially about the rewarding or painful aspects of touch (from the somatosensory cortex via the insula) (Mesulam and Mufson 1982a, b; Friedman *et al.* 1986). The amygdala also receives projections from the posterior orbitofrontal cortex (Carmichael and Price 1995) (see Fig. 4.11, areas 12 and 13).

Subcortical inputs to the amygdala include projections from the midline thalamic nuclei, the subiculum, and CA1 parts of the hippocampal formation, the hypothalamus and substantia innominata, the nucleus of the solitary tract (which receives gustatory and visceral inputs), and from olfactory structures (Amaral *et al.* 1992). Although there are some inputs from early on in some sensory pathways, for example auditory inputs from the medial geniculate nucleus (LeDoux 1987, 1992), this route is unlikely to be involved in most emotions, for which cortical analysis of the stimulus is likely to be required. Emotions are usually elicited to environmental stimuli analysed to the object level (including other organisms), and not to retinal arrays of spots or the frequency (tone) of a sound as represented in the cochlea. Consistent with this view (that neural systems involved in emotion in primates generally receive from sensory systems where analysis of the identity of the stimulus as an object is performed), neurons in the inferior temporal visual cortex do not have responses related to the association with reinforcement of visual stimuli (Rolls, Judge and Sanghera 1977); whereas such neurons are found in the amygdala and orbitofrontal cortex (see below; cf. Fig. 4.2). Similarly, processing in the taste system of primates up to and including the primary taste cortex reflects the identity of the tastant, whereas its hedonic value as influenced by hunger is reflected in the responses of neurons in the secondary taste cortex (Rolls 1989b, 1995a; see Fig. 4.2).

The outputs of the amygdala (Amaral *et al.* 1992) include the well-known projections to the hypothalamus, from the lateral amygdala via the ventral amygdalofugal pathway to the lateral hypothalamus and from the medial amygdala, which is relatively small in the primate, via the stria terminalis to the medial hypothalamus. The ventral amygdalofugal pathway includes some long descending fibres that project to the autonomic centres in the medulla oblongata, and provide a route for cortically processed signals to reach the brainstem. A further interesting output of the amygdala is to the ventral striatum (Heimer, Switzer and Van Hoesen 1982) including the nucleus accumbens, for via this route information processed in the amygdala could gain access to the basal ganglia and thus influence motor output. (The output of the amygdala also reaches more dorsal parts of the striatum.) The amygdala also projects to the medial part of the mediodorsal nucleus of the thalamus, which projects to the orbitofrontal cortex, providing another output pathway for the amygdala. In addition, the amygdala has direct projections back to many areas of the temporal, orbitofrontal, and insular cortices from which it receives inputs (Amaral *et al.*

1992). It is suggested elsewhere (Rolls 1989a,c; Rolls and Treves 1998) that the functions of these backprojections include the guidance of information representation and storage in the neocortex, and recall (when this is related to reinforcing stimuli). Another interesting set of output pathways of the amygdala are the projections to the entorhinal cortex, which provides the major input to the hippocampus and dentate gyrus, and to the ventral subiculum, which provides a major output of the hippocampus (Amaral *et al.* 1992).

These anatomical connections of the amygdala indicate that it is strategically placed to receive highly processed information from the cortex and to influence motor systems, autonomic systems, some of the cortical areas from which it receives inputs, and other limbic areas. The functions mediated through these connections will now be considered, using information available from the effects of damage to the amygdala and from the activity of neurons in the amygdala.

4.4.2 Effects of amygdala lesions

Bilateral removal of the amygdala in monkeys produces striking behavioural changes which include tameness, a lack of emotional responsiveness, excessive examination of objects, often with the mouth, and eating of previously rejected items such as meat (Weiskrantz 1956). These behavioural changes comprise much of the Kluver–Bucy syndrome which is produced in monkeys by bilateral anterior temporal lobectomy (Kluver and Bucy 1939). In analyses of the bases of these behavioural changes, it has been observed that there are deficits in some types of learning. For example, Weiskrantz (1956) found that bilateral ablation of the amygdala in the monkey produced a deficit on learning an active avoidance task. The monkeys failed to learn to make a response when a light signalled that shock would follow unless the response was made. He was perhaps the first to suggest that these monkeys had difficulty with forming associations between stimuli and reinforcers, when he suggested that "the effect of amygdalectomy is to make it difficult for reinforcing stimuli, whether positive or negative, to become established or to be recognized as such" (Weiskrantz 1956). In this avoidance task, associations between a stimulus and negative reinforcers were impaired.

Evidence soon became available that associations between stimuli and positive reinforcers (reward) were also impaired in, for example, serial reversals of a visual discrimination made to obtain food (Jones and Mishkin 1972; cf. Spiegler and Mishkin, 1981). In this task the monkey must learn that food is under one of two objects, and after he has learned this, he must then relearn (reverse) the association as the food is then placed under the other object. Jones and Mishkin (1972) showed that the stages of this task which are particularly affected by damage to this region are those when the monkeys are responding at chance to the two visual stimuli or are starting to respond more to the currently rewarded stimuli, rather than the stage when the monkeys are continuing to make perseverative responses to the previously rewarded visual stimulus. They thus argued that the difficulty produced by this anterior temporal lobe damage is in learning to associate stimuli with reinforcers, in this case with food reward.

There is evidence from lesion studies in monkeys that the amygdala is involved in learning associations between visual stimuli and rewards (see D. Gaffan 1992; D. Gaffan and Harrison 1987; E. Gaffan *et al.* 1988; D. Gaffan, Gaffan and Harrison, 1989; L. Baylis and Gaffan 1991). However, lesion studies are subject to the criticism that the effects of a lesion could be due to inadvertent damage to other brain structures or pathways close to the intended lesion site. For this reason, many of the older lesion studies are being repeated and extended with lesions in which instead of an ablation (removal) or elec- trolytic lesion (which can damage axons passing through a brain region), a neurotoxin is used to damage cells in a localized region, but to leave intact fibres of passage. Using such lesions (made with ibotenic acid) in monkeys, Malkova, Gaffan and Murray (1997) showed that amygdala lesions did not impair visual discrimination learning when the reinforcer was an auditory secondary reinforcer learned as being positively reinforcing preopera- tively. This was in contrast to an earlier study by D. Gaffan and Harrison (1987; see also D. Gaffan 1992). In the study by Malkova *et al.* (1997) the animals with amygdala lesions were somewhat slower to learn a visual discrimination task for food reward, and made more errors, but with the small numbers of animals (the numbers in the groups were 3 and 4), the difference did not reach statistical significance. It would be interesting to test such animals when the association was directly between a visual stimulus and a primary reinforcer such as taste. (In most such studies, the reward being given is usually solid food, which is seen before it is tasted, and for which the food delivery mechanism makes a noise. These factors mean that the reward for which the animal is working includes secondary reinforcing components, the sight and sound). However, in the 1997 study it was shown that amygdala lesions made with ibotenic acid did impair the processing of reward-related stimuli, in that when the reward value of one set of foods was reduced by feeding it to satiety (i.e. sensory-specific satiety), the monkeys still chose the visual stimuli associated with the foods with which they had been satiated (Malkova *et al.* 1997). Further evidence that neurotoxic lesions of the amygdala in primates affect behaviour to stimuli learned as being reward-related as well as punishment-related is that monkeys with neurotoxic lesions of the amygdala showed abnormal patterns of food choice, picking up and eating foods not normally eaten such as meat, and picking up and placing in their mouths inedible objects (Murray, E. Gaffan and Flint, 1996). These symptoms produced by selective amygdala lesions are classical Kluver-Bucy symptoms. Thus in primates, there is evidence that selective amygdala lesions impair some types of behaviour to learned reward-related stimuli as well as to learned punishment-related stimuli. However, we should not conclude that this is the only brain structure involved in this type of learning, for especially when rapid stimulus-reinforcement association learning is performed in primates, the orbitofrontal cortex is involved, as shown in Section 4.5.

Further evidence linking the amygdala to reinforcement mechanisms is that monkeys will work in order to obtain electrical stimulation of the amygdala, and that single neurons in the amygdala are activated by brain-stimulation reward of a number of different sites (Rolls 1975; Rolls, Burton and Mora 1980).

The symptoms of the Kluver–Bucy syndrome, including the emotional changes, could be a result of this type of deficit in learning stimulus-reinforcement associations (Jones and Mishkin 1972; Mishkin and Aggleton 1981; Rolls 1986a,b, 1990b, 1992b). For example, the tameness, the hypoemotionality, the increased orality, and the altered responses to food would arise because of damage to the normal mechanism by which stimuli become associated with reward or punishment. Other evidence is also consistent with the hypothesis that there is a close relationship between the learning deficit and the emotion-related and other symptoms of the Kluver–Bucy syndrome. For example, in a study of subtotal lesions of the amygdala, Aggleton and Passingham (1981) found that in only those monkeys in which the lesions produced a serial reversal learning deficit was hypoemotionality present.

In rats, there is also evidence that the amygdala is involved in behaviour to stimuli learned as being associated with reward as well as with punishment. In studies to investigate the role of the amygdala in reward-related learning in the rat, Cador, Robbins and Everitt (1989) obtained evidence consistent with the hypothesis that the learned incentive (conditioned reinforcing) effects of previously neutral stimuli paired with rewards are mediated by the amygdala acting through the ventral striatum, in that amphetamine injections into the ventral striatum enhanced the effects of a conditioned reinforcing stimulus only if the amygdala was intact (see further Everitt and Robbins 1992; Robbins *et al.* 1989). In another study, Everitt *et al.* (1989) showed that excitotoxic lesions of the basolateral amygdala disrupted appetitive sexual responses maintained by a visual conditioned reinforcer, but not the behaviour to the primary reinforcer for the male rats, copulation with a female rat in heat (see further Everitt and Robbins 1992). (The details of the study were that the learned reinforcer or conditioned stimulus was a light for which the male rats worked on a FR10 schedule (i.e. 10 responses made to obtain a presentation of the light), with access to the female being allowed for the first FR10 completed after a fixed period of 15 min. This is a second order schedule of reinforcement. For comparison, and this is relevant to Chapter 8, medial preoptic area lesions eliminated the copulatory behaviour of mounting, intromission and ejaculation to the primary reinforcer, the female rat, but did not affect the learned appetitive responding for the conditioned or secondary reinforcing stimulus, the light.) In another study demonstrating the role of the amygdala in responses to learned positive reinforcers in rats, Everitt *et al.* (1991) showed that a conditioned place preference to a place where rats were given 10% sucrose was abolished by bilateral excitotoxic lesions of the basolateral amygdala. Moreover, the output of the amygdala for this learned reinforcement effect on behaviour appears to be via the ventral striatum, for a unilateral lesion of the amygdala and a contralateral lesion of the nucleus accumbens also impaired the conditioned place preference for the place where sucrose was made available (Everitt *et al.* 1991; see further Everitt and Robbins 1992). In another study showing the importance of the basolateral amygdala for effects of learned rewards on behaviour, Whitelaw, Markou, Robbins and Everitt (1996) showed that excitotoxic lesions of the basolateral amygdala in rats impaired behavioural responses to a light associated with intravenous administration of cocaine, but not to the primary reinforcer of the cocaine itself. (A second order schedule comparable to that described above was used to show the impairment of drug-seeking behaviour, that is responses made to obtain the light associated with delivery of the drug. Self-administration of the drug in a continuous reinforcement schedule was not impaired, showing that the amygdala is not necessary for the primary reinforcing effects of cocaine.)

It has long been known that rats with lesions of the amygdala display altered fear responses. For example, Rolls and Rolls (1973) showed that rats with amygdala lesions showed less neophobia to new foods. In a model of fear conditioning in the rat, LeDoux and colleagues (see LeDoux 1994, 1995, 1996; Quirk *et al.* 1996) have shown that lesions of the amygdala attenuate fear responses learned when pure tones are associated with footshock. The learned responses include typical classically conditioned responses such as heart-rate changes and freezing to fear-inducing stimuli (see, e.g., LeDoux 1994) and also operant responses (see, e.g., Gallagher and Holland 1994). The deficits typically involve particularly the learned (emotional) responses, e.g. fear to the conditioned stimuli, rather than changes in behavioural responses to the unconditioned stimuli such as altered responses to pain per se (but see Hebert *et al.* 1997). In another type of paradigm, it has been shown that amygdala lesions impair the devaluing effect of pairing a food reward with (aversive) lithium chloride, in that amygdala lesions reduced the classically conditioned responses of the rats to a light previously paired with the food (Hatfield *et al.* 1996). In a different model of fear-conditioning in the rat, Davis and colleagues (Davis 1992, 1994; Davis *et al.* 1995), have used the fear-potentiated startle test, in which the amplitude of the acoustic startle reflex is increased when elicited in the presence of a stimulus previously paired with shock. The conditioned stimulus can be visual or a low-frequency auditory stimulus. Chemical or electrolytic lesions of either the central nucleus or the lateral and basolateral nuclei of the amygdala block the expression of fear-potentiated startle. These latter amygdala nuclei may be the site of plasticity for fear conditioning, because local infusion of the NMDA (*N*-methyl-D-aspartate) receptor antagonist AP5 (which blocks long-term potentiation, an index of synaptic plasticity) blocks the acquisition but not the maintenance of fear-potentiated startle (Davis 1992, 1994; Davis *et al.* 1995).

There are separate output pathways for the amygdala for different fear-related responses, in that lesions of the lateral hypothalamus (which receives from the central nucleus of the amygdala) blocked conditioned heart rate (autonomic) responses; lesions of the central gray of the midbrain (which also receives from the central nucleus of the amygdala) blocked the conditioned freezing but not the conditioned autonomic response (LeDoux *et al.* 1988); and lesions of the stria terminalis blocked the neuroendocrine responses (T. Gray *et al.* 1993) (see Fig. 4.12). In addition, cortical arousal may be produced by the conditioned stimuli via the central nucleus of the amygdala outputs to the cholinergic basal forebrain magnocellular nuclei of Meynert (see Kapp *et al.* 1992; Wilson and Rolls 1990a,b,c; Section 4.7.1; Rolls and Treves 1998, Section 7.1.5).

The different output routes for different effects mediated by the amygdala are complemented by separate roles of different nuclei within the amygdala in conditioned fear responses. In a study by Killcross, Robbins and Everitt (1997), rats with lesions of the central nucleus exhibited a reduction in the suppression of behaviour elicited by a conditioned fear stimulus, but were simultaneously able to direct their actions to avoid further presentations of this aversive stimulus. In contrast, animals with lesions of the basolateral amygdala were unable to avoid the conditioned aversive stimulus by their choice behaviour, but exhibited normal conditioned suppression to this stimulus. This double dissociation indicates separable contributions of different amygdaloid nuclei to different types of conditioned fear behaviour.

In summary, there is thus much evidence that the amygdala is involved in responses made to stimuli that are associated by learning with primary reinforcers, including rewards

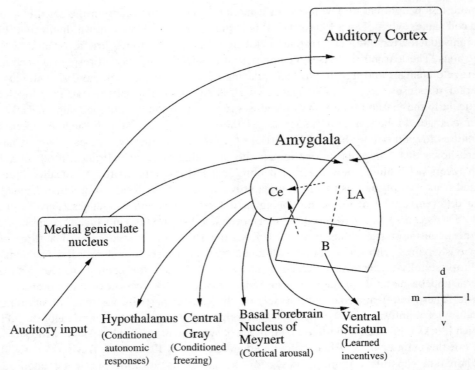

Fig. 4.12 The pathways for fear-conditioning to pure-tone auditory stimuli associated with footshock in the rat (after Quirk, Armony, Repa, Li and LeDoux 1996). The lateral amygdala (LA) receives auditory information directly from the medial part of the medial geniculate nucleus (the auditory thalamic nucleus), and from the auditory cortex. Intra-amygdala projections (directly and via the basal and basal accessory nuclei, B) end in the central nucleus (Ce) of the amygdala. Different output pathways from the central nucleus and the basal nucleus mediate different conditioned fear-related effects. d, dorsal; v, ventral; m, medial; l, lateral.

as well as punishers. The evidence is consistent with the hypothesis that the amygdala is a brain region for stimulus-reinforcement association learning. There is also evidence that it may be involved in whether novel stimuli are approached, for monkeys with amygdala lesions place novel foods and non-food objects in their mouths, and rats with amygdala lesions have decreased neophobia, in that they more quickly accept new foods (Rolls and Rolls 1973; see also Dunn and Everitt 1988; Rolls 1992b; Wilson and Rolls 1993).

4.4.3 Neuronal activity in the primate amygdala to reinforcing stimuli

Recordings from single neurons in the amygdala of the monkey have shown that some neurons do respond to visual stimuli, consistent with the inputs from the temporal lobe visual cortex (Sanghera, Rolls and Roper-Hall 1979). Other neurons responded to auditory, gustatory, olfactory, or somatosensory stimuli, or in relation to movements. In tests of whether the neurons responded on the basis of the association of stimuli with reinforcers, it was found that approximately 20% of the neurons with visual responses had responses which occurred primarily to stimuli associated with reinforcers, for example to food and to a range of stimuli which the monkey had learned signified food in a visual discrimination task (Sanghera, Rolls and Roper-Hall 1979; Rolls 1981b; Wilson and Rolls 1993, 1999) (see Fig 4.13a). However, none of these neurons (in contrast with some neurons in the hypothalamus and orbitofrontal cortex described below) responded exclusively to rewarded stimuli, in that all responded at least partly to one or more neutral, novel, or aversive stimuli. Neurons with responses which are probably similar to these have also been described by Ono *et al.* (1980), and by Nishijo, Ono and Nishino (1988) (see Ono and Nishijo 1992).

The degree to which the responses of these amygdala neurons are associated with reinforcement has been assessed in learning tasks. When the association between a visual stimulus and reinforcement was altered by reversal (so that the visual stimulus formerly associated with juice reward became associated with aversive saline and vice versa), it was found that 10 of 11 neurons did not reverse their responses, and for the other neuron the evidence was not clear) (Sanghera, Rolls and Roper-Hall 1979; see Rolls 1992b). Wilson and Rolls (1999) obtained evidence consistent with this from two more neurons that did not reverse their responses to stimuli when the reinforcement contingency was reversed in the visual discrimination task. On the other hand, in a rather simpler relearning situation in which salt was added to a piece of food such as a water melon, the responses of four amygdala neurons to the sight of the water melon diminished (Nishijo, Ono and Nishino (1988). More investigations are needed to show the extent to which amygdala neurons do alter their activity flexibly and rapidly in relearning tests such as these (see further Rolls 1992b). What has been found in contrast is that neurons in the orbitofrontal cortex do show *very rapid reversal* of their responses in visual discrimination reversal, and it therefore seems likely that the orbitofrontal cortex is especially involved when repeated relearning and re-assessment of stimulus–reinforcer associations is required, as described below, rather than initial learning, in which the amygdala may be involved.

LeDoux and colleagues (see LeDoux 1995, 1996; Quirk *et al.* 1996) have made interesting contributions to understanding the role of the amygdala and related systems in fear-conditioning in the rat. They have shown that for some classes of stimulus, such as pure tones, the association between the tone and an aversive unconditioned stimulus (a footshock) is reflected in the responses of neurons in the amygdala. Some of the circuitry involved is shown in Fig. 4.12. The auditory inputs reach the amygdala both from the subcortical, thalamic, auditory nucleus, the medial geniculate (medial part), and from the auditory cortex. These auditory inputs project to the lateral nucleus of the amygdala (LA), which in turn projects to the central nucleus of the amygdala (Ce) both directly and via the basal (B) and accessory basal nuclei of the amygdala. Le Doux has emphasized the role of the subcortical inputs to the amygdala in this type of conditioning, based on the observations that the conditioning to pure tones can take place without the cortex, and that the shortest latency of the auditory responses in the amygdala are too short to be mediated via the auditory cortex. (Although some conditioning of auditory responses has been found even in the medial geniculate to these pure tones, this conditioning is not of short latency, and LeDoux suggests that it reflects backprojections from the cortex (in which conditioning is also found) to the thalamus.)

The amygdala is well placed anatomically for learning associations between objects and primary reinforcers, for it receives inputs from the higher parts of the visual system, and from systems processing primary reinforcers such as taste, smell, and touch (see Fig. 4.2). The association learning in the amygdala may be implemented by Hebb-modifiable synapses from visual and auditory neurons on to neurons receiving inputs from taste, olfactory, or somatosensory primary reinforcers (see Figs. 4.3 and 4.6; Rolls 1986a,b, 1987, 1990b; Rolls and Treves 1998). Consistent with this, Davis and colleagues (Davis 1992, 1994; Davis et al. 1995) have shown that the stimulus–reinforcement association learning involved in fear-potentiated startle (see Section 4.4.2) is blocked by local application to the lateral amygdala of the NMDA-receptor blocking agent AP5, which blocks long-term potentiation. The hypothesis (see Figs 4.3 and 4.6 and Appendix 1) thus is that synaptic modification takes place between potential secondary reinforcers and primary reinforcers which project on to the same neurons in the amygdala. One index of synaptic modification is long-term potentiation (see Appendix 1), and consistent with this hypothesis, the potential invoked in the rat amygdala by a pure tone increased (suggesting long-term potentiation) after the tone was paired with footshock as the unconditioned stimulus (Rogan, Staubli and LeDoux1997).

LeDoux (1992, 1995, 1996) has described a theory of the neural basis of emotion which is conceptually similar to that of Rolls (1975, 1986a,b, 1990b, 1995c, and this book), except that he focuses mostly on the role of the amygdala in emotion (and not on other brain regions such as the orbitofrontal cortex, which are poorly developed in the rat); except that he focuses mainly on fear (based on his studies of the role of the amygdala and related structures in fear conditioning in the rat); and except that he suggests from his neurophysiological findings that an important route for conditioned emotional stimuli to influence behaviour is via the subcortical inputs (especially auditory from the medial part of the medial geniculate nucleus of the thalamus) to the amygdala. This latter issue, of the normal routes for sensory information about potential secondary reinforcers to reach the amygdala via subcortical pathways will now be addressed, because it raises an important issue about the stimuli that normally cause emotion, and brain design. For simple stimuli such as pure tones, there is evidence of subcortical inputs for the conditioned stimuli to the amygdala, and even of the conditioned stimulus–unconditioned stimulus association being learned prior to involvement of the amygdala (see LeDoux 1995, 1996; Quirk et al. 1996). However, as described above in the part of Section 4.3.3 entitled 'Why reward and punishment associations of stimuli are not represented early in information processing in the primate brain', we humans and other animals do not generally want to learn that a particular pure tone is associated with reward or punishment. Instead, it might be a particular complex pattern of sounds such as a vocalization (or, for example, in vision, a face expression) that carries a reinforcement signal, and this may be independent of the exact pitch at which it is uttered. Thus cases in which some modulation of neuronal responses to pure tones in parts of the brain such as the medial geniculate (the thalamic relay for hearing) where tonotopic tuning is found (LeDoux 1994) may be rather special *model* systems (i.e. simplified systems on which to perform experiments), and not reflect the way in which auditory-to-reinforcement pattern associations are normally learned. (For discrimination of more complex sounds, the auditory cortex is required.) The same is true for vision, in that we do not normally want to associate particular blobs of light at given positions on our retinae (which is what could be represented at the thalamic level in the lateral geniculate nucleus) with primary reinforcement, but instead we may want to associate an invariant representation of an object, or of a person's face, or of a facial expression, with a primary reinforcer. Such analysis *requires* cortical processing, and it is in high-order temporal lobe cortical areas (which provide major afferents to the primate amygdala) that invariant representations of these types of stimulus are found (see Rolls 1994b, 1995b, 1996b; Wallis and Rolls 1997). Moreover, it is crucial that the representation is invariant (with respect to, for example, position on the retina, size, and, for identity, even viewing angle), so that if an association is learned to the object when in one position on the retina, it can generalize correctly to the same object in different positions on the retina, in different sizes, and even with different viewing angles. For this to occur, the invariant representation must be formed before the object–reinforcer association is learned, otherwise generalization to the same object seen on different occasions would not occur, and different inconsistent associations might even be learned to the same object when seen in slightly different positions on the retina, in slightly different sizes, etc. (see Rolls and Treves 1998). Rolls and Treves (1998) also show that it is not a simple property of neuronal networks that they generalize correctly across variations of position and size; special mechanisms, which happen to take a great deal of cortical visual processing, are required to perform such computations (see also Wallis and Rolls 1997). Similar points may also be made for touch in so far as one considers associations between objects identified by somatosensory input, and primary reinforcers. An example might be selecting a food object by either hand from a whole collection of objects in the dark. These points make it unlikely that the subcortical route for conditioned stimuli to reach the amygdala, suggested by LeDoux (1992, 1995, 1996), is generally relevant to the learning of emotional responses to stimuli.

4.4.4 Responses of these amygdala neurons to novel stimuli which are reinforcing

As described above, some of the amygdala neurons that responded to rewarding visual stimuli also responded to some other stimuli that were not associated with reward. Wilson and Rolls (1999) discovered a possible reason for this. They showed that these neurons with reward-related responses also responded to relatively novel visual stimuli. This was shown in a serial recognition memory task, in which it was shown that these neurons responded the first and the second times that visual stimuli were shown in this task (see Fig. 4.13a). On the two presentations of each stimulus used in this task, the stimuli were thus either novel or still relatively novel. When the monkeys are given such relatively novel stimuli outside the task, they will reach out for and explore the objects, and in this respect the novel stimuli are reinforcing. Repeated presentation of the stimuli results in habituation of the neuronal response and of behavioural approach, if the stimuli are not associated with a primary reinforcer. It is thus suggested that the amygdala neurons described operate as filters which provide an output if a stimulus is associated with a positive reinforcer, or is positively reinforcing because of relative unfamiliarity, and which provide no output if a stimulus is familiar and has not been associated with a positive primary reinforcer or is associated with a negative reinforcer. The functions of this output may be to influence the interest shown in a stimulus, whether it is approached or avoided, whether an affective response occurs to it, and whether a representation of the stimulus is made or maintained via an action mediated through either the basal forebrain nucleus of Meynert or the backprojections to the cerebral cortex (Rolls 1987, 1989a, 1990b, 1992b). It is an important adaptation to the environment to explore relatively novel objects or situations, for in this way advantage due to gene inheritance can become expressed and selected for. This function appears to be implemented in the amygdala in this way. Lesions of the amygdala impair the operation of this mechanism, in that objects are approached and explored indiscriminately, relatively independently of whether they are associated with positive or negative reinforcers, or are novel or familiar.

An interesting observation on the neurons that respond to rewarding and to relatively novel visual stimuli was made in the recognition memory task used by Wilson and Rolls (1999). It was found that the neurons responded the first time a stimulus was shown, when the monkey had to use the rule 'Do not make a lick response to a stimulus the first time a stimulus is shown, otherwise aversive saline will be obtained', as well as the second time the stimulus was shown when the monkey had to apply the rule 'If a stimulus has been seen before today, lick to it to obtain glucose reward'. Thus these amygdala neurons do not code for reward value when this is based on a rule (e.g. first presentation aversive; second presentation reward), but instead code for reward value when it is decoded on the basis of previous stimulus–reinforcer associations, or when relatively novel stimuli are shown which are treated as rewarding and to be explored.

The details of the neuronal mechanisms that implement the process by which relatively novel stimuli are treated as rewarding in the amygdala are not currently known, but could be as follows. Cortical visual signals which do not show major habituation with repeated visual stimuli, as shown by recordings in the temporal cortical visual areas (see Rolls 1994a, 1996c; Rolls, Judge and Sanghera 1977) reach the amygdala. In the amygdala, neurons respond to these at first, and have the property that they gradually habituate unless the pattern-association mechanism in the amygdala detects co-occurrence of these stimuli with a primary reinforcer, in which case it strengthens the active synapses for that object, so that it continues to produce an output from amygdala neurons that responds to either rewarding or punishing visual stimuli. Neurophysiologically, the habituation condition would correspond in a pattern associator to long-term depression (LTD) of synapses with high presynaptic activity but low postsynaptic activity, that is to homosynaptic LTD (see Rolls and Treves 1998).

4.4.5 Neuronal responses in the primate amygdala to faces

Another interesting group of neurons in the amygdala responds primarily to faces (Rolls 1981b; Leonard, Rolls, Wilson and Baylis 1985). Each of these neurons responds to some but not all of a set of faces, and thus across an ensemble could convey information about the identity of the face (see Fig. 4.13b). These neurons are found especially in the basal

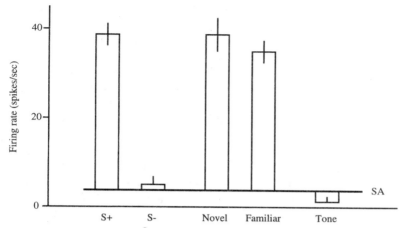

Fig. 4.13a This macaque amygdala neuron responded to the sight of a stimulus associated with food reward (S+), but not to a visual stimulus associated with aversive saline (S −) in a visual discrimination task. The same neuron responded to visual stimuli while they were relatively novel, including here on the first (Novel) and second (Familiar) presentations of new stimuli. The neuron did not respond to the tone which indicated the start of a trial. SA, spontaneous firing rate of the neuron. The mean responses and the sem to the different stimuli are shown.

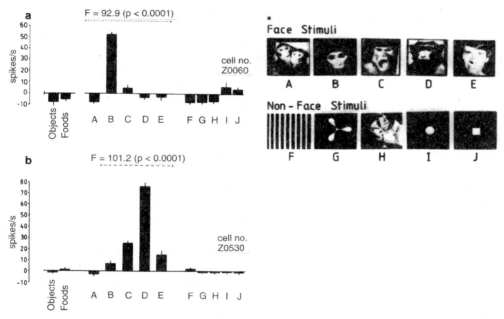

Fig. 4.13b The responses of two cells (a–b) in the amygdala to a variety of monkey and human face stimuli (A–E and K–P), and to non-face stimuli (F–J), objects, and foods. Each bar represents the mean response above baseline with the standard error calculated over 4 to 10 presentations. The F ratio for an analysis of variance calculated over the face sets indicates that the units shown range from very selective between faces (Y0809) to relatively non-selective (Z0264). Some stimuli for cells Y0801 and Y0809 produced inhibition below the spontaneous firing rate. (From Leonard, Rolls, Wilson and Baylis 1985.)

accessory nucleus of the amygdala (see Fig. 4.14; Leonard *et al.* 1985), a part of the amygdala that develops markedly in primates (Amaral *et al.* 1992). It will be of interest to investigate whether some of these amygdala face neurons respond on the basis of facial expression. Some neurons in the amygdala do respond during social interactions (Brothers and Ring 1993). It is probable that the amygdala neurons responsive to faces receive their inputs from a group of neurons in the cortex in the superior temporal sulcus which respond to faces, often on the basis of features present, such as eyes, hair, or mouth (Perrett, Rolls and Caan 1982), and consistent with this, the response latencies of the amygdala neurons tend to be longer than those of neurons in the cortex in the superior temporal sulcus (Leonard, Rolls, Wilson and Baylis 1985; Rolls 1984a). It has been suggested that this is part of a system which has evolved for the rapid and reliable identification of individuals from their faces, because of the importance of this in primate social behaviour (Rolls 1981b, 1984a, 1990b, 1992a,b,c; Perrett and Rolls 1983; Leonard, Rolls, Wilson and Baylis 1985). The part of this system in the amygdala may be particularly involved in emotional and social responses to faces. According to one possibility, such emotional and social responses would be 'looked up' by a 'key' stimulus, which consisted of the face of a particular individual (Rolls 1984a, 1987, 1990b, 1992a,b,c). Indeed, it is suggested that the tameness of the Kluver–Bucy syndrome, and the inability of amygdalectomized monkeys to interact normally in a social group (Kling and Steklis 1976; Kling and Brothers, 1992), arises because of damage to this system specialized for processing faces (Rolls 1981a,b, 1984a, 1990b, 1992a,b,c). The amygdala may allow neurons which reflect the social significance of faces to be formed using face representations received from the temporal cortical areas and information about primary reinforcers received from, for example, the somatosensory system (via the insula—Mesulam and Mufson 1982a,b), and the gustatory system (via, for example, the orbitofrontal cortex) (see Fig. 4.2).

4.4.6   Evidence from humans

The theory described above about the role of the amygdala in emotion, based largely on research in non-human primates, has been followed up by studies in humans which are producing generally consistent results. One type of evidence comes from the effects of brain damage, which though rarely restricted just to the amygdala, and almost never bilateral, does provide some consistent evidence (Aggleton 1992). For example, in some patients alterations in feeding behaviour and emotion might occur after damage to the amygdala (see Aggleton 1992; Halgren 1992). In relation to neurons in the macaque amygdala with responses selective for faces and social interactions (Leonard, Rolls, Wilson and Baylis 1985; Brothers and Ring 1993), Young *et al.* (1995, 1996) have described in patient D. R. who has bilateral damage to or disconnection of the amygdala, an impairment of face-expression matching and identification, but not of matching face identity or in discrimination. This patient is also impaired at detecting whether someone is gazing at the patient, another important social signal (Perrett *et al.* 1985). The same patient is also impaired at the auditory recognition of fear and anger (S. Scott *et al.* 1997). Adolphs *et al.* (1994) also found face expression but not face identity impairments in a patient (S. M.)

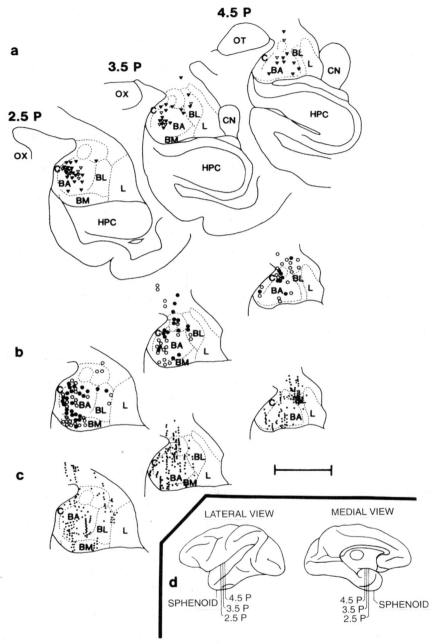

Fig. 4.14 (a) The distribution of neurons responsive to faces in the amygdala of four monkeys. The cells are plotted on three coronal sections at different distances (in mm) posterior (P) to the sphenoid (see inset). Filled triangles: cells selective for faces; open triangles: cells responding to face and hands. (b) Other responsive neurons. Closed circles: cells with other visual responses; open circles: cells responding to cues, movement, or arousal. (c) The locations of non-responsive cells. Abbreviations: BA, basal accessory nucleus of the amygdala; BL, basolateral nucleus of the amygdala; BM, basomedial nucleus of the amygdala; C, cortical nucleus of the amygdala; CN, tail of the caudate nucleus; HPC, hippocampus; L, lateral nucleus of the amygdala; OF, optic tract; OX, optic chiasm. (From Leonard, Rolls, Wilson and Baylis 1985.)

with bilateral damage to the amygdala. A similar impairment was not found in patients with unilateral amygdala damage (Adolphs *et al.* 1995). The bilateral amygdala patient S. M. was especially impaired at recognizing the face expression of fear, and also rated expressions of fear, anger, and surprise as less intense than control subjects.

For comparison, in a much more extensive series of patients it has been shown that damage to the orbitofrontal cortex can produce face expression deficits in the absence of face identification deficits, and that some patients with orbitofrontal cortex damage are impaired at the auditory identification of emotional sounds (Hornak, Rolls and Wade 1996; see Section 4.5.5). Interestingly, the visual face expression and auditory vocal expression impairments are partly dissociable in these orbitofrontal patients, indicating partially separate processing systems in the orbitofrontal cortex, and indicating that a general emotional impairment produced by these lesions is not the simple explanation of the alterations in face and voice expression processing after damage to the orbitofrontal cortex. I note that the most consistent change after orbitofrontal cortex damage in our series of patients (Rolls, Hornak, Wade and McGrath 1994; Hornak, Rolls and Wade 1996) is an alteration in face expression decoding, and that the amygdala is strongly connected to the orbitofrontal cortex.

Functional brain imaging studies have also shown activation of the amygdala by face expression. For example, Morris *et al.* (1996) found more activation of the left amygdala by face expressions of fear than of happiness in a PET study. They also reported that the activation increased as the intensity of the fear expression increased, and decreased as the intensity of the happy expression increased.

However, although in studies of the effects of amygdala damage in humans greater impairments have been reported to face expressions of fear than to some other expressions (Adolphs *et al.* 1994; S. Scott *et al.* 1997), and in functional brain imaging studies greater activation may be found to certain classes of emotion-provoking stimuli, e.g. to stimuli that provoke fear compared with those which produce happiness (Morris *et al.* 1996), it is most unlikely that the amygdala is specialized for the decoding of only certain classes of emotional stimulus, such as fear. This emphasis on fear may be related to the research in rats on the role of the amygdala in fear conditioning (LeDoux 1992, 1994, 1996). However, in contrast to that view, it is quite clear from single-neuron neurophysiological studies in non-human primates that different neurons are activated by different classes of both rewarding and punishing stimuli (Sanghera, Rolls and Roper-Hall 1979; Rolls 1992b; Ono and Nishijo 1992; Wilson and Rolls 1993, 1999) and by a wide range of different face stimuli (Leonard, Rolls, Wilson and Baylis 1985). Also, lesions of the macaque amygdala impair the learning of both stimulus–reward and stimulus–punisher associations (see above). Amygdala lesions with ibotenic acid impair the processing of reward-related stimuli, in that when the reward value of a set of foods was reduced by feeding it to satiety (i.e. sensory-specific satiety), the monkeys still chose the visual stimuli associated with the foods with which they had been satiated (Malkova, Gaffan and Murray 1997). Further, electrical stimulation of the macaque and human amygdala at some sites is rewarding and humans report pleasure from stimulation at such sites (Rolls 1975; Rolls, Burton and Mora 1980; Sem-Jacobsen 1968, 1976; Halgren 1992). Thus any differences in the magnitude of effects between different classes of emotional stimuli which appear in human functional brain imaging studies (Morris *et al.* 1996) or even after amygdala damage (Adolphs *et al.* 1994; S. Scott *et al.* 1997) should not be taken as showing that the human amygdala is involved in only some emotions, but instead may reflect differences in the efficacy of the stimuli in leading to strong emotional reactions, or differences in the magnitude per se of different emotions, making some effects more apparent for some emotions than others. Additional factors are that some expressions are much more identifiable than others. For example, we (Hornak, Rolls and Wade 1996) found that happy faces were easier to identify than other face expressions in the Ekman set, and that the orbitofrontal patients we studied were not impaired on identifying the (easy) happy face expression, but showed deficits primarily on the more difficult set of other expressions (fear, surprise, anger, sadness, etc.). Another factor in imaging studies in which the human subjects may be slightly apprehensive is that happy expressions may produce some relaxation in the situation, whereas expressions of fear may do the opposite, and this could contribute to the results found. Thus I suggest caution in interpreting human studies as showing that the amygdala (or orbitofrontal cortex) are involved only in certain emotions. It is much more likely that both are involved in emotions produced to positively as well as to negatively reinforcing stimuli. However, an interesting difference between non-human primates and humans may be found in the degree of lateralization of some types of processing related to emotions in different hemispheres evident in humans. This is discussed in Section 4.9.

4.4.7 Summary

The evidence described in Section 4.4 implicates the amygdala in the processing of a number of stimuli which are primary reinforcers, including the sight, smell, and taste of food, touch, and pain. It also receives information about potential secondary reinforcers, such as visual stimuli, including faces. Many of the deficits produced by amygdala damage are related to impairments in learning associations between stimuli and primary reinforcers, e.g. between visual or auditory stimuli and pain. The amygdala is not concerned only with aversive reinforcers, in that it receives information about food, and in that amygdala lesions impair the altered behaviour which normally occurs to foods when their reward value is reduced by feeding to satiety. The associative stimulus–reinforcer learning or conditioning in the amygdala may require NMDA receptor activation for the learning, which appears to occur by a process like long-term potentiation. We know that autonomic responses learned to conditioned stimuli can depend on outputs from the amygdala to the hypothalamus, and that the effects that learned incentives have on behaviour may involve outputs from the amygdala to the ventral striatum. We also know that there are similar neurons in the ventral striatum to some of those described in the amygdala (Williams, Rolls, Leonard and Stern 1993). All this is consistent with the hypothesis that there are neuronal networks in the amygdala that perform the required pattern association. Interestingly, there is somewhat of a gap in our knowledge here, for the microcircuitry of the amygdala has been remarkably little studied. It is known from Golgi studies (performed in young rats in which sufficiently few amygdala cells are stained that it is possible to see them individually) that there are pyramidal cells in the amygdala with large dendrites and many synapses (Millhouse and DeOlmos 1983; McDonald 1992; Millhouse 1986). What has not yet been defined is whether visual and taste inputs converge anatomically on to some cells, and whether (as might be predicted) the taste inputs are likely to be strong (e.g. large synapses close to the cell body), whereas the visual inputs are more numerous, and on a part of the dendrite with NMDA receptors. Clearly to bring our understanding fully to the network level, such evidence is required, together with further neurophysiological evidence showing the appropriate convergence at the single neuron level and evidence that the appropriate synapses on to these single neurons are modifiable by a Hebb-like rule (such as might be implemented using the NMDA receptors, see Rolls and Treves 1998), in a network of the type shown in Fig. 4.6.

At least part of the importance of the amygdala in emotion appears to be that it is involved in this type of emotional learning. However, the amygdala does not appear to provide such rapid relearning of reward-related emotional responses to stimuli as does the orbitofrontal cortex, to which we now turn. It transpires that the orbitofrontal cortex develops in primates to be very important in decoding which stimuli are primary reinforcers (e.g. taste, smell, and touch), and in rapidly learning and relearning associations of other stimuli, e.g. visual stimuli, to these primary reinforcers, as described in Section 4.5.

4.5 The orbitofrontal cortex

The prefrontal cortex is the region of cortex that receives projections from the mediodorsal nucleus of the thalamus and is situated in front of the motor and premotor cortices

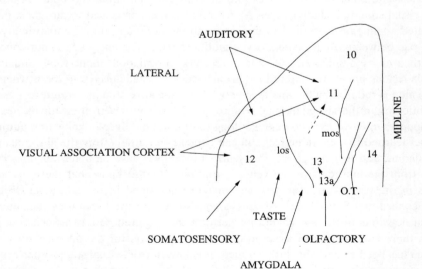

Fig. 4.15 Ventral view of the macaque orbitofrontal cortex. The midline is on the right of the diagram, and the inferior convexity is laterally, on the left. Subdivisions (after Barbas and Pandya 1989) and some afferents to the orbitofrontal cortex are shown. mos, medial orbital sulcus; los, lateral orbital sulcus.

(Areas 4 and 6) in the frontal lobe. Based on the divisions of the mediodorsal nucleus, the prefrontal cortex may be divided into three main regions (Fuster 1996). First, the magnocellular, medial, part of the mediodorsal nucleus projects to the orbital (ventral) surface of the prefrontal cortex (which includes Areas 13 and 12). It is called the orbitofrontal cortex, and is the part of the primate prefrontal cortex that appears to be primarily involved in emotion. The orbitofrontal cortex receives information from the ventral or object-processing visual stream, and taste, olfactory, and somatosensory inputs. Second, the parvocellular, lateral, part of the mediodorsal nucleus projects to the dorsolateral prefrontal cortex. This part of the prefrontal cortex receives inputs from the parietal cortex, and is involved in tasks such as spatial short-term memory tasks (see Fuster 1996; Rosenkilde 1979; Rolls and Treves 1998). Third, the pars paralamellaris (most lateral) part of the mediodorsal nucleus projects to the frontal eye fields (Area 8) in the anterior bank of the arcuate sulcus.

The orbitofrontal cortex is considered in the rest of this section. The cortex on the orbital surface of the frontal lobe includes Area 13 caudally, and Area 14 medially, and the cortex on the inferior convexity includes Area 12 caudally and Area 11 anteriorly (see Figs 4.15 and 2.20 and Carmichael and Price 1994; Petrides and Pandya 1995). This brain region is poorly developed in rodents, but well developed in primates including humans. To understand the function of this brain region in humans, the majority of the studies described were therefore performed with macaques or with humans.

4.5.1 Connections

Rolls, Yaxley and Sienkiewicz (1990) discovered a taste area in the lateral part of the orbitofrontal cortex, and showed that this was the secondary taste cortex in that it receives a major projection from the primary taste cortex (L. Baylis, Rolls and Baylis 1994). More medially, there is an olfactory area (Rolls and Baylis 1994). Anatomically, there are direct connections from the primary olfactory cortex, pyriform cortex, to area 13a of the posterior orbitofrontal cortex, which in turn has onward projections to a middle part of the orbitofrontal cortex (area 11) (Price *et al.* 1991; Morecraft *et al.* 1992; Barbas 1993; Carmichael *et al.* 1994) (see Figs 4.15 and 4.16). Visceral inputs may reach the posteromedial and lateral areas from the ventral part of the parvicellular division of the ventroposteromedial nucleus of the thalamus (VPMpc) (Carmichael and Price 1995b). Visual inputs reach the orbitofrontal cortex directly from the inferior temporal cortex, the cortex in the superior temporal sulcus, and the temporal pole (Jones and Powell 1970; Barbas 1988, 1993, 1995; Petrides and Pandya 1988; Barbas and Pandya 1989; Seltzer and Pandya 1989; Morecraft *et al.* 1992; Carmichael and Price 1995b). There are corresponding auditory inputs (Barbas 1988, 1993), and somatosensory inputs from somatosensory cortical areas 1, 2 and SII in the frontal and pericentral operculum, and from the insula (Barbas 1988; Preuss and Goldman-Rakic 1989; Carmichael and Price 1995b). The caudal orbitofrontal cortex receives strong reciprocal connections with the amygdala (e.g. Price *et al.* 1991; Carmichael and Price 1995a). The orbitofrontal cortex also receives inputs via the mediodorsal nucleus of the thalamus, pars magnocellularis, which itself receives afferents from temporal lobe structures such as the prepyriform (olfactory) cortex, amygdala and inferior temporal cortex (Nauta 1972; Krettek and Price 1974, 1977). The medial orbital

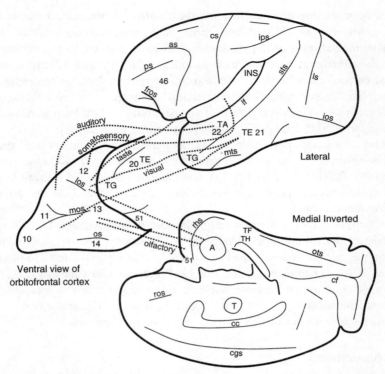

Fig. 4.16 Fig. 4.16 Schematic diagram showing some of the gustatory, olfactory, and visual pathways to the orbitofrontal cortex, and some of the outputs of the orbitofrontal cortex. The secondary taste cortex and the secondary olfactory cortex are within the orbitofrontal cortex. V1, primary visual cortex. V4, visual cortical area V4. Abbreviations: as, arcuate sulcus; cc, corpus callosum; cf., calcarine fissure; cgs, cingulate sulcus; cs, central sulcus; ls, lunate sulcus; ios, inferior occipital sulcus; mos, medial orbital sulcus; os, orbital sulcus; ots, occipito-temporal sulcus; ps, principal sulcus; rhs, rhinal sulcus; sts, superior temporal sulcus; lf, Lateral (or Sylvian) fissure (which has been opened to reveal the insula); A, amygdala; INS, insula; T, thalamus; TE (21), inferior temporal visual cortex; TA (22), superior temporal auditory association cortex; TF and TH, parahippocampal cortex; TG, temporal pole cortex; 12, 13, 11, orbitofrontal cortex; 35, perirhinal cortex; 51, olfactory (prepyriform and periamygdaloid) cortex.

areas, and parts of lateral orbital area 12, receive connections from the anterior cingulate cortex (Carmichael and Price 1995a). The medial orbitofrontal cortex receives connections from the subiculum (Carmichael and Price 1995a), which itself receives connections from the hippocampus (see Rolls and Treves 1998). The orbitofrontal cortex projects back to temporal lobe areas such as the inferior temporal cortex, and, in addition, to the entorhinal cortex (or 'gateway to the hippocampus') and cingulate cortex (Nauta 1964; Insausti *et al.* 1987). The orbitofrontal cortex also projects to the preoptic region, lateral hypothalamus and brainstem autonomic areas such as the dorsal motor nucleus of the vagus and the nucleus of the solitary tract, to the ventral tegmental area (Nauta 1964; Johnson *et al.* 1968; Van der Kooy *et al.* 1984), and to the head of the caudate nucleus (Kemp and Powell 1970). Reviews of the cytoarchitecture and connections of the or- bitofrontal cortex are provided by Petrides and Pandya (1995), Pandya (1996), Carmichael and Price (1994, 1995a,b), and Barbas (1995).

4.5.2 Effects of damage to the orbitofrontal cortex

Damage to the caudal orbitofrontal cortex in the monkey produces emotional changes. These include reduced aggression to humans and to stimuli such as a snake and a doll, a reduced tendency to reject foods such as meat (Butter, Snyder and McDonald 1970; Butter and Snyder 1972; Butter, McDonald and Snyder 1969), and a failure to display the normal preference ranking for different foods (L. Baylis and Gaffan 1991). In the human, euphoria, irresponsibility, and lack of affect can follow frontal lobe damage (see Kolb and Whishaw 1990; Damasio 1994; Eslinger and Damasio, 1985), particularly orbitofrontal damage (Rolls, Hornak, Wade and McGrath 1994a).

These changes which follow frontal-lobe damage may be related to a failure to react normally to and learn from non-reward in a number of different situations (see Fig. 2.20). This failure is evident as a tendency to respond when responses are inappropriate, e.g. no longer rewarded. In particular, macaques with lesions of the orbitofrontal cortex are impaired at tasks which involve learning about which stimuli are rewarding and which are not, and especially in altering behaviour when reinforcement contingencies change. The monkeys may respond when responses are inappropriate, e.g. no longer rewarded, or may respond to a non-rewarded stimulus. For example, monkeys with orbitofrontal damage are impaired on go/nogo task performance, in that they go on the nogo trials (Iversen and Mishkin 1970), in an object-reversal task in that they respond to the object which was formerly rewarded with food, and in extinction in that they continue to respond to an object which is no longer rewarded (Butter 1969; Jones and Mishkin 1972; Meunier, Bachevalier and Mishkin 1997). There is some evidence for dissociation of function within the orbitofrontal cortex, in that lesions to the inferior convexity produce the go/nogo and object reversal deficits, whereas damage to the caudal orbitofrontal cortex, area 13, produces the extinction deficit (Rosenkilde 1979). The visual discrimination learning deficit shown by monkeys with orbitofrontal cortex damage (Jones and Mishkin 1972; L. Baylis and Gaffan 1991), may be due to the tendency of these monkeys not to withhold responses to non-rewarded stimuli (Jones and Mishkin 1972), including foods that are not normally accepted (Butter, McDonald and Snyder 1969; L. Baylis and Gaffan 1991).

Lesions more laterally, in, for example, the inferior convexity which receives from the inferior temporal visual cortex, can influence tasks in which objects must be remembered for short periods, e.g. delayed matching to sample and delayed matching to non-sample tasks (Passingham 1975; Mishkin and Manning 1978; Kowalska *et al.* 1991), and neurons in this region may help to implement this visual object short-term memory by holding the representation active during the delay period (Rosenkilde *et al.* 1981; Wilson *et al.* 1993). Whether this inferior convexity area is specifically involved in a short-term object memory is not yet clear, and a medial part of the frontal cortex may also contribute to this function (Kowalska *et al.* 1991). It should be noted that this short-term memory system for objects (which receives inputs from the temporal lobe visual cortical areas in which objects are represented) is different from the short-term memory system in the dorsolateral part of the prefrontal cortex, which is concerned with spatial short-term memories, consistent with its inputs from the parietal cortex (see, e.g., Wilson *et al.* 1993). In any case, it is worth noting that this part of the prefrontal cortex could be involved in a function related to short-term memory for objects. This does not exclude this part of the prefrontal cortex from, in addition, being part of the more orbitofrontal system involved in visual to reinforcer association learning and reversal.

4.5.3 Neurophysiology of the orbitofrontal cortex

The hypothesis that the orbitofrontal cortex is involved in correcting behavioural responses made to stimuli previously associated with reinforcement has been investigated by making recordings from single neurons in the orbitofrontal cortex while monkeys performed these tasks known to be impaired by damage to the orbitofrontal cortex. It has been shown that some neurons respond to primary reinforcers such as taste and touch; that others respond to learned secondary reinforcers, such as the sight of a rewarded visual stimulus; and that the rapid learning of associations between previously neutral visual stimuli and primary reinforcers is reflected in the responses of orbitofrontal neurons. These types of neuron are described next.

4.5.3.1 Taste

One of the recent discoveries that has helped us to understand the functions of the orbitofrontal cortex in behaviour is that it contains a major cortical representation of taste (see Rolls 1989b, 1995a, 1997b; cf. Fig. 4.2 and Chapter 2). Given that taste can act as a primary reinforcer, that is without learning as a reward or punisher, we now have the start for a fundamental understanding of the function of the orbitofrontal cortex in stimulus–reinforcer association learning. We now know how one class of primary reinforcer reaches and is represented in the orbitofrontal cortex. A representation of primary reinforcers is essential for a system that is involved in learning associations between previously neutral stimuli and primary reinforcers, e.g. between the sight of an object, and its taste (cf. Fig. 4.6).

The representation (shown by analysing the responses of single neurons in macaques) of taste in the orbitofrontal cortex includes robust representations of the prototypical tastes sweet, salt, bitter, and sour (Rolls, Yaxley and Sienkiewicz 1990), but also separate representations of the taste of water (Rolls, Yaxley and Sienkiewicz 1990), of protein or umami as exemplified by monosodium glutamate (L. Baylis and Rolls 1991) and inosine monophosphate (Rolls, Critchley, Wakeman and Mason 1996d), and of astringency as exemplified by tannic acid (Critchley and Rolls 1996c).

The nature of the representation of taste in the orbitofrontal cortex is that the reward value of the taste is represented. The evidence for this is that the responses of orbitofrontal taste neurons are modulated by hunger (as is the reward value or palatability of a taste). In particular, it has been shown that orbitofrontal cortex taste neurons stop responding to the taste of a food with which the monkey is fed to satiety (Rolls, Sienkiewicz and Yaxley 1989b). In contrast, the representation of taste in the primary taste cortex (T. Scott, Yaxley, Sienkiewicz and Rolls 1986b; Yaxley, Rolls and Sienkiewicz 1990) is not modulated by hunger (Rolls, Scott, Sienkiewicz and Yaxley 1988; Yaxley, Rolls and Sienkiewicz 1988). Thus in the primary taste cortex, the reward value of taste is not represented, and instead the identity of the taste is represented. Additional evidence that the reward value of food is represented in the orbitofrontal cortex is that monkeys work for electrical stimulation of this brain region if they are hungry, but not if they are satiated (Mora, Avrith, Phillips and Rolls 1979). Further, neurons in the orbitofrontal cortex are activated from many brain-stimulation reward sites (Rolls, Burton and Mora 1980; Mora, Avrith and Rolls 1980). Thus there is clear evidence that it is the reward value of taste that is represented in the orbitofrontal cortex.

The secondary taste cortex is in the caudolateral part of the orbitofrontal cortex, as defined anatomically (L. Baylis, Rolls and Baylis 1994). This region projects on to other regions in the orbitofrontal cortex (L. Baylis, Rolls and Baylis 1994), and neurons with taste responses (in what can be considered as a tertiary gustatory cortical area) can be found in many regions of the orbitofrontal cortex (see Rolls, Yaxley and Sienkiewicz 1990; Rolls and Baylis 1994; Rolls, Critchley, Mason and Wakeman 1996b).

The equivalent areas in humans have been investigated using fMRI. It has been shown that there is a representation of taste not only in the insular (primary taste) cortex, but also more anteriorly in the medial part of the human orbitofrontal cortex (Rolls, Francis *et al.* 1997b; see Figs 2.21 (in the plates section) and 2.22). The orbitofrontal cortical area activated in humans by, for example, sweet taste or salt taste is distinct from the orbitofrontal cortex area activated by olfactory stimuli (see below) and by touch stimuli (see Section 4.2 and Fig. 4.5 (in the plates section)).

4.5.3.2 An olfactory representation in the orbitofrontal cortex

Takagi, Tanabe and colleagues (see Takagi 1991) described single neurons in the macaque orbitofrontal cortex that were activated by odours. A ventral frontal region has been implicated in olfactory processing in humans (Jones-Gotman and Zatorre 1988; Zatorre and Jones-Gotman 1991; Zatorre *et al.* 1992). Rolls and colleagues have analysed the rules by which orbitofrontal olfactory representations are formed and operate in primates. For 65% of neurons in the orbitofrontal olfactory areas, Critchley and Rolls (1996a) showed that the representation of the olfactory stimulus was independent of its association with taste reward (analysed in an olfactory discrimination task with taste reward). For the remaining 35% of the neurons, the odours to which a neuron responded were influenced by the taste (glucose or saline) with which the odour was associated. Thus the odour representation for 35% of orbitofrontal neurons appeared to be built by olfactory-to-taste association learning. This possibility was confirmed by reversing the taste with which an odour was associated in the reversal of an olfactory discrimination task. It was found that 73% of the sample of neurons analysed altered the way in which they responded to odour when the taste reinforcement association of the odour was reversed (Rolls, Critchley, Mason and Wakeman 1996b). (Reversal was shown by 25%, and 48% no longer discriminated after the reversal. The olfactory to taste reversal was quite slow, both neurophysiologically and behaviourally, often requiring 20–80 trials, consistent with the need for some stability of flavour representations. The relatively high proportion of neurons with modification of responsiveness by taste association in the set of neurons in this experiment was probably related to the fact that the neurons were preselected to show differential responses to the odours associated with different tastes in the olfactory discrimination task.) Thus the rule according to which the orbitofrontal olfactory representation was formed was for some neurons by association learning with taste.

To analyse the nature of the olfactory representation in the orbitofrontal cortex, Critchley and Rolls (1996b) measured the responses of olfactory neurons that responded to food while they fed the monkey to satiety. They found that the majority of orbitofrontal olfactory neurons reduced their responses to the odour of the food with which the monkey was fed to satiety. Thus for these neurons, the reward value of the odour is what is represented in the orbitofrontal cortex. We do not yet know whether this is the first stage of processing at which reward value is represented in the olfactory system (although in rodents the influence of reward–association learning appears to be present in some neurons in the pyriform cortex—Schoenbaum and Eichenbaum 1995).

Although individual neurons do not encode large amounts of information about which of 7–9 odours has been presented, we have shown that the information does increase linearly with the number of neurons in the sample (Rolls, Critchley and Treves 1996c). This ensemble encoding does result in useful amounts of information about which odour has been presented being provided by orbitofrontal olfactory neurons.

The equivalent areas in humans have been investigated in PET and fMRI studies. It has been shown that there is a representation of olfactory stimuli not only in the pyriform (primary olfactory) cortex, but also more anteriorly in the right human orbitofrontal cortex (Jones-Gotman and Zatorre 1988; Zatorre and Jones-Gotman 1991; Zatorre *et al*. 1992; Rolls, Francis *et al*. 1997b; see Figs 2.21 (in plates section) and 2.22).

4.5.3.3 Convergence of taste and olfactory inputs in the orbitofrontal cortex: the representation of flavour

In the more medial and anterior parts of the orbitofrontal cortex, not only unimodal taste neurons, but also unimodal olfactory neurons are found. In addition some single neurons respond to both gustatory and olfactory stimuli, often with correspondence between the two modalities (Rolls and Baylis 1994; cf. Fig. 4.2). It is probably here in the orbitofrontal cortex of primates that these two modalities converge to produce the representation of flavour (Rolls and Baylis 1994). Further evidence will be described below that indicates that these representations are built by olfactory–gustatory association learning, an example of stimulus–reinforcer association learning.

4.5.3.4 Visual inputs to the orbitofrontal cortex, and visual stimulus–reinforcer association learning and reversal

We have been able to show that there is a major visual input to many neurons in the orbitofrontal cortex, and that what is represented by these neurons is in many cases the reinforcement association of visual stimuli. The visual input is from the ventral, temporal lobe, visual stream concerned with 'what' object is being seen, in that orbitofrontal visual neurons frequently respond differentially to objects or images (but depending on their reward association) (Thorpe, Rolls and Maddison 1983; Rolls, Critchley, Mason and

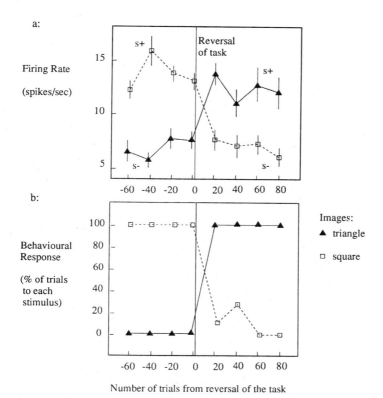

a:

b:

Images:
▲ triangle
□ square

Number of trials from reversal of the task

Fig. 4.17 Orbitofrontal cortex: visual discrimination reversal. The activity of an orbitofrontal visual neuron during performance of a visual discrimination task and its reversal. The stimuli were a triangle and a square presented on a video monitor. (a) Each point represents the mean poststimulus activity in a 500-ms period of the neuron based on approximately 10 trials of the different visual stimuli. The standard errors of these responses are shown. After 60 trials of the task the reward associations of the visual stimuli were reversed. (+ indicates that a lick response to that visual stimulus produces fruit juice reward; – indicates that a lick response to that visual stimulus results in a small drop of aversive tasting saline). This neuron reversed its responses to the visual stimuli following the task reversal. (b) The behavioural response of the monkey to the task. It is shown that the monkey performs well, in that he rapidly learns to lick only to the visual stimulus associated with fruit juice reward. (Reprinted from Rolls, Critchley, Mason and Wakeman 1996b.)

Wakeman 1996b). The primary reinforcer that has been used is taste. The fact that these neurons represent the reinforcement associations of visual stimuli has been shown to be the case in formal investigations of the activity of orbitofrontal cortex visual neurons, which in many cases reverse their responses to visual stimuli when the taste with which the visual stimulus is associated is reversed by the experimenter (Thorpe, Rolls and Maddison 1983; Rolls *et al.* 1996b). An example of the responses of an orbitofrontal cortex cell that reversed the stimulus to which it responded during reward-reversal is shown in Fig. 4.17. This reversal by orbitofrontal visual neurons can be very fast, in as little as one trial, that is a few seconds (see for example Fig. 4.18).

These cells thus reflect the information about which stimulus to make behavioural responses to during reversals of visual discrimination tasks. If a reversal occurs, then the

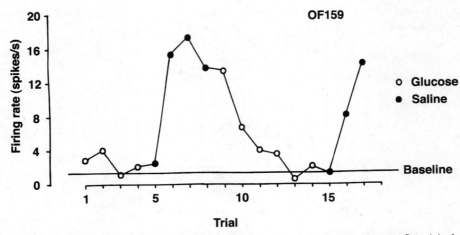

Fig. 4.18 Orbitofrontal cortex: one-trial visual discrimination reversal by a neuron. On trials 1–5, no response of the neuron occurred to the sight of a 2-ml syringe from which the monkey had been given orally glucose solution to drink on the previous trial. On trials 6–9, the neuron responded to the sight of the same syringe from which he had been given aversive hypertonic saline to drink on the previous trial. Two more reversals (trials 10–15, and 16–17) were performed. The reversal of the neuron's response when the significance of the same visual stimulus was reversed shows that the responses of the neuron only occurred to the sight of the visual stimulus when it was associated with a positively reinforcing and not with a negatively reinforcing taste. Moreover, it is shown that the neuronal reversal took only one trial. (Reprinted from Thorpe, Rolls and Maddison 1983.)

taste cells provide the information that an unexpected taste reinforcer has been obtained, another group of cells shows a vigorous discharge which could signal that reversal is in progress, and the visual cells with reinforcement association-related responses reverse the stimulus to which they are responsive. These neurophysiological changes take place rapidly, in as little as 5 s, and are presumed to be part of the neuronal learning mechanism that enables primates to alter their knowledge of the reinforcement association of visual stimuli so rapidly. This capacity is important whenever behaviour must be corrected when expected reinforcers are not obtained, in, for example, feeding, emotional, and social situations (see Rolls 1996b).

This reversal learning found in orbitofrontal cortex neurons probably occurs in the orbitofrontal cortex, for it does not occur one synapse earlier in the visual inferior temporal cortex (Rolls, Judge and Sanghera 1977) and it is in the orbitofrontal cortex that there is convergence of visual and taste pathways on to the same neurons (Thorpe, Rolls and Maddison 1983; Rolls, Critchley, Mason and Wakeman 1996b). The probable mechanism for this learning is Hebbian modification of synapses conveying visual input on to taste-responsive neurons, implementing a pattern-association network (Rolls and Treves 1998).

In addition to these neurons that encode the reward-association of visual stimuli, other neurons (3.5%) in the orbitofrontal cortex detect different types of non-reward (Thorpe, Rolls and Maddison 1983). For example, some neurons responded in extinction, immediately after a lick had been made to a visual stimulus which had previously been associated with fruit juice reward, and other neurons responded in a reversal task, immediately after the monkey had responded to the previously rewarded visual stimulus, but had obtained punishment rather than reward (see example in Fig. 4.19). Different populations of such neurons respond to other types of non-reward, including the removal of a formerly approaching taste reward, and the termination of a taste reward (Thorpe, Rolls and Maddison 1983) (see Table 4.1). These neurons did not respond simply as a function of arousal. The presence of these neurons is fully consistent with the hypothesis that they are part of the mechanism by which the orbitofrontal cortex enables very rapid reversal of behaviour by stimulus–reinforcement association relearning when the association of stimuli with reinforcers is altered or reversed (see Rolls 1986a, 1990b). The fact that the non-reward neurons respond to different types of non-reward (e.g. some to the noise of a switch which indicated that extinction of free licking for fruit juice had occurred, and others to the first presentation of a visual stimulus that was not followed by reward in a visual discrimination task) potentially enable context-specific extinction or reversal to occur. (For example, the fact that fruit juice is no longer available from a lick tube does not necessarily mean that a visual discrimination task will be operating without reward.) This information appears to be necessary for primates to rapidly alter behavioural responses when reinforcement contingencies are changed, as shown by the effects of damage to the orbitofrontal cortex described above.

It is interesting to note the proportions of different types of neuron recorded in the orbitofrontal cortex in relation to what might or might not be seen in a human brain imaging study. The proportions of different types of neuron in the study by Thorpe, Rolls and Maddison (1983) are shown in Table 4.2. It is seen that only a relatively small percentage convey information about, for example, which of two visual stimuli is currently reward-associated in a visual discrimination task. An even smaller proportion (3.5%) responds in relation to non-reward, and in any particular non-reward task, the proportion is very small, that is just a fraction of the 3.5%. The implication is that an imaging study might not reveal really what is happening in a brain structure such as the orbitofrontal cortex where quite small proportions of neurons respond to any particular condition; and, especially, one would need to be very careful not to place much weight on a failure to find activation in a particular task, as the proportion of neurons responding may be small, and the time period for which they respond may be small too. For example, non-reward neurons typically respond for 2–8 s on the first two non-reward trials of extinction or reversal (Thorpe, Rolls and Maddison 1983).

Further evidence on other types of stimulus–reinforcer association learning in which neurons in the orbitofrontal cortex are involved is starting to become available. One such example comes from learning associations between olfactory stimuli and tastes. It has been shown that some neurons in the orbitofrontal cortex respond to taste and to olfactory stimuli (Rolls and Baylis 1994). It is probably here in the orbitofrontal cortex that the representation of flavour in primates is built. To investigate whether these bimodal cells are built by olfactory-to-taste association learning, we measured the responses of these olfactory cells during olfactory-to-taste discrimination reversal (Rolls, Critchley, Mason and Wakeman 1996b). We found that some of these cells did reverse (see, for example, Fig. 4.20), others during reversal stopped discriminating between the odours, while others still did not reverse (see Table 4.3). When reversal did occur, it was quite

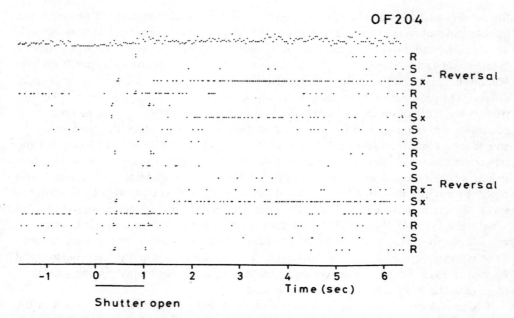

Fig. 4.19 Responses of an orbitofrontal cortex neuron that responded only when the monkey licked to a visual stimulus during reversal, expecting to obtain fruit juice reward, but actually obtaining the taste of aversive saline because it was the first trial of reversal. Each single dot represents an action potential; each vertically arranged double dot represents a lick response. The visual stimulus was shown at time 0 for 1 s. The neuron did not respond on most reward (R) or saline (S) trials, but did respond on the trials marked x, which were the first trials after a reversal of the visual discrimination on which the monkey licked to obtain reward, but actually obtained saline because the task had been reversed. (Reprinted from Thorpe, Rolls and Maddison 1983.)

slow, often needing 20–50 trials. This evidence thus suggests that although there is some pattern-association learning between olfactory stimuli and taste implemented in the orbitofrontal cortex, the mechanism involves quite slow learning, perhaps because in general it is important to maintain rather stable representations of flavours. Moreover, olfactory-to-taste association learning occurs for only some of the olfactory neurons. The olfactory neurons which do not reverse may be carrying information which is in some cases independent of reinforcement association (i.e. is about olfactory identity). In other cases, the olfactory representation in the orbitofrontal cortex may reflect associations of odours with other primary reinforcers (for example whether sickness has occurred in association with some smells), or may reflect primary reinforcement value provided by some olfactory stimuli. (For example, the smell of flowers may be innately pleasant and attractive and some other odours may be innately unpleasant—see Chapter 10.) In this situation, the olfactory input to some orbitofrontal cortex neurons may represent an unconditioned stimulus input with which other (for example visual) inputs may become associated. It is likely that auditory stimuli can be associated with primary reinforcers in the orbitofrontal cortex, though there is less direct evidence of this yet.

4.5.3.5 A representation of faces in the orbitofrontal cortex

Another type of information represented in the orbitofrontal cortex is information about

Table 4.1
Numbers of orbitofrontal cortex neurons responding in different types of extinction or reversal (after Thorpe et al. 1983)

Neuron number	1	2	3	4	5	6	7	8	9	10	11	12	13	14	15	16	17	18
Visual discrimination: Reversal	1	0	1	0	0	1	1	0						0				
Visual discrimination: Extinction	1																	
Ad lib licking: Reversal	1	1																
Ad lib licking: Extinction	0	0																
Taste of saline				0	0	0	0	0	1	0	0	0	0	0	0	0	0	0
Removal of reward			0	1	1	0	1	1	1	1	1	1	1	1	1	1	1	1
Visual arousal	1	1	0	0	0	1	0	1	0	0	0	0	0	1	1	0	0	0

The table shows the tasks (rows) in which individual orbitofrontal neurons responded (1), did not respond (0), or were not tested (blank).

faces. There is a population of orbitofrontal face-selective neurons which respond in many ways similarly to those in the temporal cortical visual areas (see Rolls 1984a, 1992a, 1994a, 1995b, 1996b, 1996d for a description of their properties). The orbitofrontal face-responsive neurons, first observed by Thorpe, Rolls and Maddison (1983), then by Rolls, Critchley and Browning (1998 in preparation), tend to respond with longer latencies than temporal lobe neurons (140–200 ms typically, compared with 80–100 ms); they also convey information about which face is being seen, by having different responses to different faces (see Fig. 4.21); and are typically rather harder to activate strongly than temporal cortical face-selective neurons, in that many of them respond much better to real faces than to two-dimensional images of faces on a video monitor (cf. Rolls and Baylis 1986). Some of the orbitofrontal face-selective neurons are responsive to face gesture or movement. The findings are consistent with the likelihood that these neurons are activated via the inputs from the temporal cortical visual areas in which face-selective neurons are found (see Fig. 4.2). The significance of the neurons is likely to be related to the fact that faces convey information that is important in social reinforcement, both by conveying face expression (cf. Hasselmo, Rolls and Baylis 1989a), which can indicate reinforcement, and by encoding information about which individual is present, also important in evaluating and utilizing reinforcing inputs in social situations.

4.5.4 A neurophysiological basis for stimulus–reinforcer association learning and reversal in the orbitofrontal cortex

The neurophysiological and lesion evidence described suggests that one function implemented by the orbitofrontal cortex is rapid stimulus–reinforcer association learning, and the correction of these associations when reinforcement contingencies in the environment change. To implement this, the orbitofrontal cortex has the necessary representation of primary reinforcers, such as taste, as described above, but also somatosensory inputs (see Sections 2.4.2 and 4.2). It also receives information about objects, e.g. visual information, and can associate this very rapidly at the neuronal level with primary reinforcers such as taste, and reverse these associations. Another type of stimulus which can be conditioned in this way in the orbitofrontal cortex is olfactory, although here the learning is slower. It is likely that auditory stimuli can be associated with primary reinforcers in the orbitofrontal cortex, though there is less direct evidence of this yet.

The orbitofrontal cortex neurons which detect non-reward in a context-specific manner are likely to be used in behavioural extinction and reversal. Such non-reward neurons may help behaviour in situations in which stimulus-reinforcer associations must be disconnected, not only by helping to reset the reinforcement association of neurons in the orbitofrontal cortex, but also by sending a signal to the striatum which could be routed by the striatum to produce appropriate behaviours for non-reward (Rolls and Johnstone 1992; Williams, Rolls, Leonard and Stern 1993; Rolls 1994b). Indeed, it is via this route, the striatal, that the orbitofrontal cortex may directly influence behaviour when the orbitofrontal cortex is decoding reinforcement contingencies in the environment, and is altering behaviour in response to altering reinforcement contingencies. Some of the evidence for this is that neurons which reflect these orbitofrontal neuronal responses are

Table 4.2
Proportion of different types of neuron recorded in the macaque orbitofrontal
cortex during sensory testing and visual discrimination reversal and related tasks.
(After Thorpe, Rolls and Maddison 1983)

Sensory testing:

Visual, non-selective	10.7%
Visual, selective (i.e. responding to some objects or images)	13.2%
Visual, food-selective	5.3%
Visual, aversive objects	3.2%
Taste	7.3%
Visual and taste	2.6%
Removal of a food reward	6.3%
Extinction of ad lib licking for juice reward	7.5%

Visual discrimination reversal task:

Visual, reversing in the visual discrimination task	5.3%
Visual, conditional discrimination in the visual discrimination task	2.5%
Visual, stimulus-related (not reversing) in the visual discrimination task	0.8%
Non-reward in the visual discrimination task	0.9%
Auditory tone cue signalling the start of a trial of the visual discrimination task	15.1%

The number of neurons analysed was 463.
Being categorized as responding in the visual discrimination task, rows 4–6, was not exclusive for being categorized in the sensory testing.
The visual neurons with conditional discrimination in the visual discrimination responded, for example, to a green discriminative stimulus when it signified reward and not to the blue stimulus when it signified aversive saline; but did not respond to either stimulus when the visual discrimination task was reversed.

found in the ventral part of the head of the caudate nucleus and the ventral striatum, which receive from the orbitofrontal cortex (Rolls, Thorpe and Maddison 1983b; Williams, Rolls, Leonard and Stern 1993); and lesions of the ventral part of the head of the caudate nucleus impair visual discrimination reversal (Divac *et al.* 1967) (see further Chapter 6).

Decoding the reinforcement value of stimuli, which involves for previously neutral (e.g. visual) stimuli learning their association with a primary reinforcer, often rapidly, and which may involve not only rapid learning but also rapid relearning and alteration of responses when reinforcement contingencies change, is then a function proposed for the orbitofrontal cortex. This way of producing behavioural responses would be important in, for example, motivational and emotional behaviour. It would be important in motivational behaviour such as feeding and drinking by enabling primates to learn rapidly about the food reinforcement to be expected from visual stimuli (see Rolls 1994c). This is important, for primates frequently eat more than 100 varieties of food; vision by visual–taste association learning can be used to identify when foods are ripe; and during the course of a meal, the pleasantness of the sight of a food eaten in the meal decreases in a sensory-specific way (Rolls, Thorpe and Maddison 1983a), a function that is probably implemented by the sensory-specific satiety-related responses of orbitofrontal visual neurons (Critchley and Rolls 1996b).

With regard to emotional behaviour, decoding and rapidly readjusting the reinforcement value of visual signals is likely to be crucial, for emotions can be described as responses elicited by reinforcing signals (Rolls 1986a,b, 1990b, 1995b; see Chapter 3). The

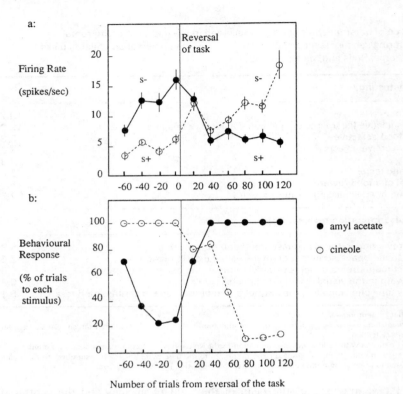

Fig. 4.20 Orbitofrontal cortex: olfactory to taste association reversal. (a) The activity of a single orbitofrontal olfactory neuron during the performance of a two-odour olfactory discrimination task and its
reversal is shown. Each point represents the mean poststimulus activity of the neuron in a 500-ms period
on approximately 10 trials of the different odourants. The standard errors of these responses are shown.
The odourants were amyl acetate (closed circle) (initially S−) and cineole (o) (initially S+). After 80 trials of
the task the reward associations of the stimuli were reversed. This neuron reversed its responses to the
odourants following the task reversal. (b) The behavioural responses of the monkey during the performance of the olfactory discrimination task. The number of lick responses to each odourant is plotted as a
percentage of the number of trials to that odourant in a block of 20 trials of the task. (Reprinted from Rolls,
Critchley, Mason and Wakeman 1996b.)

ability to perform this learning very rapidly is probably very important in social situations
in primates, in which reinforcing stimuli are continually being exchanged, and the
reinforcement value of these must be continually updated (relearned), based on the actual
reinforcers received and given. Although the operation of reinforcers such as taste, smell,
and faces are best understood in terms of orbitofrontal cortex operation, there are tactile
inputs that are likely to be concerned with reward evaluation, and in humans the rewards
processed in the orbitofrontal cortex include quite general rewards such as working for
'points', as will be described shortly.

Although the amygdala is concerned with some of the same functions as the orbitofrontal cortex, and receives similar inputs (see Figs 4.2, 4.7, and 4.16), there is evidence
that it may function less effectively in the very rapid learning and reversal of stimulus–
reinforcer associations, as indicated by the greater difficulty in obtaining reversal from

amygdala neurons (see, e.g., Rolls 1992b), and by the greater effect of orbitofrontal lesions in leading to continuing behavioural responses to previously rewarded stimuli (Jones and Mishkin 1972). In primates the necessity for very rapid stimulus–reinforcement re-evaluation, and the development of powerful cortical learning systems may result in the orbitofrontal cortex effectively taking over this aspect of amygdala functions (see Rolls 1992b).

The details of the neuronal network architecture which underlies orbitofrontal cortex reversal learning have not been fully analyzed yet, but are presumably as shown in Fig. 4.6. It is likely that NMDA receptors help to implement the modifiability of the visual inputs on to taste neurons (see Appendix, and Rolls and Treves 1998). This could be tested by using NMDA-receptor blockers applied locally to individual neurons with visual responses in the orbitofrontal cortex during visual discrimination reversal, or by perfusion of the orbitofrontal cortex with an NMDA-receptor blocker to investigate whether this interferes with behavioural visual discrimination reversal. Presumably the process during reversal would be as follows. Consider a neuron with unconditioned responses to taste in the orbitofrontal cortex. When a particular visual stimulus, say a triangle, was associated with the taste of glucose, the active synaptic connections for this visual (conditioned) stimulus would have shown long-term potentiation (LTP, a measure of synaptic strengthening, see Appendix) on to the taste neuron, which would respond to the sight of the triangle. During reversal, the same visual stimulus, the triangle, would again activate the same synaptic afferents to the neuron, but that neuron would be inactive when the taste of saline was given. Active presynaptic inputs and little postsynaptic activation is the condition for homosynaptic long-term depression (see Fig. A.1.4), which would then occur, resulting in a decline of the response of the neuron to the triangle. At the same time, visual presentation of a square would now be associated with the taste of glucose, which would activate the postsynaptic neuron, leading now to long-term potentiation of afferents on to that neuron made active by the sight of the square. The difference predicted for this system from that in the amygdala is that the orbitofrontal associativity would be more rapidly modifiable (in one trial) than that in the amygdala (which might take very many trials). Indeed, the cortical neuronal reversal mechanism in the orbitofrontal cortex may be effectively a fast version of what is implemented in the amygdala, that has evolved particularly to enable rapid updating by received reinforcers in social and other situations in primates. This hypothesis, that the orbitofrontal cortex, as a rapid learning mechanism, effectively provides an additional route for some of the functions performed by the amygdala, and is very important when this stimulus–reinforcer learning must be rapidly readjusted, has been developed elsewhere (Rolls 1990c, 1992a, 1996b).

Although the mechanism has been described so far for visual-to-taste association learning, this is because neurophysiological experiments on this are most direct. It is likely, given the evidence from the effects of lesions, that taste is only one type of primary reinforcer about which such learning occurs in the orbitofrontal cortex, and is likely to be an example of a much more general type of stimulus–reinforcer learning system. Some of the evidence for this is that humans with orbitofrontal cortex damage are impaired at visual discrimination reversal when working for a reward that consists of points (Rolls, Hornak, Wade and McGrath 1994a; Rolls 1996b). Moreover, as described above, there is

Table 4.3
Proportion of neurons in the primate orbitofrontal cortex showing reversal,
or extinction (ceasing to discriminate after the reversal), or no change of responses, during
visual or olfactory discrimination reversal (from Rolls, Critchley, Mason and Wakeman 1996b)

	Olfactory cells		Visual cells	
	Number	%	Number	%
Reversal	7	25.0	12	70.6
Extinction	12	42.9	4	23.5
No change	9	32.1	1	5.9
Total	28	100	17	100

now evidence that the representation of the affective aspects of touch is represented in the human orbitofrontal cortex (Rolls, Francis *et al.* 1997a), and learning about what stimuli are associated with this class of primary reinforcer is also likely to be an important aspect of the stimulus–reinforcement association learning performed by the orbitofrontal cortex.

4.5.5   The human orbitofrontal cortex and connected regions including the cingulate cortex[2]
4.5.5.1   The human orbitofrontal cortex

It is of interest that a number of the symptoms of frontal lobe damage in humans appear to be related to this type of function, of altering behaviour when stimulus–reinforcement associations alter, as described next. Thus, humans with frontal lobe damage can show impairments in a number of tasks in which an alteration of behavioural strategy is required in response to a change in environmental reinforcement contingencies (see Goodglass and Kaplan 1979; Jouandet and Gazzaniga 1979; Kolb and Whishaw 1990). For example, Milner (1963) showed that in the Wisconsin card sorting task (in which cards are to be sorted according to the colour, shape, or number of items on each card depending on whether the examiner says 'right' or 'wrong' to each placement) frontal patients either had difficulty in determining the first sorting principle, or in shifting to a second principle when required to. Also, in stylus mazes frontal patients have difficulty in changing direction when a sound indicates that the correct path has been left (see Milner 1982). It is of interest that, in both types of test, frontal patients may be able to verbalize the correct rules yet may be unable to correct their behavioural sets or strategies appropriately. Some of the personality changes that can follow frontal lobe damage may be related to a similar

---

[2] According to Papez's (1937) theory of emotion, a brain circuit including the loop hippocampus via fornix to mammillary bodies to anterior thalamic nuclei to cingulate and back via the cingulum bundle to the retrosplenial (posterior) hippocampus was involved in emotion. Part of the evidence came from rabid dogs, in which neuropathology was found (among other places) in the mammillary bodies. However, the hippocampal part of that circuit does not appear to be involved in emotion, in that anterograde amnesia with an episodic memory deficit and no emotional change follows hippocampo–fornical system damage in humans (Squire 1992; Squire and Knowlton 1995; D. Gaffan and Gaffan 1991; see Rolls and Treves 1998); and in that section of the fornix or hippocampal lesions in monkeys do not produce an impairment in stimulus–reinforcer association learning (Jones and Mishkin 1972; D. Gaffan *et al.* 1984).

type of dysfunction. For example, the euphoria, irresponsibility, lack of affect, and lack of concern for the present or future which can follow frontal lobe damage (see Hecaen and Albert 1978) may also be related to a dysfunction in altering behaviour appropriately in response to a change in reinforcement contingencies. Indeed, in so far as the orbitofrontal cortex is involved in the disconnection of stimulus–reinforcement associations, and such associations are important in learned emotional responses (see above), then it follows that the orbitofrontal cortex is involved in emotional responses by correcting stimulus–reinforcement associations when they become inappropriate.

We return to this issue in the following paragraph, but should at this stage remember the evidence, much of it difficult to interpret (see Valenstein 1974), from the prefrontal lobotomies or leucotomies (cutting white matter) performed in humans, in which the surgery was often intended to damage or disconnect parts of the ventral prefrontal cortex or anterior cingulate cortex. The history of these interventions is that during an investigation of the effects of frontal lobe lesions on delayed response, i.e. short-term memory, tasks, Jacobsen (1936) noted that one of his animals became calmer and showed less frustration when reward was not given after the operation. (A delayed response deficit follows damage to the dorsolateral prefrontal cortex in the monkey—Goldman et al. 1971, see Rolls and Treves 1998—with which we are not concerned here.) Hearing of this emotional change, Moniz, a neurosurgeon, argued that anxiety, irrational fears, and emotional hyperexcitability in humans might be treated by damage to the frontal lobes. He operated on twenty patients and published an enthusiastic report of his findings (Moniz 1936; Fulton 1951). This rapidly led to the widespread use of this surgical procedure, and more than 20 000 patients were subjected to prefrontal 'lobotomies' or 'leucotomies' of varying extent during the next 15 years. Although irrational anxiety or emotional outbursts were sometimes controlled, intellectual deficits and other side-effects were often apparent (Rylander 1948; Valenstein 1974). Thus these operations have been essentially discontinued. A lesson is that very careful and full assessment and follow-up of patients should be performed when a new neurosurgical procedure is considered, before it is ever considered for widespread use. In relation to pain, patients who underwent a frontal lobotomy sometimes reported that after the operation they still had pain but that it no longer bothered them (Freeman and Watts 1950; Melzack and Wall 1996).

The hypotheses about the role of the orbitofrontal cortex in the rapid alteration of stimulus–reinforcement associations, and the functions more generally of the orbitofrontal cortex in human behaviour, have been investigated in recent studies in humans with damage to the ventral parts of the frontal lobe. (The description ventral is given to indicate that there was pathology in the orbitofrontal or related parts of the frontal lobe, and not in the more dorso–lateral parts of the frontal lobe.) A task which was directed at assessing the rapid alteration of stimulus–reinforcement associations was used, because the findings above indicate that the orbitofrontal cortex is involved in this type of learning. This was used instead of the Wisconsin card sorting task, which requires patients to shift from category (or dimension) to category, e.g. from colour to shape. The task used was visual discrimination reversal, in which patients could learn to obtain points by touching one stimulus when it appeared on a video monitor, but had to withhold a response when a different visual stimulus appeared, otherwise a point was lost. After the subjects had

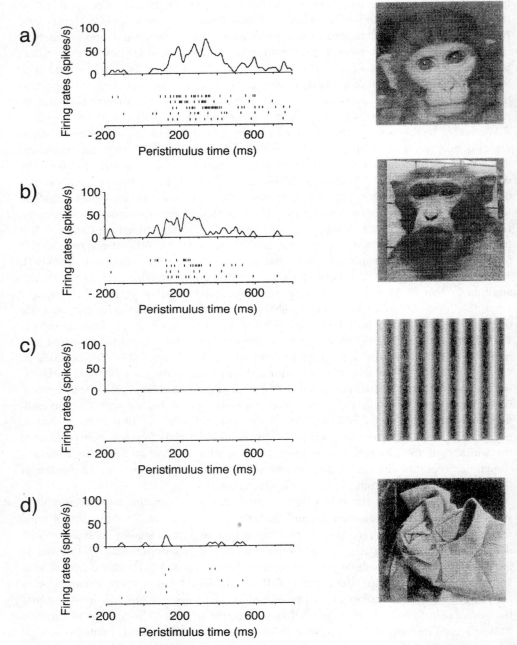

Fig. 4.21 Orbitofrontal cortex face-selective neuron as found in macaques. Peristimulus rastergrams and time histograms are shown. Each trial is a row in the rastergram. Several trials for each stimulus are shown. The ordinate is in spikes s^{-1}. The neuron responded best to face (a), also responded, though less to face (b), had different responses to other faces (not shown), and did not respond to non-face stimuli (e.g. (c) and (d)). The stimulus appeared at time 0 on a video monitor. (From Rolls, Critchley and Browning, in preparation.)

acquired the visual discrimination, the reinforcement contingencies unexpectedly reversed. The patients with ventral frontal lesions made more errors in the reversal (or in a similar extinction) task, and completed fewer reversals, than control patients with damage elsewhere in the frontal lobes or in other brain regions (Rolls, Hornak, Wade and McGrath 1994a) (see Fig. 4.22). The impairment correlated highly with the socially inappropriate or disinhibited behaviour of the patients, and also with their subjective evaluation of the changes in their emotional state since the brain damage. The patients were not impaired at other types of memory task, such as paired associate learning. The findings are being extended in current research by Rolls and Hornak in which visual discrimination acquisition and reversal are also found to be impaired in a visual discrimination task in which two stimuli are always present on the video monitor and the patient obtains points by touching the correct stimulus, and loses points by touching the incorrect stimulus. It is of interest that the patients can often verbalize the correct response, yet commit the incorrect action. This is consistent with the hypothesis that the orbitofrontal cortex is normally involved in executing behaviour when the behaviour is performed by evaluating the reinforcement associations of environmental stimuli (see below). The orbitofrontal cortex seems to be involved in this in both humans and non-human primates, when the learning must be performed rapidly, in, for example, acquisition, and during reversal.

An idea of how such stimulus–reinforcer learning may play an important role in normal human behaviour, and may be related to the behavioural changes seen clinically in these patients with ventral frontal lobe damage, can be provided by summarizing the behavioural ratings given by the carers of these patients. The patients were rated high on at least some of the following: disinhibition or socially inappropriate behaviour; violence, verbal abusiveness; lack of initiative; misinterpretation of other people's behaviour; anger or irritability; and lack of concern for their own condition (Rolls *et al.* 1994a). Such behavioural changes correlated with the stimulus–reinforcer reversal and extinction learning impairment (Rolls *et al.* 1994a). The suggestion thus is that the insensitivity to reinforcement changes in the learning task may be at least part of what produces the changes in behaviour found in these patients with ventral frontal lobe damage. The more general impact on the behaviour of these patients is that their irresponsibility tended to affect their everyday lives. For example, if such patients had received their brain damage in a road traffic accident, and compensation had been awarded, the patients often tended to spend their money without appropriate concern for the future, sometimes, for example, buying a very expensive car. Such patients often find it difficult to invest in relationships too, and are sometimes described by their family as having changed personalities, in that they care less about a wide range of factors than before the brain damage. The suggestion that follows from this is that the orbitofrontal cortex may normally be involved in much social behaviour, and the ability to respond rapidly and appropriately to social reinforcers is, of course, an important aspect of primate social behaviour. When Goleman (1996) writes about emotional intelligence, the functions being performed may be those that we are now discussing, and also those concerned with face-expression decoding which are described below. Bechara and colleagues also have findings which are consistent with these in patients with frontal lobe damage when they perform a gambling task (Bechara *et al.* 1994, 1996, 1997; see also Damasio 1994). The patients could choose cards from two

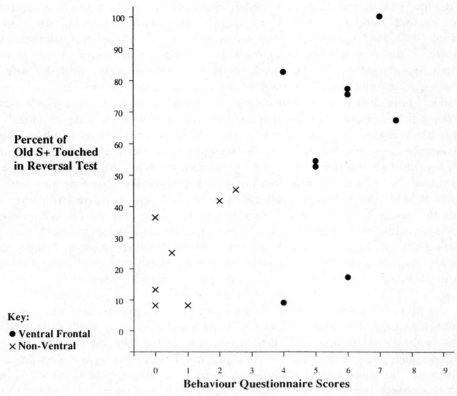

Fig. 4.22 Visual discrimination reversal performance in humans with damage to the ventral part of the frontal lobe. The task was to touch the screen when one image, the S+, was shown in order to obtain a point; and to refrain from touching the screen when a different visual stimulus, the S−, was shown in order to obtain a point. The scattergraph shows that during the reversal the group with ventral damage were more likely to touch the previously rewarded stimulus (Old S+), and that this was related to the score on a Behaviour Questionnaire. Each point represents one patient in the ventral frontal group or in a control group. The Behaviour Questionnaire rating reflected high ratings on at least some of the following: disinhibited or socially inappropriate behaviour; misinterpretation of other people's moods; impulsiveness; unconcern about or underestimation of the seriousness of his condition; and lack of initiative. (From Rolls, Hornak, Rolls and McGrath 1994.)

piles. The patients with frontal damage were more likely to choose cards from a pile which did give rewards with a reasonable probability, but also had occasional very heavy penalties resulting in lower net gains than choices from the other pile. In this sense, the patients were not affected by the negative consequences of their actions: they did not switch from the pile of cards which was providing significant rewards even when large punishments were incurred.

To investigate the possible significance of face-related inputs to orbitofrontal visual neurons described above, we also tested the responses of these patients to faces. We included tests of face (and also voice) expression decoding, because these are ways in which the reinforcing quality of individuals is often indicated. Impairments in the identification of facial and vocal emotional expression were demonstrated in a group of patients with ventral frontal lobe damage who had socially inappropriate behaviour (Hornak, Rolls and Wade 1996) (see Fig. 4.23). The expression identification impairments could occur independently of perceptual impairments in facial recognition, voice discrimination, or environmental sound recognition. The face and voice expression problems did not necessarily occur together in the same patients, providing an indication of separate processing. Poor performance on both expression tests was correlated with the degree of alteration of emotional experience reported by the patients. There was also a strong positive correlation between the degree of altered emotional experience and the severity of the behavioural problems (e.g. disinhibition) found in these patients. A comparison group of patients with brain damage outside the ventral frontal lobe region, without these behavioural problems, was unimpaired on the face expression identification test, was significantly less impaired at vocal expression identification, and reported little subjective emotional change (Hornak, Rolls and Wade1996). In current studies, these findings are being extended, and it is being found that patients with face expression decoding problems do not necessarily have impairments at visual discrimination reversal, and vice versa. This is consistent with some topography in the orbitofrontal cortex (see, e.g., Rolls and Baylis 1994).

To elucidate the role of the human orbitofrontal cortex in emotion further, Rolls, Francis *et al.* (1997a) performed the investigation described in Section 4.2 to determine where the pleasant affective component of touch is represented in the brain. Touch is a primary reinforcer that can produce pleasure. They found with functional magnetic resonance imaging (fMRI) that a weak but very pleasant touch of the hand with velvet produced much stronger activation of the orbitofrontal cortex than a more intense but affectively neutral touch of the hand with wood. In contrast, the affectively neutral but more intense touch produced more activation of the primary somatosensory cortex than the pleasant stimuli. It is concluded that part of the orbitofrontal cortex is concerned with representing the positively affective aspects of somatosensory stimuli (see Figs 4.4 and 4.5). The significance of this finding is that a primary reinforcer that can produce affectively positive emotional responses is represented in the human orbitofrontal cortex. This provides one of the bases for the human orbitofrontal cortex to be involved in the stimulus–reinforcement association learning that provides the basis for emotional learning. I assume that there is also a representation of the affectively negative aspects of touch in the human orbitofrontal cortex, for humans with damage to the ventral part of the frontal lobe are said to report that they know that a stimulus is pain-producing, but that the pain does not feel very bad to them (see Freeman and Watts 1950; Valenstein 1964; Melzack and Wall 1996). It will be of interest to determine whether the regions of the human orbitofrontal cortex that represent pleasant touch and pain are close topologically or overlap. Even if fMRI studies show that the areas overlap, it would nevertheless be the case that different populations of neurons would be being activated, for this is what recordings from single cells in monkeys indicate about positively vs negatively affective taste, olfactory and visual stimuli.

It is also of interest that nearby, but not overlapping, parts of the human orbitofrontal cortex are activated by taste stimuli (such as glucose) and by olfactory stimuli (such as vanilla) (Rolls, Francis *et al.* 1997b) (Fig. 2.21). It is not yet known from human fMRI studies whether it is the reinforcing aspects of taste and olfactory stimuli that are

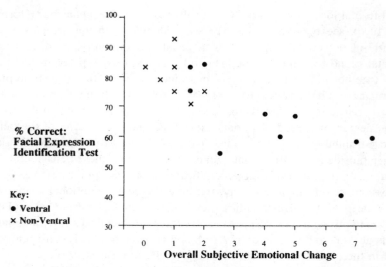

Fig. 4.23 Face expression identification deficit in humans with damage to the ventral part of the frontal lobe, and its relation to the patient's own rating of Subjective Emotional Change since the brain damage, based on sadness (or regret), anger (or frustration), fear (or anxiety), disgust, and excitement or enjoyment. (From Hornak, Rolls and Wade 1996.)

represented here, but this is likely in view of the findings in non-human primates (see Rolls 1997b).

4.5.5.2 Human brain imaging investigations of mood and depression

Brain regions involved in mood and in depression have been investigated by mood induction in normal subjects; and by measuring the changes in activity associated with depression, and its treatment by antidepressant drugs (see Mayberg 1997; Drevets and Raichle 1992; Dolan *et al*. 1992; George *et al*, 1996; Dolan, 1997). In one example of this approach, Drevets *et al*. (1997) showed that positron emission tomography (PET) measures of regional blood flow and glucose metabolism and magnetic resonance imaging (MRI)-based measures of gray matter volume are abnormally reduced in the 'subgenual pre-frontal cortex' in depressed subjects with familial major depressive disorder ('unipolar depression' and bipolar disorder ('manic-depressive illness'). This cortex is situated on the anterior cingulate gyrus lying ventral to the genu of the corpus callosum and may also be described as the subgenual or subcallosal anterior cingulate cortex (see Fig. 4.24, area 25). In another example, which implicates a similar area although apparently in the opposite direction, the recovery of depression associated with fluoxetine treatment is associated with a decrease of glucose metabolism (as indicated by fluorodeoxyglucose PET) in the ventral (subgenual) cingulate area 25, while the induction of a mood of sadness in normal subjects increased glucose metabolism in the same area (see Mayberg 1997; Mayberg, Brannan, Mahurin *et al*. 1997) (see Fig. 4.25 in the plates section; it is notable that the area indicated as Cg25 is very close to the caudal orbitofrontal cortex). At the same time, the sadness was associated with reduced glucose metabolism in more dorsal areas such as the dorsal prefrontal cortex (labelled F9 in Fig. 4.25—see plates section), the inferior parietal cortex, and the dorsal anterior cingulate and the posterior cingulate cortex (Mayberg 1997). These dorsal areas are involved in processing sensory and spatial stimuli, in spatial attention, and in sensori–motor responses (see Rolls and Treves 1998), and the reduced metabolism in these dorsal areas during sadness might reflect less interaction with the environment and less activity which normally accompanies such a change of mood. In contrast, the changes in the more ventral areas such as the ventral (i.e. subgenual) cingulate cortex may be more closely related to the changes in mood per se.

4.5.5.3 Pain and the cingulate cortex

Vogt, Derbyshire and Jones (1996) showed that pain produced an increase in regional cerebral blood flow (rCBF, measured with positron emission tomography, PET) in an area of perigenual cingulate cortex which included parts of areas 25, 32, 24a, 24b and/or 24c. Vogt et al. suggested that activation of this area is related to the affective aspect of pain. In terms of connections (see Van Hoesen, Morecraft and Vogt 1993; Vogt, Pandya and Rosene 1987; Vogt and Pandya 1987), the anterior cingulate cortex is connected to the medial orbitofrontal areas, parts of lateral orbitofrontal area 12 (Carmichael and Price 1995a), the amygdala (which projects strongly to cingulate subgenual area 25) and the temporal pole cortex, and also receives somatosensory inputs from the insula and other somatosensory cortical areas (see Fig. 4.24). The anterior cingulate cortex has output projections to the periaqueductal gray in the midbrain (which is implicated in pain processing), to the nucleus of the solitary tract and dorsal motor nucleus of the vagus (through which autonomic effects can be elicited), and to the ventral striatum and caudate nucleus (through which behavioural responses could be produced). Consistent with this anterior cingulate region being involved in affect, it is close to (just above) the area activated by the induction of a sad mood in the study described by Mayberg (1997). Also consistent with this region being involved in affect, Lane et al. (1997) found increased regional blood flow in a PET study in a far anterior part of the cingulate cortex where it adjoins prefrontal cortex when humans paid attention to the affective aspects of pictures they were being shown which contained pleasant images (e.g. flowers) and unpleasant pictures (e.g. a mangled face and a snake). Vogt et al. also found a mid-cingulate area (i.e. further back than the perigenual cingulate region) that was also activated by pain but, because this area is also activated in response selection in tasks such as divided attention and Stroop tasks, they suggested that activation of this mid-cingulate area by painful stimuli was related to the response selection effect of painful stimuli. Further evidence consistent with this possibility is that Derbyshire, Vogt and Jones (1998) showed that the perigenual cingulate area activated by pain was anterior to the mid-cingulate area activated in a Stroop attention task.

 Given the inputs to the anterior cingulate cortex from somatosensory cortical areas including the insula, and the orbitofrontal cortex and amygdala (see Fig. 4.24), and its output connections to brainstem areas such as the periaqueductal (or central) gray in the midbrain (which is implicated in pain, see Section 6.6.1 and Melzack and Wall 1996), the ventral striatum, and the autonomic brainstem nuclei (see Van Hoesen, Morecraft and

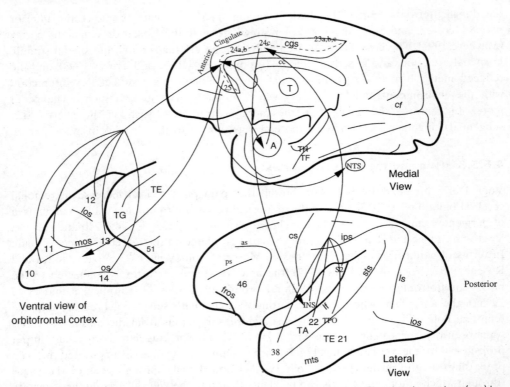

Fig. 4.24 Connections of the anterior and middle cingulate cortical areas. The cingulate sulcus (cgs) has been opened to reveal the cortex in the sulcus, with the dashed line indicating the depths (fundus) of the sulcus. The anterior cingulate cortex extends from cingulate areas 24a and 24b to subgenual cingulate area 25. (The cortex is called subgenual because it is below the genu (knee) formed by the anterior end of the corpus callosum, cc.) The anterior cingulate cortex tends to have connections with the amygdala and orbitofrontal cortex, whereas the mid-cingulate cortex (e.g. area 24c) tends to have connections with the somatosensory insula (INS), the auditory association cortex (22, TA), and with the temporal pole cortex (38). Abbreviations: as, arcuate sulcus; cc, corpus callosum; cf., calcarine fissure; cgs, cingulate sulcus; cs, central sulcus; ls, lunate sulcus; ios, inferior occipital sulcus; mos, medial orbital sulcus; os, orbital sulcus; ps, principal sulcus; sts, superior temporal sulcus; lf, Lateral (or Sylvian) fissure (which has been opened to reveal the insula); A, amygdala; INS, insula; NTS, autonomic areas in the medulla, including the nucleus of the solitary tract and the dorsal motor nucleus of the vagus; T, thalamus; TE (21), inferior temporal visual cortex; TA (22), superior temporal auditory association cortex; TF and TH, parahippocampal cortex; TPO, multimodal cortical area in the superior temporal sulcus; 38, TG, temporal pole cortex; 12, 13, 11, orbitofrontal cortex; 51, olfactory (prepyriform and periamygdaloid) cortex.

Vogt 1993), the anterior cingulate cortex may be part of an executive, output, response selection system for some emotional states, perhaps those especially related to somatosensory stimuli, and perhaps especially when they are aversive.

4.5.6 Executive functions of the orbitofrontal cortex

The research described indicates that the orbitofrontal cortex is involved in the execution of behavioural responses when these are computed by reward or punisher association learning, a function for which the orbitofrontal cortex is specialized, in terms of representations of primary (unlearned) reinforcers, and in rapidly learning and readjusting associations of stimuli with these primary reinforcers. The fact that patients with ventral frontal lesions often can express verbally what the correct responses should be, yet cannot follow what previously obtained rewards and punishments indicate is appropriate behaviour, is an indication that when primates (including humans) normally execute behavioural responses on the basis of reinforcement evaluation, they do so using the orbitofrontal cortex. Eliciting behaviour on the basis of rewards and punishments obtained previously in similar situations is of course a simple and adaptive way to control behavioural responses that has been studied and accepted for very many years (see e.g. the history of psychology; and in terms of brain mechanisms, see, e.g., Rolls 1975, 1986a,b, 1990b, 1994b, 1995b), and has been recently emphasized by Damasio (1994). The particular utility of one of the alternative routes to behaviour (there are, of course, many routes to behaviour) made possible by language is that this enables long-term planning, where the plan involves many syntactic arrangements of symbols (e.g. many if ... then statements). It is suggested that when this linguistic (in terms of syntactic manipulation of symbols) system needs correction, being able to think about the plans (higher-order thoughts), enables the plans to be corrected, and that this process is closely related to explicit, conscious, processing (Rolls 1995b, 1997a; cf. Rosenthal 1993; see Chapter 9). It follows that the functions performed by the orbitofrontal cortex need not be performed with explicit (conscious) processing, but can be performed with implicit processing. It is in this way that it is suggested that the orbitofrontal cortex is involved in some, but certainly not all, types of executive function.

In that the orbitofrontal cortex may retain as a result of synaptic modification in a pattern associator (see Appendix and Rolls and Treves 1990, 1998) the most recent reinforcement association for large numbers of different stimuli, it could perhaps be fitted into a view that the frontal cortical areas are in general concerned with different types of working memory. However, the term working memory is normally used in neurophysiology to refer to a memory in which the memoranda are held in the memory by continuing neuronal activity, as in an autoassociator or attractor network which has recurrent collateral connections (see, e.g., Rolls and Treves 1998). It should be realized that although there may be a functional similarity between such a working memory and the ability of the orbitofrontal cortex to retain the most recent reinforcement association of many stimuli, the implementations are very different. The different implementations do in fact have strong functional consequences: it is difficult to retain more than a few items active in an autoassociative memory, and hence in practice individual items are retained typically only for short periods in such working memories; whereas in pattern associators, because synaptic modification has taken place, the last reinforcement association of a very large number of stimuli can be stored for long periods, and recalled whenever each stimulus is seen again in the future, without any neuronal firing to hold the representation active (see, e.g., Rolls and Treves 1998).

It is perhaps useful to note how the orbitofrontal cortex may link to output systems to control behaviour, for the occasions when the orbitofrontal cortex does control behaviour. Rolls has proposed elsewhere (Rolls 1984b, 1994b; Rolls and Johnstone 1992; Rolls and Treves 1998, Chapter 9) the outline of a theory of striatal function according to which all areas of the cerebral cortex gain access to the striatum, compete within the striatum and the rest of the basal ganglia system for behavioural output depending on how strongly each part of the cerebral cortex is calling for output, and the striatum maps (as a result of slow previous habit or stimulus–response learning) each particular type of input to the striatum to the appropriate behavioural output (implemented via the return basal ganglia connections to premotor/prefrontal parts of the cerebral cortex). This is one of the ways in which reinforcing stimuli can exert their influence relatively directly on behavioural output. The importance of this route is attested to by the fact that restricted striatal lesions impair functions implemented by the part of the cortex which projects to the lesioned part of the striatum (see Rolls 1984b, 1994b; Rolls and Johnstone 1992; Section 6.4).

Another set of outputs from the orbitofrontal cortex enables it to influence autonomic function. The fact that ventral prefrontal lesions block autonomic responses to learned reinforcers (Damasio 1994) (actually known since at least the 1950s, e.g. Elithorn *et al.* 1955 in humans; Grueninger *et al.* 1965 in macaques) is of course consistent with the hypothesis that learned reinforcers elicit autonomic responses via the orbitofrontal cortex and amygdala (see, e.g., Rolls 1986a,b, 1990b). It is worth emphasizing here that this does not prove the hypothesis that behavioural responses elicited by conditioned reinforcers are mediated via peripheral changes, themselves used as 'somatic markers' to determine which response to make. The question of whether there is any returning information from the periphery which is necessary for emotion, as the somatic marker hypothesis postulates, has been considered in Section 3.1.6. The present hypothesis is, in contrast, that somatic markers are not part of the route by which emotions are felt or emotional decisions are taken, but that instead the much more direct neural route from the orbitofrontal cortex and amygdala to the basal ganglia provides a pathway which is much more efficient, and is directly implicated in producing, the behavioural responses to learned incentives (Divac *et al.* 1967; Everitt and Robbins 1992; Williams, Rolls, Leonard and Stern 1993; Rolls 1994b) (see Section 4.6.2, and for explicit verbal outputs see Chapter 9 also).

4.6   Output pathways for emotional responses

4.6.1   The autonomic and endocrine systems

The first output system introduced above in Section 4.1 is the autonomic and endocrine system. Through it changes such as increased heart rate and the release of adrenaline, which prepare the body for action, are produced by emotional stimuli. There are brainstem routes through which peripheral stimuli can produce reflex autonomic responses. In addition, there are outputs from the hypothalamus to the autonomic brainstem centres (Schwaber *et al.* 1982). Structures such as the amygdala and orbitofrontal cortex can produce autonomic responses to secondary reinforcing (or classically conditioned) stimuli both directly, for example by direct connections from the amygdala to the dorsal motor nucleus of the vagus (Schwaber *et al.* 1982), and via the lateral hypothalamus. For example, LeDoux, Iwata, Cichetti and Reis (1988) showed that lesions of the lateral hypothalamus (which receives from the central nucleus of the amygdala) blocked conditioned heart rate (autonomic) responses (see also Kapp *et al.* 1992). The outputs of the orbitofrontal cortex are also involved in learned autonomic responses, in that ventral prefrontal lesions block autonomic responses to learned reinforcers (Elithorn *et al.* 1955 and Damasio 1994, in humans; Grueninger *et al.* 1965 in macaques).

4.6.2 Motor systems for implicit responses, including the basal ganglia

The second type of output is to brain systems concerned with performing actions unconsciously or implicitly, in order to obtain rewards or avoid punishers. These brain systems include the basal ganglia. For example, Cador, Robbins and Everitt (1989) obtained evidence consistent with the hypothesis that the learned incentive (conditioned reinforcing) effects of previously neutral stimuli paired with rewards are mediated by the amygdala acting through the ventral striatum (which includes the nucleus accumbens), in that amphetamine injections into the ventral striatum enhanced the effects of a conditioned reinforcing stimulus only if the amygdala was intact (see further Everitt and Robbins 1992). To analyse the functions of the ventral striatum, the responses of more than 1000 single neurons were recorded in a region which included the nucleus accumbens and olfactory tubercle in five macaque monkeys in test situations in which lesions of the amygdala, hippocampus and inferior temporal cortex produce deficits, and in which neurons in these structures respond (Rolls and Williams 1987b; Rolls 1990b,d, 1992a,b; Rolls, Cahusac *et al.* 1993; Williams, Rolls, Leonard and Stern 1993). While the monkeys performed visual discrimination and related feeding tasks, the different populations of neurons found included neurons which responded to novel visual stimuli; to reinforcement-related visual stimuli such as (for different neurons) food-related stimuli, aversive stimuli, or faces; to other visual stimuli; in relation to somatosensory stimulation and movement; or to cues which signalled the start of a task. The neurons with responses to reinforcing or novel visual stimuli may reflect the inputs to the ventral striatum from the amygdala and hippocampus, and are consistent with the hypothesis that the ventral striatum provides a route for learned reinforcing and novel visual stimuli to influence behaviour. The output for the shell, limbic-related, part of the nucleus accumbens is directed towards the ventral pallidum, and thus to the mediodorsal nucleus of the thalamus, which in turn projects to the prefrontal cortex. In primates, the outputs from brain regions such as the amygdala and orbitofrontal cortex spread though much beyond the ventral striatum, to the ventral parts of the head of the caudate nucleus (Kemp and Powell 1970). This other part of the striatum is important as an output route to behaviour for the amygdala and orbitofrontal cortex, in that damage to the head of the caudate nucleus can impair the performance of monkeys on tasks also affected by lesions of, for example, the orbitofrontal cortex, such as visual discrimination reversal (Divac *et al.* 1967; Divac and Oberg 1979; Oberg and Divac 1979; Iversen 1984). For example, in the monkey lesions of the ventrolateral part of the head of the caudate nucleus (as of the orbitofrontal cortex which projects to it) impaired object reversal performance, which measures the ability to reverse stimulus–reinforcement associations. In contrast, lesions of the anterodorsal part of the head of the caudate nucleus disrupted delayed spatial alternation performance, a task which requires spatial short-term memory, which is also impaired by lesions of the corresponding cortical region, the dorsolateral prefrontal cortex. Lastly, lesions of the tail of the caudate nucleus (as of the inferior temporal visual cortex which projects to this part of the caudate) produced a visual pattern discrimination deficit (Divac *et al.* 1967; cf. Iversen 1979). A fuller description of the functions of the ventral striatum as an output system for the effects of learned incentives decoded by the amygdala and orbitofrontal cortex to influence behaviour is provided in Chapter 6. More evidence on the functions of the basal ganglia, and a computational theory of how they may operate, is provided by Rolls and Treves (1998).

Other outputs for learned implicit behavioural responses may proceed from the amygdala through the midbrain, in that lesions of the central gray of the midbrain (which also receives from the central nucleus of the amygdala) blocked the conditioned freezing but not the conditioned autonomic response to an aversive conditioned stimulus (LeDoux *et al.* 1988).

4.6.3 Output systems for explicit responses to emotional stimuli

The third type of output is to a system capable of planning many steps ahead and, for example, deferring short-term rewards in order to execute a long-term plan. This system may use syntactic processing in order to perform the planning, and is therefore part of a linguistic system which performs explicit processing. This system, discussed in Chapter 9, is the one in which explicit, declarative, processing occurs. Processing in this system is frequently associated with reason and rationality, in that many of the consequences of possible actions can be taken into account. The actual computation of how rewarding a particular stimulus or situation is, or will be, probably still depends on activity in the orbitofrontal and amygdala, in that the reward value of stimuli is computed and represented in these regions, and in that it is found that verbalized expressions of the reward (or punishment) value of stimuli are dampened by damage to these systems. (For example, damage to the orbitofrontal cortex renders painful input still identifiable as pain, but without the strong affective, 'unpleasant', reaction to it.)

4.7 Basal forebrain and hypothalamus

It was suggested above that the hypothalamus and basal forebrain may provide one output system for the amygdala and orbitofrontal cortex for autonomic and other responses to emotional stimuli. Consistent with this, there are neurons in the lateral hypothalamus and basal forebrain of monkeys that respond to visual stimuli associated with rewards such as food (Rolls 1975, 1981a,c, 1982, 1986a,b,c, 1990b, 1993a; Rolls, Burton and Mora 1976; Burton, Rolls and Mora 1976a,b; Mora, Rolls and Burton 1976b; Wilson and Rolls 1990a). These neurons show rapid reversal of their responses during the reversal of stimulus–reinforcer associations. Other neurons in the hypothalamus responded only to stimuli associated with punishment, that is to aversive visual stimuli (Rolls, Sanghera and Roper-Hall 1979b). The responses of these neurons with reinforcement-related activity would be appropriate for producing autonomic responses to emotional stimuli, via pathways which descend from the hypothalamus towards the brainstem autonomic motor nuclei (Saper *et al.* 1976; Schwaber *et al.* 1982). It is also possible that these outputs could influence emotional behaviour, through, for example, the connections from the hypothalamus to the amygdala (Aggleton *et al.* 1980), to the substantia nigra (Nauta and Domesick 1978), or even by the connections to the neocortex (Divac 1975; Kievit and Kuypers 1975). Indeed, it is suggested that the latter projection, by releasing acetylcholine in the cerebral cortex when emotional stimuli (including reinforcing and novel stimuli) are seen, provides one way in which emotion can influence the storage of memories in the cerebral cortex (Rolls 1987; Wilson and Rolls 1990a,b). In this case, the basal forebrain magnocellular neurons may act as a 'cortical strobe' which facilitates memory storage and processing when the neurons are firing fast.

4.7.1 Basal forebrain cholinergic neurons

Before leaving the learning systems in the amygdala and orbitofrontal cortex, it is useful to consider the role in memory of one of the systems to which they project, the basal forebrain magnocellular nuclei of Meynert. The cells in these nuclei lie just lateral to the lateral hypothalamus in the substantia innominata, and extend forward through the preoptic area into the diagonal band of Broca (see Mesulam 1990). These cells, many of which are cholinergic, project directly to the cerebral cortex (Divac 1975; Kievit and Kuypers 1975; Mesulam 1990). These cells provide the major cholinergic input to the cerebral cortex, in that if they are lesioned the cortex is depleted of acetylcholine (Mesulam 1990). Loss of these cells does occur in Alzheimer's disease, and there is consequently a reduction in cortical acetylcholine in this disease (Mesulam 1990). This loss of cortical acetylcholine may contribute to the memory loss in Alzheimer's disease, although it may well not be the primary factor in the aetiology.

In order to investigate the role of the basal forebrain nuclei in memory, Aigner *et al.* (1991) made neurotoxic lesions of them in monkeys. Some impairments on a simple test of recognition memory, delayed non-match-to-sample, were found. Analysis of the effects of similar lesions in rats showed that performance on memory tasks was impaired, perhaps because of failure to attend properly (Muir *et al.* 1994). There are quite limited numbers of these basal forebrain neurons (in the order of thousands). Given that there are relatively few of these neurons, it is not likely that they carry the information to be stored in cortical memory circuits, for the number of different patterns that could be represented and stored is so small. (The number of different patterns that could be stored is dependent in a leading way on the number of input connections on to each neuron in the pattern associator, see Chapter 2). With this few neurons distributed throughout the cerebral cortex, the memory capacity of the whole system would be impractically small. This argument alone indicates that they are unlikely to carry the information to be stored in cortical memory systems. Instead, they could modulate information storage in the cortex of information derived from what provides the numerically major input to cortical cells, the glutamatergic terminals of other cortical cells. This modulation may operate by setting thresholds for cortical cells to the appropriate value, or by more directly influencing the cascade of processes involved in long-term potentiation (see Appendix). There is indeed evidence that acetylcholine is necessary for cortical synaptic modifiability, as shown by studies in which depletion of acetylcholine and noradrenaline impaired cortical LTP/synaptic modifiability (Bear and Singer 1986).

The question then arises of whether the basal forebrain cholinergic neurons tonically release acetylcholine, or whether they release it particularly in response to some external influence. To examine this, recordings have been made from basal forebrain neurons, at least some of which will have been the cholinergic neurons just described. It has been found that some of these neurons respond to visual stimuli associated with rewards such as food (Rolls 1975, 1981b, 1986a,b,c, 1990c; Burton, Rolls and Mora 1976a,b; Mora, Rolls and Burton 1976b; Rolls, Burton and Mora 1976; Wilson and Rolls 1990b,c), or with punishment (Rolls, Sanghera and Roper-Hall 1979b), that others respond to novel visual stimuli (Wilson and Rolls 1990a), and that others respond to a range of visual stimuli. For example, in one set of recordings, one group of these neurons (1.5%) responded to novel visual stimuli while monkeys performed recognition or visual discrimination tasks (Wilson and Rolls 1990a). A complementary group of neurons more anteriorly responded to familiar visual stimuli in the same tasks (Wilson and Rolls 1990a; Rolls and Rolls 1982). A third group of neurons (5.7%) responded to positively reinforcing visual stimuli in visual discrimination and in recognition memory tasks (Wilson and Rolls 1990b,c). In addition, a considerable proportion of these neurons (21.8%) responded to any visual stimuli shown in the tasks, and some (13.1%) responded to the tone cue which preceded the presentation of the visual stimuli in the task, and was provided to enable the monkey to alert to the visual stimuli (Wilson and Rolls 1990a). These neurons did not respond to touch to the leg which induced arousal, so their responses did not simply reflect arousal. Neurons in this region receive inputs from the amygdala (see Mesulam 1990; Aggleton 1992), and it is probably via the amygdala that the information described here reaches the basal forebrain neurons, for neurons with similar response properties have been found in the amygdala and the amygdala appears to be involved in decoding visual stimuli that are associated with reinforcers, or are novel (Rolls 1990c, 1992a; Wilson and Rolls 1993, 1999).

It is therefore suggested that the normal physiological function of these basal forebrain neurons is to send a general activation signal to the cortex when certain classes of environmental stimulus occur. These stimuli are often stimuli to which behavioural activation is appropriate or required, such as positively or negatively reinforcing visual stimuli, or novel visual stimuli. The effect of the firing of these neurons on the cortex is excitatory, and in this way produces activation. This cortical activation may produce behavioural arousal, and may thus facilitate concentration and attention, which are both impaired in Alzheimer's disease. The reduced arousal and concentration may themselves contribute to the memory disorders. But the acetylcholine released from these basal magnocellular neurons may in addition be more directly necessary for memory formation, for Bear and Singer (1986) showed that long-term potentiation, used as an indicator of the synaptic modification which underlies learning, requires the presence in the cortex of acetylcholine as well as noradrenaline. For comparison, acetylcholine in the hippocampus makes it more likely that LTP will occur, probably through activation of an inositol phosphate second messenger cascade (Markram and Siegel 1992; see Siegel and Auerbach

1996; see also Hasselmo and Bower 1993; Hasselmo *et al*. 1995). The adaptive value of the cortical strobe provided by the basal magnocellular neurons may thus be that it facilitates memory storage especially when significant (e.g. reinforcing) environmental stimuli are detected. This means that memory storage is likely to be conserved (new memories are less likely to be laid down) when significant environmental stimuli are not present. In that the basal forebrain projection spreads widely to many areas of the cerebral cortex, and in that there are relatively few basal forebrain neurons (in the order of thousands), the basal forebrain neurons do not determine the actual memories that are stored. Instead the actual memories stored are determined by the active subset of the thousands of cortical afferents on to a strongly activated cortical neuron (cf. Treves and Rolls 1994; Rolls and Treves 1998). The basal forebrain magnocellular neurons would then according to this analysis simply when activated increase the probability that a memory would be stored. Impairment of the normal operation of the basal forebrain magnocellular neurons would be expected to interfere with normal memory by interfering with this function, and this interference could contribute in this way to the memory disorder in Alzheimer's disease.

Another property of cortical neurons emphasized recently (Markram and Tsodyks 1996; Abbott *et al*. 1997) is that they tend to adapt with repeated input. However, this adaptation is most marked in slices, in which there is no acetylcholine. One effect of acetylcholine is to reduce this adaptation. When recordings are made from single neurons operating in physiological conditions in the awake behaving monkey, peristimulus time histograms of inferior temporal cortex neurons to visual stimuli show only some adaptation. There is typically an onset of the neuronal response at 80–100 ms after the stimulus, followed within 50 ms by the highest firing rate. There is after that some reduction in the firing rate, but the firing rate is still typically more than half maximal 500 ms later (see example in Rolls and Treves 1998, Fig. 10.13). Thus under normal physiological conditions, firing rate adaptation can occur, but does not involved a major adaptation, even when cells are responding fast (at e.g. 100 spikes s^{-1}) to a visual stimulus. One of the factors that keeps the response relatively maintained may however be the presence of acetylcholine. Its depletion in some disease states could lead to less sustained neuronal responses (i.e. more adaptation), and this may contribute to the symptoms found.

4.7.2 Noradrenergic neurons

The source of the noradrenergic projection to the neocortex is the locus coeruleus (noradrenergic cell group A6) in the pons (see Green and Costain 1981). (Note that noradrenaline is the same as norepinephrine.) There are a few thousand of these neurons that innervate the whole of the cerebral cortex, as well as the amygdala and other structures, so it is unlikely that the noradrenergic neurons convey the specific information stored in synapses that specifies each memory. Instead, to the extent that the noradrenergic neurons are involved in memory (including pattern association), it is likely that they would have a modulatory role on cell excitability, which would influence the extent to which the voltage-dependent NMDA receptors are activated, and thus the likelihood that information carried on specific afferents would be stored (cf. Siegel and Auerbach 1996). Evidence that this may be the case comes from a study in which it was shown that neocortical LTP is impaired if noradrenergic and simultaneously cholinergic inputs to cortical cells are blocked pharmacologically (Bear and Singer 1986). Further, in a study designed to show whether the noradrenergic modulation is necessary for memory, Borsini and Rolls (1984) showed that intra-amygdaloid injections of noradrenergic receptor blockers did impair the type of learning in which rats gradually learned to accept novel foods. The function implemented by this noradrenergic input may more be general activation, rather than a signal that carries information about whether reward vs punishment has been given, for noradrenergic neurons in rats respond to both rewarding and punishing stimuli, and one of the more effective stimuli for producing release of noradrenaline is placing the feet in cool water (see McGinty and Szymusiak 1988).

4.8   Effects of emotion on cognitive processing

The analyses above of the neural mechanisms of emotion have been concerned primarily with how stimuli are decoded to produce emotional states, and with how these states can influence behaviour. In addition, current mood state can affect the cognitive evaluation of events or memories (see Blaney 1986). For example, happy memories are more likely to be recalled when happy. Why does this occur?

It is suggested that whenever memories are stored, part of the context is stored with the memory. This is very likely to happen in associative neuronal networks such as those in the hippocampus (Rolls 1987, 1989a, 1990c, 1996a, Treves and Rolls 1994). The CA3 part of the hippocampus may operate as a single autoassociative memory capable of linking together almost arbitrary co-occurrences of inputs, including inputs about emotional state that reach the entorhinal cortex from, for example, the amygdala. Recall of a memory occurs best in such networks when the input key to the memory is nearest to the original input pattern of activity which was stored (see Rolls 1989a,c,d; Rolls and Treves 1990, 1998; Treves and Rolls 1994). It thus follows that a memory of, for example, a happy episode is recalled best when in a happy mood state. This is a special case of a general theory of how context is stored with a memory, and of how context influences recall (see Treves and Rolls 1994). The effect of emotional state on cognitive processing and memory is thus suggested to be a particular case of a more general way in which context can affect the storage and retrieval of memories, or can affect cognitive processing.

Another brain system where effects of mood on storage and recall could be instantiated is in the backprojection system from structures important in emotion such as the amygdala and orbitofrontal cortex to parts of the cerebral cortex important in the representation of objects, such as the inferior temporal visual cortex (see Fig. 4.26). It is suggested (Rolls 1989a,c; Treves and Rolls 1994; Rolls and Treves 1998) that co-activity between forward inputs and backprojecting inputs to strongly activated cortical pyramidal cells would lead to both sets of synapses being modified (see Fig. 4.27). This could result in facilitation or recall of cortical representations (for example of particular faces) that had become associated with emotional states, represented by activity in the amygdala (see further Rolls 1990b).

Thus emotional states may affect whether or how strongly memories are stored using

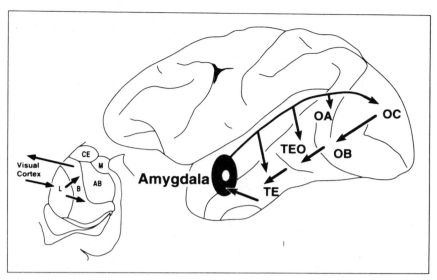

Fig. 4.26 The backprojections from the primate amygdala to the cortex spread more widely than the afferent connections, which for vision come mainly from the inferior temporal visual cortical areas, e.g. area TE. OC, striate cortex; OB, OA, prestriate visual cortical areas; TEO, posterior inferior temporal visual cortex. The insert to the left shows a coronal section of the primate amygdala, with lateral on the left, to indicate that many of the visual cortical afferents reach the lateral nucleus of the amygdala (L), and that many of the backprojections arise from the basal nucleus of the amygdala (B). CE, central nucleus of the amygdala; AB, accessory basal nucleus; M, medial nucleus. (Reproduced with permission from Amaral *et al.* 1992.)

the basal forebrain memory strobe (see Section 4.7.1); be stored as part of many memories; and may influence both the recall of such memories, and the operation of cognitive processing, in the way described in the preceding paragraphs.

4.9 Laterality effects in human emotional processing

In humans, there is some lateralization of function of emotional processing, with the right hemisphere frequently being implicated in processing face expressions. Some of the evidence for this is reviewed next.

A first type of evidence comes from the effects of brain damage in humans. Damage to the left hemisphere (in right handed people) is more likely to affect language, and to the right hemisphere is more likely to affect emotional processing. This may be evident, for example, in the greater probability of impairments in recognizing facial expressions after right rather than left hemisphere damage (see Etcoff 1989). A second type of evidence comes from split brain patients (with the corpus callosum sectioned to prevent epilepsy on one side affecting the other side of the brain). These patients may respond behaviourally to an emotion-provoking stimulus which reaches the right hemisphere, even though they cannot specify verbally (with the left hemisphere) what they saw (Gazzaniga 1988). Third, when faces are flashed rapidly on a screen, there may be better performance in identifying the expression on the face when the stimulus is projected to the right than to the left

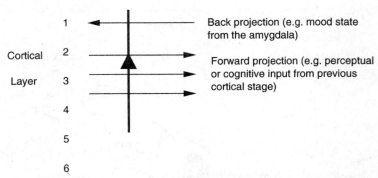

Fig. 4.27 Pyramidal cells in, for example, layers 2 and 3 of the temporal lobe association cortex receive forward inputs from preceding cortical stages of processing, and also backprojections from the amygdala. It is suggested that the backprojections from the amygdala make modifiable synapses on the apical dendrites of cortical pyramidal cells during learning when amygdala neurons are active in relation to a mood state; and that the backprojections from the amygdala via these modified synapses allow mood state to influence later cognitive processing, for example by facilitating some perceptual representations.

hemisphere (Strauss and Moscovitsch 1981). These effects on face expression identification are not produced just because face-processing modules are lateralized to the right hemisphere: face identification deficits are not necessarily associated with face expression identification impairments.

For other types of emotional processing, there may also be some lateralization. Davidson *et al.* (1990) and Davidson (1992) have some evidence from EEG recording that for negative emotional episodes there is more activation of the right side of the brain; and for positive episodes there is more activation of the left side of the brain. Another type of evidence comes from patients who are more likely to be depressed by a stroke if it is to the left than to the right hemisphere (see Starkstein and Robinson 1991). This may indicate that to feel depressed, the right hemisphere is normally involved.

Why should there be some lateralization of emotional processing in humans? One argument is that whenever a function does not need to be represented bilaterally due to the topology of the body (e.g. we have left and right hands, and separate representations of each hand are needed), then it is more efficient to place the group of neurons concerned with that processing close together. One advantage of placing neurons concerned with similar processing close together is that the length of the connections between the neurons will be minimized. This is important for minimizing brain size and weight, which is a significant factor in evolution. If half the neurons concerned with a particular function were on one side of the brain, and the other half were on the contralateral side, then the total length of the connections between the neurons would be large. Neurons concerned with the same function are frequently interconnected for a number of reasons. One is that there are recurrent collateral axons between nearby cortical neurons concerned with the same function. One of the functions performed by these excitatory recurrent collaterals is to enable the network to act as a local attractor or autoassociation memory, so that the output of the module can take into account not only the activation produced in any one neuron, but also the activations received by the other connected neurons (see Rolls and Treves 1998, Chapters 3 and 10). Another way in which this is performed is by using feedback inhibitory interneurons, which are activated by many of the cortical pyramidal cells in a region. This helps not only autoassociation (and pattern association) networks to remain stable, but also is important for competitive networks, in which categorization of stimuli occurs, by effectively allowing the neurons in a population with the strongest activation by a particular stimulus to remain active (see Rolls and Treves 1998, Chapter 4). A second advantage of placing neurons concerned with the same function close together is that this may simplify the wiring rules between neurons which must be implemented genetically. Given that there are in the order of 100 000 genes in the human genome, and more than 10^{14} synapses, it is clearly impossible for genes to specify all the connections between every neuron. Instead, the genetic rules may specify, for example, neurons of type y make approximately 12 000 excitatory synapses with associative long-term potentiation and heterosynaptic long-term depression to other neurons of type y in the surrounding 2 mm (this forms a recurrent collateral pathway); make approximately 12 000 excitatory synapses with associative long-term potentiation and heterosynaptic long-term depression with neurons of type z up to 4 mm away (which might be the next cortical area); make approximately 500 synapses with neurons of type I within 2 mm (which might be GABA-containing inhibitory feedback neurons); and receive approximately 6000 inputs from neurons of type x up to 4 mm away (which might be the pyramidal cells in the preceding cortical area). This type of specification would build many of the networks found in different brain regions (see Rolls and Treves 1998). An advantage of this type of specification, and of keeping neurons concerned with the same computation close together, is that this minimizes the problems of guidance of axons towards their targets. If neurons concerned with the same function were randomly distributed in the brain, then finding the distant correct neurons with which to connect would be an impossible guidance problem. (As it is, some distant parts of the brain which are connected in adults are connected because the connections can be made early in development, before the different brain regions have migrated to become possibly distant.)

All these constraints imply that wherever possible neurons performing the same computation should be close together. Where there is no body-symmetry reason to have separate representations for each side of the body, then the representation would optimally be lateralized. This appears to be the case for certain aspects of emotional processing. However, it is of interest that this lateralization of function may itself give rise to lateralization of performance. It may be because the brain mechanisms concerned with face expression identification are better represented in the right hemisphere that expression identification is better for the left half of the visual field (which might correspond to the left half of a centrally fixated face).

Another possible reason for partial lateralization of human emotion may be that language is predominantly in the left hemisphere (for right-handed people). The result of this may be that although explicit (conscious, verbal) processing related to emotion (see Chapter 6) may take place in the left hemisphere, the implicit type of processing may take place where there is room in the brain, that is in the left hemisphere. The suggestion that there are these two types of output route for emotional behaviour is made in Section 4.6, and in Chapter 6. The fact that they are to some extent separate types of output processing may account for the fact that they can be placed in different modules, which happen to be in different hemispheres.

5 Brain-stimulation reward

5.1 Introduction

Electrical stimulation at some sites in the brain is rewarding, in that animals including humans will work to obtain the stimulation. This phenomenon has been very useful in helping to understand the brain mechanisms that implement reward.

The discovery that rats would learn to stimulate electrically some regions of the brain was reported by J. Olds and Milner (1954). Olds noticed that rats would return to a corner of an open field apparatus where stimulation had just been given. He stimulated the rat whenever it went to the corner and found that the animals rapidly learned to go there to obtain the stimulation, by making delivery of it contingent on other types of behaviour, such as pressing a lever in a Skinner box or crossing a shock grid (see J. Olds 1977) (see Fig. 5.1).

The electrical stimulation is usually delivered through electrodes insulated to within 0.1–0.5 mm of the tip and permanently implanted so that the tip is in a defined location in the brain. The stimulation usually consists of pulses at a frequency of 50–100 Hz delivered in a train 300–500 ms long. At self-stimulation sites the animal will repeatedly perform the operant response to obtain one train of stimulation for each press. The rate of lever pressing provides a measure of the self-stimulation behaviour. The phenomenon can be called brain-stimulation reward because the animal will work to obtain the stimulation of its brain. Brain-stimulation reward has been found in all vertebrates tested. For example, it occurs in the goldfish, pigeon, rat, cat, dog, monkey, and humans (Rolls 1975). Brain-stimulation reward can also refer to reward produced by injections of pharmacological agents into the brain. For example, animals will learn to inject small amounts of amphetamine to certain parts of the brain. Pharmacological aspects of reward are described in Chapter 6.

5.2 The nature of the reward produced

One way in which the nature of the reward produced by brain stimulation can be tested in animals is by altering the drive (e.g. the hunger) of the animal to determine how this influences the reward produced by the stimulation. At some brain sites, for example in the lateral hypothalamus, a reduction of hunger can reduce the self-stimulation rate (Hoebel 1969, 1976). As a reduction of hunger reduces both food reward (in that the animal will no longer work for food), and brain-stimulation reward at some brain sites, it is suggested that the stimulation at these brain sites is rewarding because it mimics the effect of food for a hungry animal (Hoebel 1969; Rolls 1975). This modulation of brain-stimulation reward by hunger is found at lateral hypothalamic sites (Rolls, Burton and Mora 1980) and

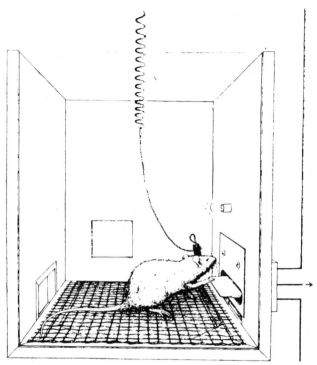

Fig. 5.1 A rat pressing a lever in order to obtain brain-stimulation reward. The reward is provided by a 0.5-s train of pulses of stimulation at typically 50–100 Hz delivered each time the rat presses the bar. (After Olds 1956.)

of all sites I have tested, most profoundly in the orbitofrontal cortex (Mora, Avrith, Phillips and Rolls 1979).

It is important to note that this effect is not just a general effect on performance of, for instance, drowsiness, because a reduction of hunger may reduce self-stimulation at some sites but not at others (Rolls 1975). Further, at some sites hunger may facilitate self-stimulation, while at other sites thirst may facilitate self-stimulation. For example, in an experiment by Gallistel and Beagley (1971) rats chose stimulation on one electrode if they were hungry and on a different electrode if they were thirsty (see Fig. 5.2). One interesting and useful feature of this experiment is that a choice rather than a rate measure of the reward value of the brain stimulation was used. The advantage of the choice measure is that any general effect such as arousal or drowsiness produced by the treatment which could affect response rate has a minimal effect on the outcome of the experiment. The experiment shows that at some sites brain-stimulation reward can be equivalent to a specific natural reward, such as food for a hungry animal or water for a thirsty animal. Support for this view that brain-stimulation reward can mimic the effects of a natural reward such as food comes from neurophysiological experiments described below in which brain-stimulation reward and food reward have been shown to activate the same neurons in the hypothalamus. At some other sites, the brain-stimulation reward produces effects

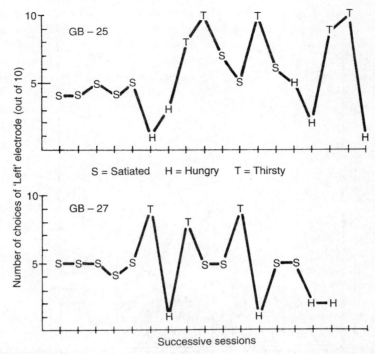

Fig. 5.2 Water and food reward effects produced by electrical stimulation of the brain in two rats. If the rats were thirsty (T) they chose to press a lever which delivered electrical stimulation to one brain site, and if they were hungry (H) they chose to press the other lever which delivered stimulation to another brain site. If the rats were satiated (S) for both food and water, then the preference for the two sites was approximately equal. (Reprinted with permission from Gallistel and Beagley 1971.)

which mimic those of sexual rewards. For example, at sites in the posterior hypothalamus but not in the lateral hypothalamus in male rats, castration decreases the self-stimulation, and subsequent androgen replacement injections produced a differential facilitation of the posterior hypothalamic self-stimulation (Caggiula 1970; see also J. Olds 1958, 1961). At other sites natural drives such as hunger and thirst do not modulate self-stimulation, so that some other reward process, perhaps more related to emotion as described next, must underlie the reward produced (Rolls 1975).

A different type of evidence on the nature of the reward produced by electrical stimulation of the brain comes from direct reports of the sensations elicited by the stimulation in humans. During the investigation of, or treatment of, epilepsy, tumours or Parkinson's disease, electrical stimulation has been given to localized brain regions to evaluate the functioning of particular regions. Sem-Jacobsen (1968, 1976) reported on the effects of stimulation at 2639 sites in 82 patients. Pleasant smells were evoked by the stimulation at nine sites, and unpleasant at six. Pleasant tastes were evoked at three sites, and unpleasant at one. Sexual responses were elicited at two sites. These types of finding are consistent with the food-related and other effects of the stimulation at some sites inferred from experiments with animals. The relative paucity of reports of this type in man may be because brain sites in the temporal and frontal lobes are usually investigated and the electrodes do not normally reach the basal regions such as the hypothalamus that are often investigated in animals. More common in humans are reports that mood changes are elicited by stimulation at some sites. In Sem-Jacobsen's series, at 360 points the patients became relaxed, at ease, had a feeling of well-being and/or were a little sleepy (classed as Positive I). At 31 sites the patients in addition showed enjoyment, frequently smiled and might want more stimulation (Positive II). At eight sites (in seven patients) the patients laughed out loud, enjoyed themselves, positively liked the stimulation and wanted more (Positive III). These and other reports of mood changes were produced by the stimulation. Thus at some brain sites in humans electrical stimulation can produce mood changes, stimulation may be desired, and this may be associated with self-stimulation (see further Heath 1954, 1963, 1972; Bishop *et al.* 1963; Stevens *et al.* 1969; Delgado 1976; Sem-Jacobsen 1976; Valenstein 1974; Halgren 1992). Examples of some of the effects produced by electrical stimulation in tracks made into the temporal lobe during neurosurgery are illustrated in Fig. 5.3.

The evidence available from animals and humans thus suggests that the nature of the reward produced at different self-stimulation sites depends on the site: at some sites (e.g. the lateral hypothalamus and the secondary taste cortex in the orbitofrontal region) the stimulation may be equivalent to a specific natural reward such as food for a hungry animal; at other sites the stimulation may produce more general changes in mood and may thus be desired. At other sites (e.g. some parts of the orbitofrontal cortex and amygdala) it is possible that the stimulation taps into brain systems concerned with learning about stimulus–reinforcement associations, where of course primary reinforcers must be represented, and where the output pathways must be capable of signalling (secondary) reinforcement if they are to implement the effects that secondary reinforcers have. This analysis makes it clear that brain self-stimulation may occur for any one of a number of reasons and that a single basis for self-stimulation should not be expected.

It is now to the neural bases of brain-stimulation reward that we turn. We will be concerned not only with the neural mechanisms of brain-stimulation reward at different sites, but also with what can be learned about reward processes in the brain from studies of brain-stimulation reward. For example, one question before us will be how it happens that animals will only work for food (i.e. find it rewarding) when they are hungry. Another question is why brain-stimulation reward continues for hours on end with no appearance of satiety. Is the elicitation of a reward by a sensory stimulus something that normally can continue indefinitely, and if so, how does the system normally arrange for any one reward not to be continue for so long, at the cost of allowing other behaviours to occur? Another question, examined in Chapter 6, will be how studies of the pharmacology of brain-stimulation reward relate to our understanding of the control of mood, and what they tell us about the neural basis of addiction.

5.3 The location of brain-stimulation reward sites in the brain

To understand the neural mechanisms of brain-stimulation reward it is first necessary to

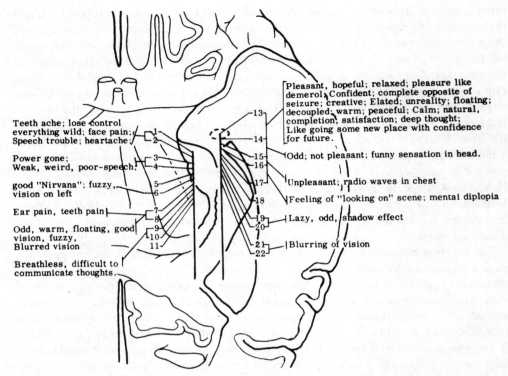

Teeth ache; lose control everything wild; face pain; Speech trouble; heartache;

Power gone; Weak, weird, poor-speech;

good "Nirvana"; fuzzy, vision on left

Ear pain, teeth pain

Odd, warm, floating, good vision, fuzzy, Blurred vision

Breathless, difficult to communicate thoughts.

Pleasant, hopeful; relaxed; pleasure like demerol; Confident; complete opposite of seizure; creative; Elated; unreality; floating; decoupled; warm; peaceful; Calm; natural, completion; satisfaction; deep thought; Like going some new place with confidence for future.

Odd; not pleasant; funny sensation in head.

Unpleasant; radio waves in chest

Feeling of "looking on" scene; mental diplopia

Lazy, odd, shadow effect

Blurring of vision

Fig. 5.3 Summary of subjective states evoked by electrical stimulation at different sites along two tracks in the human temporal lobe on a diagrammatic representation of the stimulating points. (Reprinted from Stevens, Mark, Ervin, Pacheco and Suematsu 1969.)

know where brain self-stimulation sites are located. One group is located along the general course of the medial forebrain bundle, passing lateral to the midline from the ventral tegmental area of the midbrain posteriorly, through the lateral hypothalamus, preoptic area and nucleus accumbens, toward the prefrontal cortex (orbitofrontal cortex in the monkey) anteriorly (Fig. 5.4) (see J. Olds and Olds 1965; Rolls 1971b, 1974, 1975, 1976a; Rolls and Cooper 1974; Mora, Avrith and Rolls 1980; Rolls, Burton and Mora 1980). Many cell groups and neural pathways follow this path or much of this general course. For example, there is the medial forebrain bundle itself, interconnecting forebrain and brainstem regions with hypothalamic and other diencephalic systems. There are fibres connected to neurons in prefrontal self-stimulation sites, which pass many self-stimulation sites in their course through the brain (Routtenberg et al. 1971; Rolls and Cooper 1973, 1974). In addition there are dopamine-containing fibres in the mesolimbic and mesocortical systems ascending from cell group A10 in the ventral tegmental region to the ventral striatum and orbitofrontal cortex, as well as in the substantia nigra (cell group A9) coursing to the striatum (see Chapter 6). It is likely that many neural systems are activated by electrodes in this group of sites and it is possible that stimulation of any one of a number of systems in this region may support self-stimulation. A second group of self-stimulation sites is in limbic and related areas such as the amygdala, nucleus accumbens, and prefrontal cortex (orbitofrontal cortex in the monkey) (Rolls 1974, 1975, 1976a; Rolls, Burton and Mora, 1980; Mora, Avrith and Rolls 1980). This group of sites is highly interconnected neurophysiologically with the first group lying along the general course of the medial forebrain bundle, in that stimulation in any one of these reward sites activates neurons in the others in primates (Rolls, Burton and Mora 1980; see below).

5.4   The effects of brain lesions on intracranial self-stimulation

Lateral or posterior hypothalamic self-stimulation rate is decreased (but not abolished) by small lesions in or near the medial forebrain bundle, particularly if the lesions are caudal to (i.e. behind) the self-stimulation electrode (Boyd and Gardner 1967; M. Olds and Olds 1969; Stellar and Stellar 1985). Ipsilateral, but not contralateral, lesions are effective. Thus a unilaterally organized system that can be disrupted particularly by posterior lesions at least modulates hypothalamic self-stimulation. Lesions which destroy most of the locus coeruleus do not abolish self-stimulation from regions anterior to it through which its fibres pass, so that it is unlikely that the cells of the locus coeruleus support self-stimulation even from these sites (Clavier 1976; Clavier and Routtenberg 1976). Cells in the dopamine A10 pathway are important for self-stimulation of some sites such as the ventral tegmentum, but not for self-stimulation of all sites, in that neurotoxic lesions of the dopamine inputs to the nucleus accumbens abolish self-stimulation of only some sites (A. Phillips and Fibiger 1989).

It is interesting to note that self-stimulation can occur after ablation of most of the forebrain in rats. Huston and Borbely (1973) were able to show this by requiring only a simple response of tail-raising (or lowering) which their forebrain-ablated rats were able to learn in order to obtain posterior hypothalamic stimulation (although extinction was impaired). This finding underlines the view that self-stimulation can occur because of the activation of one of a number of systems, and suggests that the basic mechanisms for rewarded behaviour must be represented at a low level in the brain. Forebrain areas may be related to reward, not because they are essential for all rewarded behaviour, but because they are concerned with decoding complex sensory inputs and determining whether these inputs are associated as a result of previous learning with reward; and with executing complex, instrumental, motor responses to obtain reward (see below).

Evidence that neurons with cell bodies in the lateral hypothalamus are involved in the reward effects produced by stimulation there comes from studies in which neurotoxic lesions of the lateral hypothalamus (which damage cell bodies there but not fibres of passage such as the dopaminergic fibres) attenuate self-stimulation of the lateral hypothalamus (and of sites anterior to it) (Lestang *et al.* 1995). It is possible that descending lateral hypothalamic neurons that mediate reward synapse on to dopamine neurons in the ventral tegmental area, and that the dopamine connection is important in the reward produced (Wise 1989; Shizgal and Murray 1989). However, the dopamine connection does not appear to be an essential part of the substrate of lateral hypothalamic brain-stimulation reward, for unilateral 6-OHDA lesions of the dopamine cell bodies in the ventral

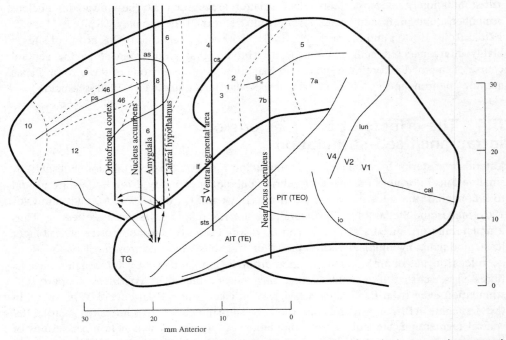

Fig. 5.4 Some brain sites in primates at which electrical stimulation of the brain can produce reward. The arrows indicate that stimulation at any one of these sites activates neurons in all of the other sites connected by arrows, as shown by Rolls, Burton and Mora (1980). The scales show the stereotaxic base planes. Abbreviations as in Fig. 4.1.

tegmentum did not attenuate lateral hypothalamic self-stimulation (A. Phillips and Fibiger 1976; Fibiger *et al.* 1987).

5.5   The neurophysiology of reward

By recording from single neurons while stimulation is delivered at the threshold current to self-stimulation electrodes[1], it is possible to determine which neural systems are actually activated by brain-stimulation reward. In the rat it is clear that during hypothalamic self-stimulation, neurons in the prefrontal cortex, amygdala and some areas of the brainstem, as well as in the hypothalamus itself, are activated (see Rolls 1974, 1975, 1976a; Ito 1976). In the monkey it has been found that neurons in the lateral hypothalamus, orbitofrontal cortex, amygdala, nucleus accumbens, and ventral tegmental area are activated during self-stimulation of any one of these sites or of the nucleus accumbens (see Fig. 5.4 and Rolls 1974, 1975, 1976a; Rolls, Burton and Mora 1980). Thus in the monkey,

---

[1] The threshold current for self-stimulation is the minimum amount of current for a given stimulation pulse-width required to produce self-stimulation at a given self-stimulation site.

there is a highly interconnected set of structures, stimulation in any one of which will support self-stimulation and will activate neurons in the other structures.

5.5.1 Lateral hypothalamus and substantia innominata

Mainly in the monkey, it has been possible to record in the alert, behaving animal from neurons activated by brain-stimulation reward, and to determine whether these neurons are also activated by natural rewards such as food given to the hungry animal or during learning. When recording in the lateral hypothalamus and substantia innominata (which is lateral and rostral to the lateral hypothalamus) from neurons activated by brain-stimulation reward, it was found that some neurons (approximately 13% in one sample of 764 neurons) altered their activity in relation to feeding (Rolls 1975, 1976b, 1979; Rolls, Burton and Mora 1980). These are the same population of hypothalamic neurons with feeding-related responses described in Chapter 2. Indeed, the neurons with feeding-related responses were discovered originally when we sought to determine what functions the hypothalamic neurons activated by brain-stimulation reward perform. In the original sample of 764 neurons, some altered their activity only during the ingestion of some substances, so that their activity appeared to be associated with the taste of food. Many more of these neurons (approximately 11% of the total sample) altered their activity before ingestion started, while the animal was looking at the food (Rolls, Burton and Mora, 1976; Rolls, Sanghera and Roper-Hall 1979b). The activity of this second set of neurons only occurred to the sight of food if the monkey was hungry (Burton, Rolls and Mora 1976b), and becomes associated with the sight of food during learning (Mora, Rolls and Burton 1976b). Thus the activity of these neurons is associated with the sight and/or taste of food in the hungry animal, that is with the presentation of food reward. To determine whether the activity of these neurons precedes, and could thus mediate, the responses of the hungry animal to food reward, their latency of activation was measured using a shutter which opened to reveal a food or a non-food-related visual stimulus (Rolls, Sanghera and Roper-Hall 1979b). The latency for different neurons was 150–200 ms, and compared with a latency of 250–300 ms for the earliest electrical activity recorded from the genioglossus muscle associated with the motor responses of a lick made to obtain food when the food-related visual stimulus was shown (see Fig. 2.9). (Upper motor neuron firing would occur in close temporal relation to the electromyogram recorded from this muscle.) Thus the motor response to the food could not result in the food-related activity of the hypothalamic neurons. This is consistent with the view that these neurons activated both by food reward and brain-stimulation reward are involved in mediating the reactions of the animal to food. These reactions to the food reward include the initiation of feeding behaviour, as well as endocrine and autonomic responses to the food (Fig. 2.8).

These neurons only respond to the sight or taste of food when the monkey is hungry (Burton, Rolls and Mora 1976b; Rolls, Murzi *et al.* 1986). This is part of the evidence that implicates these neurons in the reward produced by the sight or taste of food if hunger is present. It is also thus very interesting that self-stimulation in the lateral hypothalamus is reduced by feeding the monkey to satiety (Rolls, Burton and Mora 1980). As noted earlier, this indicates that the reward produced by the electrical stimulation of the lateral

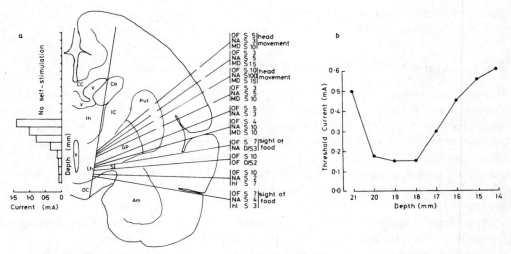

Fig. 5.5 Neurons activated by both brain-stimulation reward and the sight of food were found at the lower end of this microelectrode track in the monkey hypothalamus. Neurons higher up the track in the globus pallidus were activated by brain-stimulation reward and also by head movements. The neurons were trans-synaptically (S) or possibly in some cases directly (D/S) activated with the latencies shown in ms from self-stimulation sites in the orbitofrontal cortex (OF), nucleus accumbens (NA), mediodorsal nucleus of the thalamus (MD), or lateral hypothalamus (hl). Self-stimulation through the recording microelectrode occurred with low currents if the microelectrode was in the hypothalamus close to the neurons activated by the sight of food. (From Rolls 1975; Rolls, Burton and Mora 1980.)

hypothalamus is like food for a hungry monkey, in that the reward value of each is reduced by feeding the monkey to satiety. In an additional experiment, it was shown that the current passed through the microelectrode that had recorded from food-related neurons in the lateral hypothalamus was lowest when the electrode was at the depth of the feeding-related neurons (see Fig. 5.5) (Rolls 1975; Rolls, Burton and Mora 1980). Taken together, these results show that brain-stimulation reward of the lateral hypothalamus occurs because it activates and thus mimics the effects which food reward has on these neurons. In a reciprocal way, the fact that self-stimulation of a number of brain sites, including the lateral hypothalamus, activates these neurons also activated by food when the food is rewarding provides useful evidence that the firing of these neurons actually produced reward. This is one of the valuable outcomes of research on brain-stimulation reward—it helps to show whether the firing of neurons activated by natural rewards is causally related to producing reward, and does not reflect some other process produced by food, such as salivation to food.

It is also worth noting that hypothalamic self-stimulation does not depend on activation of dopamine neurons, in that the refractory periods of directly activated neurons that mediate lateral hypothalamic reward are in the region of 0.6–1.2 ms, whereas the refractory periods of the dopamine neurons, which are small and unmyelinated, are in the range 1.2–2.5 ms (Rolls 1971a,b; Yeomans 1990). Further, dopamine does not appear to be an essential part of the substrate of lateral hypothalamic brain-stimulation reward, for unilateral 6-OHDA lesions of the dopamine cell bodies in the ventral tegmentum did not attenuate lateral hypothalamic self-stimulation (Phillips and Fibiger 1976; Fibiger *et al.* 1987).

5.5.2 Orbitofrontal cortex

The orbitofrontal cortex is one of the brain regions in which excellent self-stimulation is produced in primates (Mora, Avrith, Phillips and Rolls 1979; A. Phillips, Mora and Rolls 1979, 1981; Rolls, Burton and Mora 1980; Mora, Avrith and Rolls, 1980). The self-stimulation is like lateral hypothalamic self-stimulation in that it is learned rapidly, and occurs at a high rate. It has been shown that the self-stimulation of the orbitofrontal cortex is hunger-dependent, in that feeding a monkey to satiety produces great attenuation of orbitofrontal cortex self-stimulation (Mora, Avrith, Phillips and Rolls 1979). Of all the brain-stimulation reward sites studied in the monkey, it is the one at which feeding to satiety has the most profound effect in reducing self-stimulation (Rolls, Burton and Mora 1980). The orbitofrontal self-stimulation pulses have also been shown to drive neurons strongly in the lateral hypothalamus with latencies of only a few ms (Rolls 1975, 1976a; Rolls, Burton and Mora 1980). On the basis of these findings, it was suggested that orbitofrontal cortex stimulation in primates is rewarding because it taps into food-reward mechanisms.

This proposal has been greatly elaborated by the discovery of the way in which the primate orbitofrontal cortex analyses the stimuli that implement food reward (and other types of reward too). The investigations of the neurophysiology of the orbitofrontal cortex that led to these discoveries were prompted by the fact that the orbitofrontal cortex is a good site for brain-stimulation reward, and that lateral hypothalamic food-related neurons are activated by rewarding stimulation of the lateral hypothalamus (Rolls 1974, 1975, 1976a,b; Rolls, Burton and Mora 1980). The discoveries included the following, considered in more detail in Chapters 2 and 4:

1 The secondary taste cortex is in the orbitofrontal cortex (Rolls, Yaxley and Sienkiewicz 1990; L. Baylis, Rolls and Baylis 1994).

2 The representation in the secondary taste cortex is of the reward value of taste, in that the responses of taste neurons here (but not in the primary taste cortex) are reduced to zero when the monkey feeds himself or herself to normal, physiological satiety (Rolls, Sienkiewicz and Yaxley 1989b; Rolls, Scott, Sienkiewicz and Yaxley 1988; Yaxley, Rolls and Sienkiewicz, 1988). There is also a representation of the reward value of the 'taste' of water in the primate orbitofrontal cortex (Rolls, Sienkiewicz and Yaxley, 1989b).

3 The reward value of olfactory stimuli is represented in the secondary and tertiary cortical olfactory areas in the primate orbitofrontal cortex (Critchley and Rolls 1996b), representations which are themselves built for some orbitofrontal olfactory neurons by association with the primary reinforcer of taste (Rolls, Critchley, Mason and Wakeman 1996b; Critchley and Rolls 1996a).

4 The reward value of visual stimuli such as the sight of food is represented in the primate orbitofrontal cortex (Critchley and Rolls 1996b), and the learning of the representation of which visual stimuli are rewarding is built in the orbitofrontal cortex by visual-to-taste reward learning (Rolls, Critchley, Mason and Wakeman 1996b), which can occur in one trial, and be reversed in one trial, by neurons in the

orbitofrontal cortex (Thorpe, Rolls and Maddison 1983; Rolls, Critchley, Mason and Wakeman 1996b).

5 There is a representation of the mouth feel of food, including information about the presence of fat, in the orbitofrontal cortex, mediated through the somatosensory system (see Chapter 2; Rolls 1997b). These sensory inputs converge on to some orbitofrontal neurons that represent the pleasantness or reward value of taste, and are themselves likely to make a major contribution to the evaluation of the palatability (reward value) of food in the mouth (Rolls 1997b).

6 The pleasantness of touch is represented in the human orbitofrontal cortex (Rolls, Francis *et al.* 1997a).

These discoveries thus extend the explanation of why orbitofrontal cortex electrical stimulation can produce reward. It does so by activating representations concerned with the reward value of a whole spectrum of rewarding sensory stimuli, including the taste, smell, and texture of food, the reward value of water, and also the reward value of touch. The fact that brain-stimulation reward of the orbitofrontal cortex occurs supports the evidence that this region implements the reward value of sensory stimuli related to food, as well as to other stimuli. The orbitofrontal cortex may be related to reward not only because it represents the reward value of a number of primary reinforcers (e.g. taste and touch), but also because it is involved in learning associations between primary reinforcers and the stimuli (such as the sight of food) with which they are associated. For this pattern-association learning (and reversal) process, the orbitofrontal cortex must contain a representation of both the primary reinforcer and the to-be-associated (e.g. visual) stimulus (see Appendix; Rolls and Treves 1998). Moreover, the firing of neurons that convey the fact that a secondary reinforcer is reinforcing must themselves if activated produce reward, and this, as well as the activation of representations of primary reinforcers such as taste and touch, implements the reward value of electrical stimulation of the orbitofrontal cortex. It is noted that in rats the reward value of what may be a corresponding though less developed region, the sulcal prefrontal cortex, does not depend on the integrity of the dopamine inputs to this region (see A. Phillips and Fibiger 1989). This suggests that activation of neurons in the orbitofrontal cortex is sufficient to produce reward.

Moreover, the findings considered above are consistent with the possibility that one way in which dopaminergic activation produced by the psychomotor stimulants such as amphetamine and cocaine produces reward is by activating the reward mechanisms just discussed in the orbitofrontal cortex and regions to which it projects such as the nucleus accumbens (see A. Phillips *et al.* 1989; A. Phillips and Fibiger 1990).

5.5.3 Amygdala

Self-stimulation pulses applied to the monkey amygdala activate lateral hypothalamic and orbitofrontal cortex neurons also activated by the taste, sight or smell of food when it is rewarding (Rolls 1976a; Rolls, Burton and Mora 1980). This is one explanation of why electrical stimulation of the amygdala can produce reward. Another, consistent, explanation is that neurons in the amygdala can be activated by the taste of food, or by the sight of food (Sanghera, Rolls and Roper-Hall 1979; Ono *et al.* 1980; Rolls 1992b; Nishijo, Ono and Nishino 1988; Wilson and Rolls 1993, 1999). The underlying conceptual reason though for an involvement of activation of amygdala neurons in brain-stimulation reward is that the amygdala is a region, evolutionarily old, implicated in stimulus-reward association learning (see Chapter 4). For its output to be interpreted as a secondary reinforcer, some part of the output of the amygdala must be interpretable by the rest of the brain as being positively reinforcing; and for the amygdala to play a role in such pattern association learning, the primary reward (e.g. the taste of food) must be represented in the amygdala. Electrical stimulation of the amygdala could also tap into this representation of primary reward. In addition, electrical stimulation of the amygdala may produce reward because it taps into systems concerned more generally with rewards, including those produced by facial expression (see Chapter 4).

5.5.4   Nucleus accumbens

The nucleus accumbens is a self-stimulation site in primates and rats (Rolls 1971b, 1974; Rolls, Burton and Mora 1980). The rewarding electrical stimulation here produces activation of neurons in the lateral hypothalamus and orbitofrontal cortex also activated by the sight and taste of food (Rolls, Burton and Mora 1980). This may be a sufficient explanation for self-stimulation of the nucleus accumbens. However, a more conceptual explanation follows. The accumbens may be a system through which conditioned incentives (secondary reinforcers) learned about in the orbitofrontal cortex and amygdala are connected to behavioural output. Such a connecting role would imply that the animal would work to obtain electrical stimulation of the output, which has to be interpretable as being rewarding if the secondary reinforcing properties of stimuli are to be interpreted by this route by the rest of the brain.

It may be that because dopamine inputs to this region enhance the secondary reinforcing properties of incentive stimuli (Cador, Robbins and Everitt 1989; Everitt and Robbins 1992[2]), presumably by facilitating transmission through the nucleus accumbens, that psychomotor stimulants such as amphetamine and cocaine come to produce their rewarding properties (see Chapter 6). Moreover, brain-stimulation reward of some sites such as the ventral tegmental area where dopamine cell bodies are located occurs because of activation of nucleus accumbens neurons through the dopaminergic ascending connections see (Chapter 6).

5.5.5   Central gray of the midbrain

Electrical stimulation of some regions of the brain can lead to analgesia in animals

---

[2] They showed that amphetamine injections into the nucleus accumbens enhanced the reinforcing properties of conditioned incentive stimuli.

ranging from rats to humans and can be equivalent in its pain-reducing properties to large doses of morphine (Liebeskind and Paul 1977). These analgesic effects can last for hours after only seconds of stimulation. The analgesia is often for only part of the body, so that a strong pinch to one side but not to the other might be ignored. This shows that the stimulation-produced analgesia is not simply some general interference with the animal's ability to respond to stimulation. The effective stimulation sites are in the medial brainstem, and extend from the rostral medulla (nucleus raphe magnus), through the midbrain central grey matter, towards the hypothalamus. There is no clear relation with brain-stimulation reward mechanisms, because at some sites analgesia and self-stimulation are found and at others the stimulation is aversive but is followed by analgesia (see Koob and LeMoal 1997). It has been shown that naloxone, a specific morphine antagonist, reverses, at least partly, stimulation-produced analgesia in both the rat and in humans (Akil, Mayer and Liebeskind 1976; Adams 1976). The endogenous morphine-like peptide enkephalin (Hughes 1975; Hughes *et al.* 1975) injected intraventricularly yields analgesia (Beluzzi *et al.* 1976), and central grey matter stimulation releases this substance or a peptide similar to it (Stein *et al.*, unpublished results, Liebeskind *et al.* 1976). Further, there are stereospecific opiate-binding sites in the central grey matter, and elsewhere in the brain (Kuhar *et al.* 1973). These findings raise the possibility that stimulation-produced analgesia is effective because it causes the release of a naturally occurring morphine-like substance which acts on opiate receptors in the central grey matter and elsewhere to induce analgesia.

The stimulation at these brainstem sites may be rewarding because of activation of enkephalin-containing neurons which make synapses on to the dopamine neurons in the ventral tegmental area (A. Phillips *et al.* 1989). The central gray stimulation may be rewarding because it is part of an endogenous opiate-containing system which controls the threshold for pain, which in emergency situations might be elevated, presumably to avoid being disabled by severe pain in situations which threaten survival.

5.6 Some of the properties of brain-stimulation reward

There are several properties of brain-stimulation reward that seemed surprising when they were discovered. However, these are properties of natural rewards, and by understanding these properties of brain-stimulation reward, we enhance our understanding of some properties of natural rewards.

5.6.1 Lack of satiety with brain-stimulation reward

One of the most striking properties of brain-stimulation reward is its persistence and lack of satiety. A record of a rat working for brain-stimulation reward for 24 h essentially without stopping is shown in Fig. 5.6. At the time that this was first discovered (see, e.g., J. Olds 1958) it seemed quite extraordinary, because normally we do not work for a reward for that long. With eating, for example, we like the taste of food but during the course of a meal its reward value drops to zero, and we no longer work for it. The folk psychology was

48 Hours
Anterior Hypothalamic Electrode # 253

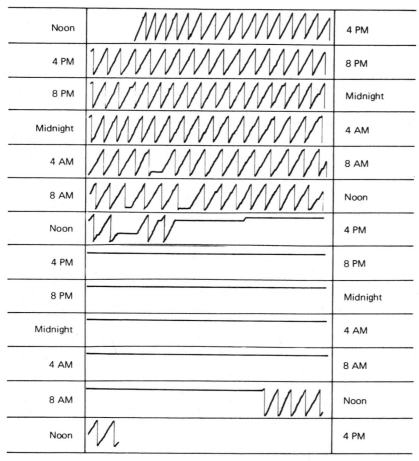

Fig. 5.6 This cumulative record shows that intracranial self-stimulation can be very vigorous and persistent. Each time the rat bar-pressed (for a 0.5-s train of electrical stimulation) the pen stepped once vertically. After 500 steps, it resets to 0. A four-hour time period is shown along the horizontal axis. (From J. Olds 1958.)

that reward somehow produced satiety, so we never worked for a reward for long. But the evidence from brain-stimulation reward showed that reward per se does *not* produce satiety. This finding was useful, because it led to reconsideration of what happens with food reward (see Rolls 1975), which does not, of course, itself produce satiety either, as the sham feeding experiments described in Section 2.2 show very clearly. The point with respect to feeding is that normally when food accumulates in the stomach and intestine it does produce peripheral satiety signals, and these via brain mechanisms reduce the reward value of sensory stimulation produced by the sight, smell, and taste of food, as shown in

Chapter 2. But there is little about food reward per se that produces satiety. The only respect in which giving food reward does affect satiety is that there is some sensory-specific satiety, which, as described in Chapter 2, is sufficient to produce variety effects in food reward, but is not sufficient to reduce food reward to zero, and stop feeding. So the finding of little satiety produced by brain-stimulation reward is actually in line with other rewards, and the persistence of brain-stimulation reward helped to underline this. It is just that normally when we have a food or water reward, we ingest the food or water, and thereby close the loop and produce negative feedback to reduce the reward value of the food. As discussed in Chapter 8, there may be special mechanisms to turn off the rewards associated with sexual behaviour in males just after ejaculation.

The conclusion is that in general reward itself does not produce satiety, apart from some sensory-specific satiety to help behaviour to switch after some time to another reward, and there are special mechanisms usually associated with the rewarded behaviour (such as the ingestion of food) that act to neurally turn off the reward.

5.6.2 Rapid extinction

Extinction from self-stimulation can be very rapid (Seward *et al.* 1959) even when the manipulandum is withdrawn, so that non-rewarded responses are prevented (Howarth and Deutsch 1962). A factor which determines the number of responses in extinction is the time elapsed since the last reward (Howarth and Deutsch 1962) which was not found to be true for thirsty rats trained for water (Quartermain and Webster 1968). Perhaps the major factor which accounts for the rapid extinction of self-stimulation often reported is that no relevant drive is present. If rats are hungry, extinction from brain-stimulation reward is very prolonged (Deutsch and DiCara 1967). Thus one conclusion which can be made from studies with brain-stimulation reward is that resistance to extinction depends on the presence of an appropriate drive. This has probably been demonstrated for conventional reinforcers by Panksepp and Trowill (1967b), who found a trend towards rapid extinction in satiated rats previously rewarded with chocolate milk (insufficient rats were run for a definite conclusion, see Gallistel 1973). Another factor which contributes to rapid extinction is the short time between pressing the manipulandum and receiving brain-stimulation reward, in contrast to the one or two seconds delay between pressing a manipulandum and then finding food or water reward available in a cup (Gibson *et al.* 1965; see also Panksepp and Trowill 1967a). Keesey (1964) also found that errors in learning a brightness discrimination are increased when the brain-stimulation reward is delayed.

5.6.3 Priming

Rats will run along a runway to obtain electrical stimulation at the end of the runway. If some of the electrical stimulation is given in addition at the start of the runway, then the rats will run faster (Gallistel 1969a). The stimulation given at the start of the runway is said to have a priming effect, which decays gradually (see Fig. 5.5—the priming effect decayed over a particularly long time in this rat). Priming stimulation (given by the

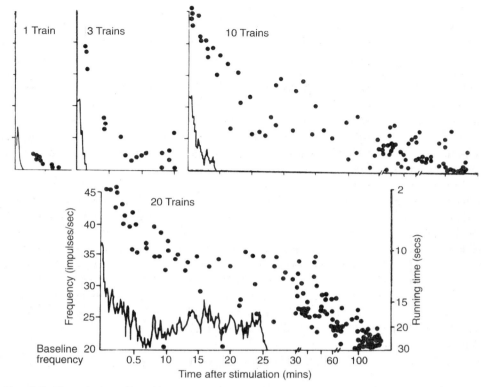

Fig. 5.7 The priming effect of brain-stimulation reward. Running speed (closed circles) for brain-stimulation reward as a function of time after different numbers of priming trains of stimulation given before the first trial (after Gallistel 1969b). The firing rate of a neuron in the reticular activating system of the midbrain as a function of time after different numbers of trains of stimulation delivered at a lateral hypothalamic self-stimulation site is shown for comparison (after Rolls 1971a,c, 1975).

experimenter) can also cause a rat to return to a self-stimulation lever and start self-stimulating. This may be useful if the rat does not bar-press at once when it is put in a self-stimulation box, i.e. if it shows an 'overnight decrement effect'.

One factor that may contribute to the priming effect is arousal. It has been shown that arousal, measured by EEG desynchronization and by increased locomotor activity, is produced by stimulation of reward sites along the medial forebrain bundle (MFB) (Rolls 1971a,c, 1975; Rolls and Kelly 1972). This arousal decays in a very similar way to the priming effect, as shown, for example, in Fig. 5.7. The arousal must at least influence MFB self-stimulation. Because of its similarities to the priming effect, it may well mediate the priming effect, at least in part. Similarities include the temporal nature of the decay, the greater magnitudes and durations of the effects produced by more stimulation trains (see Fig. 5.7), and the refractory periods of the neurons through which the effects are produced (Rolls 1971a,b, 1974). Arousal may contribute not only to priming effects, but also to differences between some self-stimulation sites. For example, arousal is elicited by rewarding stimulation of MFB, but not nucleus accumbens sites, and differences between these sites include hyperactivity and fast rates of self-stimulation at MFB self-stimulation sites (see Rolls 1971c, 1974, 1975).

A second factor that may contribute to priming effects is incentive motivation, that is the motivation that can be produced by giving a reward. For example, if satiated animals are primed with an intraoral reward of chocolate milk, then they will resume bar-pressing to obtain more chocolate milk (Panksepp and Trowill 1967b). It is important that this effect is seen most markedly under zero-drive conditions, e.g. when an animal is neither hungry nor thirsty. These are the conditions under which self-stimulation experiments are often run. Incentive motivation is seen in other situations with natural reward, e.g. as the salted-nut phenomenon (Hebb 1949), and as the increase in the rate of ingestion seen at the start of a meal (LeMagnen 1971).

A third factor that may contribute to priming effects is conflict. Kent and Grossman (1969) showed that only some rats needed priming after an interval in which self-stimulation was prevented by withdrawal of the lever. In the 'primer' rats the stimulation seemed to produce reward and aversion in that self-stimulation was accompanied by squeaking and defecation. It was suggested that during the time away from the bar the reward decayed more rapidly than the aversion, so that self-stimulation was not resumed without priming. It was also found that 'non-primer' rats could be converted into 'primers' by pairing painful tail shock with the brain-stimulation reward. Although Kent and Grossman labelled one group of their rats as 'non-primers', a priming effect can be demonstrated in this type of animal using, for example, a runway (Reid et al. 1973).

Thus there are several explanations of the priming effect which are not necessarily contradictory and which may all contribute to the priming effect.

5.7 Stimulus-bound motivational behaviour

Electrical stimulation at some brain sites can elicit feeding, drinking and other consummatory types of behaviour (see Valenstein et al. 1970). The behaviour may be called 'stimulation-bound' because it occurs during the electrical stimulation or 'stimulus-bound' because the behaviour is associated with a particular goal object, for example food pellets. If small-tipped stimulation electrodes are used relatively specific behaviours are elicited, such as drinking with electrodes near the zona incerta and feeding with electrodes in the lateral hypothalamus (J. Olds et al. 1971; Huang and Mogenson 1972). A frequently observed feature of such behaviour is plasticity, that is stimulus-bound feeding can develop into stimulus-bound drinking if food is removed from the environment and replaced with water (Valenstein et al. 1970). It is as if the stimulation activates the animal and the behaviour which is elicited depends on which environmental stimuli are available for the animal to respond to, for example, food to chew or water to lap. This type of interpretation receives support from the observation that a mild continuous tail-pinch (with, for example, a paper clip) leads to 'stimulus-bound' types of behaviour such as eating in the rat (Antelman and Szechtman 1975). Because of such findings, it is difficult to interpret stimulus-bound behaviour produced by brain stimulation as a proof of activation of a hunger or thirst mechanism—rather it could be a more general type of behavioural activation. It is worth noting that although stimulus-bound behaviour may not represent activation of a specific drive (e.g. hunger), there is evidence that reward elicited by electrical stimulation can be relatively specific. For example, it may be equivalent to food for a hungry animal or water for a thirsty animal (see Section 5.2).

5.8 Conclusions

Animals, including humans, will learn to stimulate electrically certain areas of the brain. At some sites the stimulation may be equivalent to a natural reward such as food for a hungry animal, in that hunger increases working for brain-stimulation reward at these (but not at other) sites. It has been found in the monkey that one population of neurons activated by the brain-stimulation reward at these sites is in the region of the lateral hypothalamus and substantia innominata. Some of these neurons are also activated by the sight and/or taste of food if the monkey is hungry, that is when the food is rewarding. The latency of the responses of these neurons to the sight of food is 150–200 ms. This is longer than the responses of sensory neurons to visual stimuli in the inferotemporal cortex and dorsolateral amygdala, but shorter than the latency of the animal's behavioural responses to the sight of food, as shown by electrographic recording of the muscles that implement the motor responses. Thus it is possible that these hypothalamic neurons mediate some of the reactions of the hungry animal to food reward, such as the initiation of feeding and/or autonomic and endocrine responses. In a comparable way, brain-stimulation reward of the primate orbitofrontal cortex occurs because it is activating systems normally concerned with decoding and representing taste, olfactory and tactile rewards. In this way reward-related processes can be identified and studied by analysing the operations (from sensory input through central control processes to motor output) which are involved in the responses of animals to rewarding stimuli. Self-stimulation of some sites may occur because neurons whose activity is associated with food reward are activated by stimulation at these sites. At other sites, brain-stimulation reward may be produced because the stimulation mimics other types of natural reward such as, in the nucleus accumbens, the effects of secondary reinforcers. At other sites, as shown by verbal reports in humans, the electrical stimulation is rewarding because it is producing mood states such as a feeling of happiness normally produced by emotional stimuli.

The findings with brain-stimulation reward are helpful, because they provide additional evidence about whether a particular part of the brain is involved in reward processes. Consistent with this point, in general brain-stimulation reward does not occur early in sensory processing (e.g. in visual cortical areas up to and including the inferior temporal visual cortex), where on independent grounds it is believed that in primates the reward value of stimuli is not represented (see Chapter 4). Nor does brain-stimulation reward occur in general in motor structures such as the globus pallidus (see Fig. 5.5), nor in motor cortical areas (see Rolls 1974, 1975). Thus the evidence from brain-stimulation reward complements the other evidence described in this book that it is at special stages of the pathways which lead from sensory input to motor output that reward is represented, and that this is part of brain design (see further Chapters 2, 4, and 10).

Brain-stimulation reward also historically helped to draw attention to important points, such as the fact that reward per se does not produce satiety (Section 5.6.1); and that the time between the operant response and the delivery of the reward (or a stimulus associated with the reward) has important implications for what happens when the reward is no longer available (Section 5.6.2).

5.9 Apostasis[3]

There was a great deal of research on electrical brain-stimulation reward in the years after its discovery (reported by J. Olds and Milner in 1954) until 1980. After that, research on brain-stimulation reward tailed off. Why was this? I think that one reason was that by the middle 1970s it was becoming possible to study reward mechanisms in the brain directly, by recording from single neurons, in order to provide a fundamental understanding of how natural rewards are being processed by the brain (see Rolls 1974, 1975, and this book). This led to the analysis of the neural mechanisms involved in the sensory processing, and eventually the decoding of the reward value, in the taste, olfactory, visual, and touch systems of primates. In the case of visual processing, this involved investigating the learning mechanisms that enable visual stimuli to be decoded as rewarding based on pattern-association learning between visual stimuli and primary reinforcers such as taste (see Rolls and Treves 1998). By analysing such sensory information processing, an explanation of why electrical stimulation of some parts of the brain could produce reward became evident. At the same time, the investigations of brain-stimulation reward were very helpful, because they provided additional evidence that neurons putatively involved in reward because of the nature of their responses (e.g. hypothalamic, orbitofrontal cortex, or amygdala neurons responding to the sight, smell, or taste of food) were actually involved in food reward, because electrical stimulation which activated these neurons could produce reward (see Rolls 1975; this chapter; Chapters 2 and 4). In a comparable way, electrical brain-stimulation reward was also of significance because it pointed the way towards brain regions such as the ventral tegmental area dopamine neurons, which, via their projections to the nucleus accumbens, can influence brain processing normally involved in connecting stimuli in the environment decoded as being rewarding by the amygdala and orbitofrontal cortex, to behavioural output. The implication of this brain system in reward led eventually to the discoveries that this neural system, and its projections to the orbitofrontal cortex, are involved in the rewarding and indeed addictive properties of drugs of abuse such as amphetamine and cocaine (A. Phillips, Mora and Rolls 1981; A. Phillips and Fibiger 1989; Koob and LeMoal 1997; see Chapter 6).

A second reason why research on electrical brain-stimulation reward decreased after about 1980 is that it then became possible to study the pharmacological substrates of

---

[3] Apostasis, from the Greek, meaning standing apart or away from; hence a meta-statement (literally an 'about' statement) or a comment. Different from the Latin p.s. (post-script) which means written after, which an apostatic statement might not be.

reward not only by investigating how pharmacological agents affect electrical brain-stimulation reward, which required very careful controls to show that the drugs did not affect rewarded behaviour just because of motor or arousal side effects (see Chapter 6), but also by investigating directly the self-administration of pharmacological agents, both systemically, and even directly to the brain (e.g. A. Phillips, Mora and Rolls 1981). The results of these investigations, described in Chapter 6, taken together with the increasing understanding of brain mechanisms involved in natural reward processing and learning (see Chapters 4 and 2), led directly to rapid advances in understanding the processing in the neural systems that provides the neural basis of the self-administration of drugs (see Chapter 6).

Brain-stimulation reward, though less investigated today, does nevertheless provide a way to present repeatedly for hours on end a reward which does not satiate. Indeed, the persistence of responding to obtain brain-stimulation reward was one of the startling facts that led to the clear exposition of how reward and satiety signals are very distinct in their sensory origin, and how motivational signals such as hunger and thirst actually modulate the reward value of sensory input produced, for example, by the taste of food (see Chapter 2). Studies with brain-stimulation reward emphasized the fact that (apart from some sensory-specific satiety), the delivery of reward per se does not produce satiety.

6 Pharmacology and neurochemistry of reward, and neural output systems for reward

6.1 Introduction

It is well established that pharmacological manipulations of the catecholamine transmitters in the brain (dopamine and noradrenaline) alter self-stimulation rate (see Rolls 1975). For example, amphetamine, which enhances the release of dopamine and noradrenaline from axon terminals at synapses, increases hypothalamic self-stimulation rate. Drugs which reduce catecholamine levels (e.g. α-methyl-p-tyrosine) or which block catecholamine receptors (e.g. the 'neuroleptic' or 'anti-psychotic' drugs chlorpromazine, haloperidol, and spiroperidol) reduce self-stimulation rates. These catecholamine systems have been teased apart, and it is now clear that dopamine and not noradrenaline is involved in brain-stimulation reward (Section 6.2), but that dopamine is involved in brain-stimulation reward at only some sites (Section 6.3.1).

This evidence is complemented by findings with self-administration of the psychomotor stimulant addictive drugs amphetamine and cocaine, which produce their reward by acting on the dopaminergic projection to the nucleus accumbens (see Section 6.3.2), itself implicated in the secondary reinforcing properties of stimuli.

Dopamine appears to modulate transmission which links reward systems in structures such as the amygdala and orbitofrontal cortex via their connections to the ventral striatum to behavioural response selection and execution systems. This leads to an examination in Section 6.4 of the functions of the basal ganglia in behavioural output.

In the remainder of this section, an introduction to some of the pharmacology of the dopamine systems in the brain is provided, because of its importance in understanding the pharmacology of reward.

The two catecholamines found in the brain with which we are concerned are dopamine (DA) and noradrenaline (NA) (which is also known by its Greek name norepinephrine). A schematic view of a dopaminergic synapse showing some of the ways in which pharmacological agents used to analyse self-stimulation affect its function is shown in Fig. 6.1 (see also Cooper, Bloom and Roth 1996). Tyrosine is converted to dihydroxyphenylalanine (DOPA) in the presence of the enzyme tyrosine hydroxylase. The drug α-methyl-p-tyrosine blocks this step, and thus inhibits the synthesis of DA. DOPA is then converted to DA. (In noradrenergic synapses, DA is converted to NA in the presence of the enzyme dopamine-β-hydroxylase. This latter step is inhibited by disulfiram, so that the administration of disulfiram prevents the synthesis of NA but not of DA.) Dopamine is normally released from the presynaptic membrane in vesicles when an action potential occurs. The

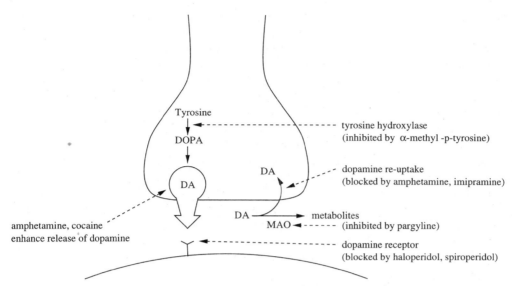

Fig. 6.1 Schematic diagram showing how pharmacological agents affect a dopaminergic synapse. The presynaptic terminal above is shown separated by the synaptic cleft from the postsynaptic cell below. DOPA, dihydroxyphenylalanine; DA, dopamine; MAO, monoamine oxidase.

released dopamine travels across the synaptic cleft to activate dopamine receptors (of which there are several types) in the postsynaptic membrane. The pharmacological agents haloperidol, spiroperidol, and pimozide block the DA receptors in the postsynaptic membrane. The drug amphetamine enhances the release of DA from the presynaptic membrane.

After dopamine is released into the synapse, and some of it activates the postsynaptic receptors, the remaining dopamine is removed from the synapse quickly by a number of mechanisms. One is reuptake into the presynaptic terminal. This process involves dopamine transporter (DAT), and is blocked by amphetamine and by cocaine, which both thus increase the concentration of dopamine in the synapse. Another mechanism for removing DA from the synapse is by monoamine oxidase (MAO), which destroys the DA. MAO is present in the synapse, and also in the presynaptic mechanism. MAO inhibitors (MAOI) thus also increase the concentration of DA in the synapse (and also of NA in noradrenergic synapses, and 5-hydroxytryptamine (5-HT, serotonin) in serotonergic synapses). Another mechanism is diffusion out of the synaptic cleft.

A number of comparisons between noradrenergic and dopaminergic mechanisms can usefully be remembered when interpreting the actions of pharmacological agents on self-stimulation. α-Methyl-p-tyrosine inhibits the synthesis of NA and DA, while disulfiram inhibits the synthesis of NA but not DA. Amphetamine releases both NA and DA. Phentolamine blocks NA-receptors but not DA-receptors. Spiroperidol and pimozide block DA-receptors and not NA-receptors. Chlorpromazine and haloperidol block both DA- and NA-receptors to some extent (as well as having other actions). The drug 6-hydroxydopamine can cause degeneration of both NA and DA nerve terminals. Some of the antidepressant drugs (such as the tricyclic reuptake inhibitors, and the MAOIs) facilitate both NA and DA mechanisms, but also considerably 5-HT mechanisms.

The catecholamines DA and NA (norepinephrine) are located in brain cells whose course has been traced using histofluorescence techniques (see Dahlström and Fuxe 1965; Ungerstedt 1971; Bjorklund and Lindvall 1986; Cooper *et al.* 1996). The mesostriatal dopamine projection (see Fig. 6.2) originates mainly (but not exclusively) from the A9 dopamine cell group in the substantia nigra, pars compacta, and projects to the (dorsal or neo-) striatum, in particular the caudate nucleus and putamen. The mesolimbic dopamine system originates mainly from the A10 cell group, and projects to the nucleus accumbens and olfactory tubercle, which together constitute the ventral striatum (see Fig. 6.2). In addition there is a mesocortical dopamine system projecting mainly from the A10 neurons to the frontal cortex, but especially in primates also to other cortical areas, including parts of the temporal cortex. However, these pathways are not completely separate from the mesostriatal projection system, in that the A10 neurons project into the ventromedial part of the striatum, and in that a dorsal and medial set of neurons in the A9 region with horizontally oriented dendrites project into the olfactory tubercle and amygdala (see A. Phillips and Fibiger 1989).

The ascending noradrenergic pathways, at one time suggested to be involved in brain-stimulation reward, are as follows. Noradrenaline cell bodies in the locus coeruleus (cell group A6 according to nomenclature of Dahlström and Fuxe 1965) give rise to ascending pathways which form a dorsal bundle in the pons and midbrain, ascend through the medial forebrain bundle, and innervate the cortex and hippocampus (Fig. 6.3). The 'ventral NA pathway' arises from cell groups A1, A2, A5, and A7, and has terminals in the lower brain stem, midbrain, and hypothalamus and preoptic area.

6.2 The noradrenergic hypothesis

Stein (1967, 1969), noting the points made in the first paragraph of Section 6.1, and that many self-stimulation sites occurred along the course of the dorsal noradrenergic bundle from its origin in the locus coeruleus (cell group A6) through the hypothalamus towards its termination in the neocortex, formulated the noradrenergic theory of reward. According to this theory, activation of noradrenergic axons in this pathway by electrical stimulation at self-stimulation sites and the consequent release of noradrenaline at its terminals, mediates brain-stimulation reward (Stein 1967, 1969; Crow 1976). Evidence against this theory comes from several sources. Rolls (1974) found that rats treated with disulfiram, which depletes the brain of noradrenaline, could self-stimulate if aroused, but were usually too drowsy to do so. Rolls, Kelly and Shaw (1974) came to a similar conclusion when they found that the doses of disulfiram required to reduce hypothalamic self-stimulation rates produced a major attenuation of spontaneous locomotor activity. Interestingly, the dopamine receptor-blocking agents pimozide or spiroperidol (used following an earlier study by Wauquier and Niemegeers 1972) produced a much greater attenuation of self-stimulation rate than of locomotor activity, suggesting that dopamine was more closely related to brain-stimulation reward at these sites than was noradrenaline. Clavier and

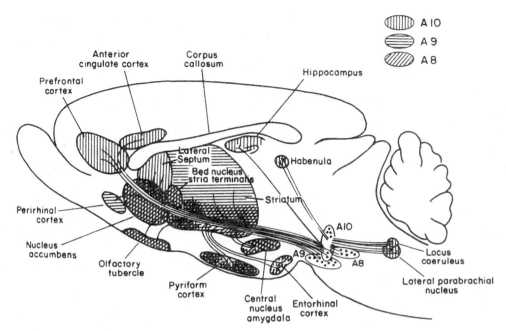

A 10
A 9
A 8

Anterior cingulate cortex

Corpus callosum

Hippocampus

Prefrontal cortex

Lateral Septum

Bed nucleus stria terminalis

Habenula

Striatum

A10

Perirhinal cortex

A9

A8

Nucleus accumbens

Locus coeruleus

Olfactory tubercle

Pyriform cortex

Central nucleus amygdala

Entorhinal cortex

Lateral parabrachial nucleus

Fig. 6.2 Schematic diagram illustrating the distribution of the main central neuronal pathways containing dopamine. The stippled regions indicate the major nerve-terminal areas and their cell groups of origin. The cell groups in this figure are named according to the nomenclature of Dahlström and Fuxe (1965). The A9 cell group in the substantia nigra pars compacta is one of the main DA-containing cell groups, and gives rise mainly to the nigro-striatal dopamine pathway terminating in the striatum. The A10 cell group in the ventral tegmental area is the other main DA-containing cell group, and gives rise mainly to the meso-limbic DA pathway which terminates in the nucleus accumbens and the olfactory tubercle (together known as the ventral striatum), and the meso-cortical DA pathway which terminates in prefrontal, anterior cingulate, and some other cortical areas. (Reprinted with permission from Cooper, Bloom and Roth 1996.)

Routtenberg's finding (1976; see also Clavier 1976) that lesions to the locus coeruleus did not attenuate self-stimulation along the course of the dorsal noradrenergic bundle also argues strongly against the noradrenergic theory of reward.

6.3 Dopamine and reward

6.3.1 Dopamine and electrical self-stimulation of the brain

There is better evidence that dopamine is involved in self-stimulation of some brain sites. Following the observation described above, that dopamine-receptor blockade with spiroperidol attenuated hypothalamic self-stimulation without producing an arousal deficit (Rolls, Kelly and Shaw 1974a), it was shown that spiroperidol attenuated self-stimulation at different sites in the rat (Rolls, Kelly and Shaw 1974a, Rolls, Rolls, Kelly, Shaw and Dale 1974b). It was also shown that spiroperidol attenuated self-stimulation even when the motor response required to obtain the stimulation was made simple in order to minimize

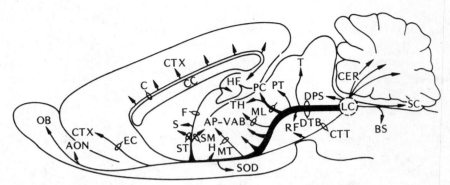

Fig. 6.3 Diagram of the projections of the locus coeruleus noradrenergic pathways viewed in the sagittal plane. Abbreviations: AON, anterior olfactory nucleus; AP-VAB, ansa peduncularis–ventral amygdaloid bundle system; BS, brainstem nuclei; C, cingulum; CC, corpus callosum; CER, cerebellum; CTT, central tegmental tract; CTX, cerebral neocortex; DPS, dorsal periventricular system; DTB, dorsal catecholamine bundle; EC, external capsule; F, fornix; H, hypothalamus; HF, hippocampal formation; LC, locus coeruleus; ML, medial lemniscus, MT, mammillothalamic tract; OB, olfactory bulb; PC, posterior commissure; PT, pretectal area; RF, reticular formation; S, septal area; SC, spinal cord; SM, stria medullaris; SOD, supraoptic decussations; ST, stria terminalis; T, tectum; TH, thalamus. (Reprinted with permission from Cooper, Bloom and Roth 1996.)

the effect of motor impairment (Mora, Sanguinetti, Rolls and Shaw 1975). Spiroperidol also attenuates self-stimulation in the monkey (Mora, Rolls, Burton and Shaw 1976c). These findings were consistent with the observation that self-stimulation in the rat can be obtained in the ventral mesencephalon near the A10 dopamine-containing cell bodies (Crow *et al.* 1972), and in the monkey from the nucleus accumbens (Rolls, Burton and Mora 1980). However, strong supporting evidence is needed in view of the situation emphasized by Rolls and his colleagues that it is difficult to exclude the possibility that dopamine-receptor blockade interferes with self-stimulation by producing a motor impairment (see also Fibiger 1978). Evidence supporting a role for dopamine in brain-stimulation reward came from experiments with apomorphine, which directly stimulates dopamine receptors. It was found that apomorphine attenuates self-stimulation of the prefrontal cortex in the rat and of the comparable region in the monkey, the orbitofrontal cortex (Mora, Phillips, Koolhaas and Rolls 1976a). Both areas are rich in dopamine-containing terminals of the mesocortical (A10) dopamine system. An attenuation of self-stimulation by the dopamine-receptor stimulant apomorphine would be predicted in a system in which the release of dopamine influenced the reward produced by stimulation of the prefrontal cortex.

In these experiments, self-stimulation with electrodes in the caudate nucleus was not attenuated by the apomorphine, so that this self-stimulation could not depend on dopamine (even though dopamine is present in this region), and the attenuation of prefrontal self-stimulation produced by the apomorphine could not have been due to a general disruption of behaviour. In a further investigation of the role of dopamine in brain-stimulation reward in the prefrontal cortex, it has been found that the administration of apomorphine intravenously decreases the firing rate of neurones in the medial prefrontal cortex of the rat (Mora, Sweeney, Rolls and Sanguinetti 1976d) (as does the local iontophoretic administration of dopamine—Bunney and Aghajanian 1976), and that dopamine is released from this region during electrical stimulation of medial prefrontal reward sites (Mora and Myers 1977). This evidence thus suggests that the mesocortical dopamine system can influence brain-stimulation reward of the prefrontal cortex in the rat and the corresponding orbitofrontal cortex in the monkey, but dopamine may not be essential for self-stimulation of the prefrontal cortex, as lesions of the dopaminergic fibres which ascend to the prefrontal cortex may not abolish prefrontal self-stimulation (A. Phillips and Fibiger 1978).

In studies with unilateral lesions of the dopamine pathways, it has been found that damage to the dopamine pathways attenuates brain-stimulation reward of the far lateral hypothalamus where the dopamine pathways project, but not in a more central part of the lateral hypothalamus, nor in the nucleus accumbens, and only partly in the medial prefrontal cortex (Fibiger *et al.* 1987; see A. Phillips and Fibiger 1989). This again indicates that activation of dopamine pathways may be sufficient for brain-stimulation reward, but is not involved in brain-stimulation reward of all brain sites. When electrodes are activating the dopaminergic A10 system, for example when the electrodes are in the ventral tegmental area, the system through which the reward is mediated appears to be via the dopamine terminals in the nucleus accumbens, in that injections of the dopamine receptor-blocking agent spiroperidol into the nucleus accumbens attenuated the tegmental self-stimulation (Mogenson *et al.* 1979). Thus, when dopamine is involved in brain-stimulation reward, the reward appears to be mediated by tapping into the nucleus accumbens system, a system which is involved in learned incentive effects on behaviour (see Sections 4.6.2, 5.5.4, and 6.4). The evidence described in Section 6.3.2 implicates this ventral striatal system also in the reward produced by systemic self-administration of the psychomotor stimulant drugs such as amphetamine and cocaine.

Thus there is reasonable evidence that dopamine is involved in brain-stimulation reward of some sites, for example of the ventral tegmental area where the A10 dopamine neuron cell bodies are located, but that dopamine is not involved in self-stimulation at all sites. Analyses of the pharmacology of brain-stimulation reward do need to show that reward, rather than performance, is affected by experimental variables. Effects on self-stimulation rate are difficult to interpret unless (as shown above) controls for side effects on performance are included. Also, as emphasized by Fibiger (1978), drug effects may depend on the initial rate of bar-pressing shown by the animal. But to equalize initial self-stimulation rates at different sites does not help, because although the self-stimulation rate at some sites may be low, stimulation at these sites may be preferred to stimulation at other sites (Valenstein 1964), and this could influence the effects of drugs. With rate measures, it is at least necessary to determine how the rate of bar-pressing is affected by the stimulation current intensity and to determine how this relation is affected by experimental variables. This has led to the use in more recent studies (see A. Phillips and Fibiger 1989) of graphs which show how the rate of self-stimulation is related to the current intensity (see e.g. Fig. 6.4). If this rate-intensity curve is moved to the left by a treatment, the implication is that the treatment has resulted in more reward for each lever press (because less current per press is needed). Conversely, if the curve moves to the right, this is interpreted as less reward per press, in that more current for each press is required to maintain responding at half its maximal rate. Other measures of reward are time spent in the side of the box in which stimulation is given and a runway in which reward can be measured independently of performance (Edmonds and Gallistel 1977; A. Phillips and Fibiger 1989; Stellar and Rice 1989).

Self-stimulation of sites in the ventral tegmental area (VTA, where there are cell bodies of the A10 dopamine neurons that project to the nucleus accumbens) increases the release of dopamine in the nucleus accumbens (Fiorino et al. 1993), and VTA self-stimulation (but not substantia nigra pars compacta self-stimulation) was abolished by dopamine depleting lesions at the hypothalamic level (A. Phillips et al. 1982). Consistently, blocking dopamine receptors in the nucleus accumbens with spiroperidol reduced self-stimulation of the ipsilateral (but not in an elegant control of the contralateral) VTA (Mogenson et al. 1979). Moreover, dopamine-depleting lesions of the nucleus accumbens (with 6-hydroxydopamine) attenuate self-stimulation of the ventral tegmental area (see A. Phillips and Fibiger 1989). A conclusion from these studies is that dopamine neurons in the VTA can support self-stimulation behaviour, but that non-dopaminergic neurons can also support brain-stimulation reward even in forebrain areas such as the nucleus accumbens and medial prefrontal cortex to which the dopamine neurons project (A. Phillips and Fibiger 1989). The unsurprising implication of the latter conclusion is that in the regions in which dopamine fibres make synapses, electrical stimulation of the postsynaptic neurons can produce reward.

Amphetamine can increase the reward value of brain-stimulation reward in regions such as the ventral tegmental area and posterior hypothalamus where the stimulation activates the dopamine system (see A. Phillips and Fibiger 1989; Koob 1992). The facilitation is measured in a rate of lever pressing vs current intensity curve, which shifts to the left when amphetamine or cocaine is present (see Fig. 6.4). This implies that each press produces more reward, because each train of electrical stimulation produced by a lever press releases more dopamine when amphetamine is present.

6.3.2 Self-administration of dopaminergic substances

In this section evidence is summarized that a major class of drug, the psychomotor stimulants such as amphetamine and cocaine, produce their reward by acting on a dopaminergic mechanism in the nucleus accumbens (see Liebman and Cooper 1989; A. Phillips and Fibiger 1990; Koob 1992, 1996; Koob and LeMoal 1997; Everitt, 1997), which receives a dopaminergic input from the A10 cell group in the ventral tegmental area. These drugs are addictive, and understanding their mode of action in the brain helps to clarify how these drugs produce their effects.

i) Amphetamine (which increases the release of dopamine and noradrenaline) is self-administered intravenously by humans, monkeys, rats, etc.

ii) Amphetamine self-injection intravenously is blocked by dopamine receptor blockers such as pimozide and spiroperidol (Yokel and Wise 1975). The implication is that the psychomotor stimulants produce their reward by causing the release of dopamine

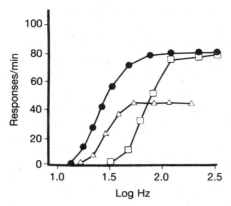

Fig. 6.4 Amphetamine can increase the reward value of brain-stimulation reward in regions such as the ventral tegmental area and posterior hypothalamus where the stimulation activates the dopamine system (see Koob 1992; A. Phillips and Fibiger 1989). Pimozide or spiroperidol, which block dopamine receptors, can reduce the reward value of brain-stimulation reward. This can be measured in graphs showing the rate of lever pressing (responses/min) vs the frequency (in Hz) of the brain stimulation pulses obtained for each lever press. Such a graph is shown with no drug as filled circles. After pimozide, the curve (open squares) moves to the right, interpreted as showing that more pulses of brain stimulation are needed with pimozide to produce the same amount of reward. If the curve is shifted down (open triangles), this indicates that the drug interferes with performance, e.g. the ability of the animal to work, and this can be produced by high doses of pimozide. Amphetamine has the effect of shifting the baseline curve to the left (not shown). This implies that each press produces more reward, because each train of electrical stimulation produced by a lever press releases more dopamine when amphetamine is present. (After Stellar and Rice 1989.)

which acts on dopamine receptors. The receptor blocker at first increases the rate at which the animal will work for the intravenous injection. The reason for this is that with each lever press for amphetamine less reward is produced than without the receptor blockade, so the animal works more to obtain the same net amount of reward. This is typical of what happens with low rate operant response behaviour when the magnitude of the reward is reduced. The rate increase is a good control which shows that the dopamine receptor blockade at the doses used does not produce its reward reducing effect by interfering with motor responses.

iii) Apomorphine (which activates D2 dopamine receptors) is self-administered intravenously.

iv) Intravenous self-administration of indirect DA-agonists such as d-amphetamine and cocaine is much decreased by 6-OHDA lesions of the nucleus accumbens (see Lyness *et al.* 1979; Roberts *et al.* 1980; Koob 1992, 1996). In a complementary way, the self-administration of the psychomotor stimulants increases the release of dopamine in the nucleus accumbens (Di Chiara *et al.* 1992).

v) Rats will learn to self-administer very small quantities of amphetamine to the nucleus accumbens. This effect is abolished by 6-OHDA lesions of the meso-limbic dopamine pathway.

vi) It is however notable that the self-administration of opiates and alcohol occurs even when the meso–limbic dopamine system is lesioned (Koob 1992; Koob and LeMoal 1997).

All these points of evidence combine to show that the psychomotor stimulants (though not other self-administered drugs) produce their effects by an action on the nucleus accumbens (see further Koob and LeMoal 1997). The neural substrate for this reward effect in the nucleus accumbens will be considered later in the light of the evidence described in the next few sections. The nucleus accumbens may however not be the only place in the primate brain where dopamine release can produce reward, for A. Phillips, Mora and Rolls (1981) showed that monkeys will learn to self-administer very small quantities of amphetamine to the orbitofrontal cortex, which receives a strong projection from the dopamine pathways. Presumably dopaminergic substances produce reward in the orbitofrontal cortex by influencing the reward systems known to be present in this region. The reward signals processed in the orbitofrontal cortex include the sight, smell, and taste of food, pleasure produced by touch, and probably the reward value of face expression (see Chapters 2 and 4).

6.3.3 Behaviours associated with the release of dopamine

The functional role of dopamine can be investigated by determining what factors influence its release. The release can be assayed by push–pull techniques in which a slow stream of fluid is transfused through a small cannula in the ventral striatum, and fluid is at the same time sucked out through another tube, allowing chemical assay of substances in the transfusate. Another method is to use in vivo chronoamperometry using stearate-modified graphite paste electrodes to monitor changes in dopamine release (A. Phillips *et al.* 1991). Preparatory behaviours for feeding, including foraging for food, food hoarding, and performing instrumental responses to obtain food, are more associated with dopamine release than is the consummatory behaviour of feeding itself (A. Phillips *et al.* 1991). In a complementary way, dopamine-depleting lesions of the nucleus accumbens disrupt appetitive behaviour produced by food-related stimuli at doses that do not affect eating itself. Similarly, Everitt *et al.* (1989) showed in rats that neurotoxic lesions of the basolateral amygdala reduced the rate of operant responding for a secondary sexual reward but not copulatory behaviour itself, and that infusions of amphetamine to the nucleus accumbens restored rates of working for the secondary sexual reward. In another study, Pfaus *et al.* (1990) showed that dopamine release in the nucleus accumbens increased in male rats during a 10 min period in which a male and female rat were placed in the same enclosure but were separated by a wire mesh screen, and increased further when the rats were allowed to copulate (see also A. Phillips *et al.* 1991). The dopamine release decreased after the first ejaculation. If a new female was placed behind the mesh screen, the dopamine release increased again, and sexual behaviour was reinstated (Fiorini, Coury and Phillips 1997). (The reinstatement is known as the Coolidge effect.) In a whole series of studies, Robbins *et al.* (1989) showed that conditioned reinforcers (for food) increase the release of dopamine in the nucleus accumbens, and that dopamine-depleting lesions of the nucleus accumbens attenuate the effect of conditioned (learned) incentives on behaviour.

Although the majority of the studies have focused on rewarded behaviour, there is also evidence that dopamine can be released by stimuli that are aversive. For example, Rada, Mark and Hoebel (1998) showed that dopamine was released in the nucleus accumbens when rats worked to escape from aversive hypothalamic stimulation (see also Hoebel 1997; Leibowitz and Hoebel 1998). Also, Gray, Young and Joseph (1997) describe evidence that dopamine can be released in the nucleus accumbens during stress, unavoidable foot-shock, and by a light or a tone associated by Pavlovian conditioning with footshock which produces fear. The necessary condition for the release of dopamine may actually be that an active behavioural response, such as active avoidance of punishment, or working to obtain food, is performed. It may not be just the delivery of reward or stimuli which signal reward. Although the most likely process to enhance the release of dopamine in the ventral striatum is an increase in the firing of dopamine neurons, another process is the release of dopamine by a presynaptic influence on the dopamine terminals in the nucleus accumbens. Also consistent with a rather non-specific, activation-related, condition for dopamine release, dopamine release from the meso-cortical dopamine system can be produced by simple manipulations such as stress (Abercrombie *et al.* 1989; Thierry *et al.* 1976).

6.3.4 The activity of dopaminergic neurons and reward

Schultz *et al.* (1995b) have argued from their recordings from dopamine neurons that the firing of these neurons might be involved in reward. For example, dopamine neurons can respond to the taste of a liquid reward in an operant task. However, these neurons may stop responding to such a primary (unlearned) reinforcer quite rapidly as the task is learned, and instead respond only to the earliest indication that a trial of the task is about to begin (Schultz *et al.* 1995b). Thus they could not convey information about a primary reward obtained if the trial is successful, but instead appear to convey information which would be much better suited to a preparation or 'Go' role for dopamine release in the striatum. The evidence that is needed on this issue is whether dopamine neurons respond when the animal has to initiate behaviour actively to escape from or avoid aversive (e.g. painful) stimuli. Although Mirenowicz and Schultz (1996) did record from presumed dopamine neurons when an aversive stimulus such as a puff of air was delivered, and found little activation of dopamine neurons, the monkeys were performing passive avoidance, that is shutting down action. If the neurons do respond when the monkey must initiate action, for example by making several operant responses to escape from or avoid an aversive stimulus, then this would be evidence that the firing of dopamine neurons is related to 'Go' rather than to reward. Some of the evidence reviewed in Section 6.3.3 that the dopamine projection does not convey a specific 'reward' signal is that dopamine release occurs not only to rewards (such as food or brain-stimulation reward, or later in training to an indication that a reward might be given later), but also to aversive stimuli such as aversive stimulation of the medial hypothalamus, foot-shock, and stimuli associated with footshock (see Hoebel *et al.* 1996; Rada, Mark and Hoebel 1998; Hoebel 1997; Leibowitz and Hoebel 1998; Gray, Young and Joseph 1997). (The dopamine release might in this case be related to the firing of dopamine neurons, or to presynaptic terminals on to the dopamine terminals in the nucleus accumbens which cause the release of dopamine.) These findings are much more consistent with the hypothesis that instead of acting as the reinforce or error signal in a reinforcement learning system, as suggested by Houk *et al.*

(1995), the dopamine projection to the striatum may act as a 'Go' or 'preparation' signal to set the thresholds of neurons in the striatum, and/or as a general modulatory signal that could help to strengthen synapses of conjunctively active pre- and postsynaptic neurons. In such a system, what is learned would be dependent on the presynaptic firing of all the input axons and the postsynaptic activation of the neuron, and would not be explicitly guided by a reinforce/teacher signal that would provide feedback *after* each trial on the degree of success of each trial as in the reinforcement learning algorithm (see Appendix section A.3 and Rolls and Treves 1998, Chapters 5 and 9). The facts that many of the neurons in the head of the caudate nucleus, and in some other parts of the striatum, respond in relation to signals which indicate that behaviour should be initiated (see Section 6.4.3), and that connections from these striatal regions as well as from the hypothalamus reach the dopamine neurons in the substantia nigra, pars compacta, and ventral tegmental area, are fully consistent with the hypothesis that the dopamine neurons are not activated only by reward-related stimuli, but more generally by stimuli including punishing stimuli that can lead to the initiation of behaviour.

6.4 The basal ganglia as an output system for emotional and motivational behaviour, and the pharmacology of this system in relation to reward

To provide a foundation for understanding how dopamine in the basal ganglia is related to the operation of reward systems in the brain, we now consider some aspects of the operation of the basal ganglia. However, in addition, we consider more generally the operation of the basal ganglia, for they provide one of the important output information processing systems in the brain concerned with emotion and motivation (see Section 4.6).

One key issue is the type of information which reaches the basal ganglia from systems such as the amygdala and orbitofrontal cortex, and whether this includes information about rewards and punishments. A second key issue is what the basal ganglia do with the various signals that they receive. A third key issue is whether dopamine inputs to the basal ganglia carry a 'reward', 'reinforce', or 'Go' signal to the basal ganglia, and how this input affects the operation of the neuronal systems in the basal ganglia.

The basal ganglia are parts of the brain that include the striatum, globus pallidus, substantia nigra, and subthalamic nucleus and that are necessary for the normal initiation of movement. For example, depletion of the dopaminergic input to the striatum leads to the lack in the initiation of voluntary movement that occurs in Parkinson's disease. The basal ganglia receive inputs from all parts of the cerebral cortex, including the motor cortex, and have outputs directed strongly towards the premotor and prefrontal cortex via which they could influence movement initiation. There is an interesting organization of the dendrites of the neurons in the basal ganglia which has potentially important implications for understanding how the neuronal network architecture of the basal ganglia enables it to perform its functions (see Rolls and Treves 1998, Chapter 9).

6.4.1 Systems-level architecture of the basal ganglia

The point-to-point connectivity of the basal ganglia as shown by experimental anterograde and retrograde neuroanatomical path tracing techniques in the primate is indicated in Figs 9.5 and 9.6. The general connectivity is for cortical or limbic inputs to reach the striatum, which then projects to the globus pallidus and substantia nigra, which in turn project via the thalamus back to the cerebral cortex. Within this overall scheme, there is a set of at least partially segregated parallel processing streams, as illustrated in Figs 6.5 and 6.6 (see reviews by DeLong *et al.* 1984; Alexander *et al.* 1990; Rolls and Johnstone 1992; Strick *et al.* 1995; Middleton and Strick 1996a,b). First, the motor cortex (area 4) and somatosensory cortex (areas 3, 1, and 2) project somatotopically to the putamen, which has connections through the globus pallidus and substantia nigra to the ventral anterior thalamic nuclei and thus to the supplementary motor cortex. Recent experiments with a virus transneuronal pathway tracing technique have shown that there might be at least partial segregation within this stream, with different parts of the globus pallidus projecting via different parts of the ventrolateral (VL) thalamic nuclei to the supplementary motor area, the primary motor cortex (area 4), and to the ventral premotor area on the lateral surface of the hemisphere (Middleton and Strick 1996b). Second, there is an oculomotor circuit (see Fig. 6.5). Third, the dorsolateral prefrontal and the parietal cortices project to the head and body of the caudate nucleus, which has connections through parts of the globus pallidus and substantia nigra to the ventral anterior group of thalamic nuclei and thus to the dorsolateral prefrontal cortex. Fourth, the inferior temporal visual cortex and the ventrolateral (inferior convexity) prefrontal cortex to which it is connected project to the posterior and ventral parts of the putamen and the tail of the caudate nucleus (Kemp and Powell 1970; Saint-Cyr *et al.* 1990; Graybiel and Kimura 1995). Moreover, part of the globus pallidus, perhaps the part influenced by the temporal lobe visual cortex, area TE, may project back (via the thalamus) to area TE (Middleton and Strick 1996a). Fifth, and of especial interest in the context of reward mechanisms in the brain, limbic and related structures such as the amygdala, orbitofrontal cortex, and hippocampus project to the ventral striatum (which includes the nucleus accumbens), which has connections through the ventral pallidum to the mediodorsal nucleus of the thalamus and thus to the prefrontal and cingulate cortices (Strick *et al.* 1995). It is notable that the projections from the amygdala and orbitofrontal cortex are not restricted to the nucleus accumbens, but also occur to the adjacent ventral part of the head of the caudate nucleus (Amaral and Price 1984; Seleman and Goldman-Rakic 1985). These same regions may also project to the striosomes or patches (in for example the head of the caudate nucleus), which are set in the matrix formed by the other cortico-striatal systems (Graybiel and Kimura 1995).

6.4.2 Systems-level analysis of the basal ganglia: effects of striatal lesions

6.4.2.1 Ventral striatum

There is evidence linking the ventral striatum and its dopamine input to reward, for manipulations of this system alter the incentive effects which learned rewarding stimuli have on behaviour in the rat (Robbins *et al.* 1989; Everitt and Robbins 1992). The type of task affected is one in which a visual or auditory stimulus is delivered at or just before the delivery of food for which an animal is working. The tone or light becomes associated by learning with the food. Its effects can be measured by whether the rat learns a new operant response to obtain the conditioned reinforcer (the tone or light). This effect in

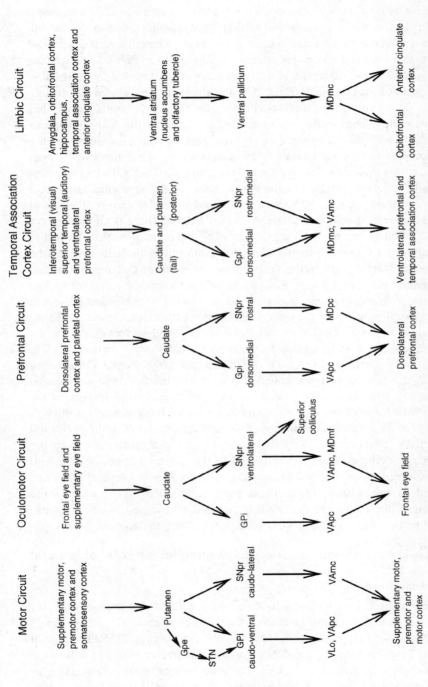

Fig. 6.5 A synthesis of some of the anatomical studies (see text) of the connections of the basal ganglia. GPe, Globus Pallidus, external segment; GPi, Globus Pallidus, internal segment; MD, nucleus medialis dorsalis; SNpr, Substantia Nigra, pars reticulata; VAmc, n. ventralis anterior pars magnocellularis of the thalamus; VApc, n. ventralis anterior pars compacta; VLo, n. ventralis lateralis pars oralis; VLm, n. ventralis pars medialis. An indirect pathway from the striatum via the external segment of the globus pallidus and the subthalamic nucleus (STN) to the internal segment of the globus pallidus is present for the first four circuits (left to right in Fig. 6.5) of the basal ganglia.

rats is probably produced via the inputs of the amygdala to the ventral striatum, for the effect is abolished by dopamine-depleting lesions of the nucleus accumbens, and amphetamine injections to the nucleus accumbens (which increase the release of dopamine) increase the effects which these learned or secondary reinforcers have on behaviour (see Robbins *et al.* 1989).

In primates, Stern and Passingham (1996) found that neurotoxic lesions of the ventral striatum produced some changes in emotionality, including increased activity and violent and aggressive behaviour when reward was no longer available during extinction (frustrative non-reward); but some of the changes found in rats were not apparent, perhaps because Stern and Passingham's lesions (1995, 1996) were small, and in any case in primates the amygdala projects not only to the ventral striatum, but also to the adjoining part of the caudate nucleus.

Further evidence linking the ventral striatum to some types of reward is that rats will self-administer amphetamine into the nucleus accumbens (a part of the ventral striatum), and lesions of the nucleus accumbens attenuate the intravenous self-administration of cocaine (A. Phillips and Fibiger 1990). In addition to this role in reward, related probably to inputs to the ventral striatum from the amygdala and orbitofrontal cortex (Rolls 1990b, see Chapter 4), the ventral striatum is also implicated in effects which could be mediated by the hippocampal inputs to the ventral striatum. For example, spatial learning (Schacter *et al.* 1989) and locomotor activity elicited by novel stimuli (see Iversen 1984) are influenced by manipulations of the nucleus accumbens.

6.4.2.2 Dorsal striatum

Damage to other parts of the striatum produces effects which suggest that they are involved in orientation to stimuli and in the initiation and control of movement. Lesions of the dopamine pathways in animals which deplete the striatum of dopamine lead to a failure to orient to stimuli, a failure to initiate movements, which is associated with catalepsy, and to a failure to eat and drink (Marshall *et al.* 1974). In humans, depletion of dopamine in the striatum is found in Parkinson's disease, in which there is akinesia, that is a lack of voluntary movement, bradykinesia, rigidity, and tremor (Hornykiewicz 1973). However, consistent with the anatomical evidence, the effects of damage to different regions of the striatum also suggest that there is functional specialization within the striatum (Divac and Oberg 1979; Oberg and Divac 1979; Iversen 1984). The selective effects may be related to the function of the cortex or limbic structure from which a region of the striatum receives inputs. For example, in the monkey, lesions of the anterodorsal part of the head of the caudate nucleus disrupted delayed spatial alternation performance, a task which requires spatial short-term memory, which is also impaired by lesions of the corresponding cortical region, the dorsolateral prefrontal cortex. Lesions of the ventrolateral part of the head of the caudate nucleus (as of the orbitofrontal cortex which projects to it), impaired object reversal performance, which measures the ability to reverse stimulus-reinforcement associations (see Chapter 3). Lesions of the tail of the caudate nucleus (as of the inferior temporal visual cortex which projects to this part of the caudate) produced a visual pattern discrimination deficit (Divac *et al.* 1967; Iversen 1979).

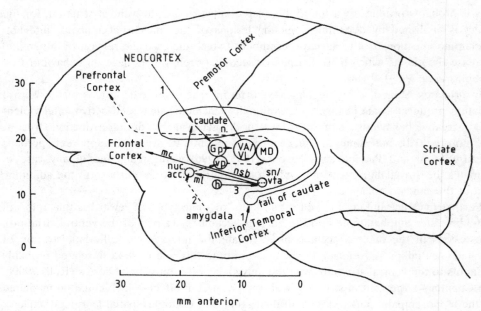

Fig. 6.6 Some of the striatal and connected regions in which the activity of single neurons is described shown on a lateral view of the brain of the macaque monkey. Gp, globus pallidus; h, hypothalamus; sn, substantia nigra, pars compacta (A9 cell group), which gives rise to the nigrostriatal dopaminergic pathway, or nigrostriatal bundle (nsb); vta, ventral tegmental area, containing the A10 cell group, which gives rise to the mesocortical dopamine pathway (mc) projecting to the frontal and cingulate cortices and to the mesolimbic dopamine pathway (ml), which projects to the nucleus accumbens (nuc acc). There is a route from the nucleus accumbens to the ventral pallidum (vp) which then projects to the mediodorsal nucleus of the thalamus (MD) which in turn projects to the prefrontal cortex. Correspondingly, the globus pallidus projects via the ventral anterior and ventrolateral (VA/VL) thalamic nuclei to cortical areas such as the premotor cortex.

Analogously, in the rat, lesions of the anteromedial head of the caudate nucleus (or of the medial prefrontal cortex, which projects to it) impaired spatial habit reversal, while lesions of the ventrolateral part of the head of the caudate nucleus (or of the orbital prefrontal cortex from which it receives) impaired the withholding of responses in a go/no-go task or in extinction (Dunnett and Iversen 1981; Iversen 1984). Further, in the rat a sensori-motor orientation deficit was produced by damage to a part of the dorsal striatum which receives inputs from lateral cortical areas (Dunnett and Iversen 1982b; Iversen 1984). Similar deficits are produced by selective depletion of dopamine in each of these areas using 6-hydroxydopamine (Dunnett and Iversen 1982a,b; Iversen 1984).

6.4.3 Systems-level analysis of the basal ganglia—neuronal activity in different parts of the striatum

We will focus first on neuronal activity in the ventral striatum, because it is particularly relevant to the processing of rewards by the basal ganglia.

6.4.3.1 Ventral striatum

To analyse the functions of the ventral striatum, the responses of more than 1000 single neurons were recorded (Rolls and Williams 1987b; Williams, Rolls, Leonard and Stern 1993) in a region which included the nucleus accumbens and olfactory tubercle in five macaque monkeys in test situations in which lesions of the amygdala, hippocampus, and inferior temporal cortex produce deficits, and in which neurons in these structures respond (Rolls 1990b,c,d,e, 1992a,b; Rolls, Cahusac et al. 1993; Rolls and Treves 1998; see Chapters 2 and 4). One population of neurons was found to respond differently in a visual discrimination task to visual stimuli which indicate that if a lick response is made, the taste of glucose reward will be obtained, and to other visual stimuli which indicate that if a lick response will be made, the taste of aversive saline will be obtained (Rolls 1990b). Responses of an example of a neuron of this type are shown in Fig. 6.7. The neuron increased its firing rate to the visual stimulus which indicated that saline would be obtained if a lick was made (the S−), and decreased its firing rate to the visual stimulus which indicated that a response could be made to obtain a taste of glucose (the S+). The differential response latency of this neuron to the reward-related and to the saline-related visual stimulus was approximately 150 ms (see Fig. 6.7), and this value was typical.

Of the neurons which responded to visual stimuli that were rewarding, relatively few responded to all the rewarding stimuli used. That is, only few (1.8%) ventral striatal neurons responded both when food was shown and to the positive discriminative visual stimulus, the S+ (e.g. a triangle shown on a video monitor), in a visual discrimination task. Instead, the reward-related neuronal responses were typically more context or stimulus-dependent, responding for example to the sight of food but not to the S+ which signified food (4.3%), differentially to the S+ or S− but not to food (4.0%), or to food if shown in one context but not in another context. Some neurons were classified as having taste or olfactory responses to food (see Table 6.1; Williams, Rolls, Leonard and Stern 1993). Some other neurons (1.4%) responded to aversive stimuli. These neurons did not respond simply in relation to arousal, which was produced in control tests by inputs from different modalities, for example by touch of the leg. Schultz et al. (1992) also found neurons in the ventral striatum with activity related to the expectation of reward.

Another population of ventral striatal neurons responded to novel visual stimuli. An example is shown in Fig. 6.8. Other ventral striatal neurons responded to faces; to other visual stimuli than discriminative stimuli and faces; in relation to somatosensory stimulation and movement; or to cues which signalled the start of a task (see Table 6.1) (Rolls and Williams 1987b; Williams, Rolls, Leonard and Stern 1993).

The neurons with responses to reinforcing or novel visual stimuli may reflect the inputs to the ventral striatum from the amygdala, orbitofrontal cortex, and hippocampus, and are consistent with the hypothesis that the ventral striatum provides a route for learned reinforcing and novel visual stimuli to influence behaviour. It was notable that although some neurons responded to visual stimuli associated with reward (see Table 6.1), 1.4% responded to visual stimuli associated with punishment, and 12% responded to arousing visual stimuli or non-specifically to visual stimuli (see Table 6.1). It was also notable that these neurons were not restricted to the nucleus accumbens, but were found also in the adjacent ventral part of the head of the caudate nucleus (Rolls and Williams 1987b; Williams, Rolls, Leonard and Stern 1993), which also receives projections from both the amygdala (Amaral and Price 1984) and orbitofrontal cortex (Seleman and Goldman-Rakic 1985).

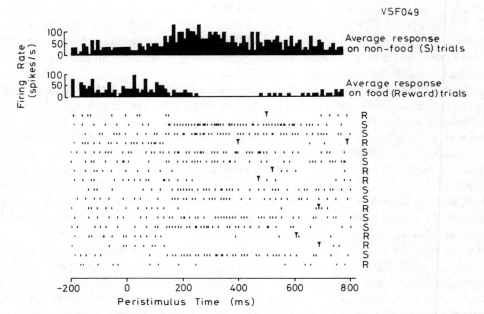

Fig. 6.7 Responses of a ventral striatal neuron in a visual discrimination task. The neuron reduced its firing rate to the S+ on food reward trials (R), and increased its firing rate to the S− on non-food trials (S) on which aversive saline was obtained if a lick was made. Rastergrams and peristimulus time histograms are shown. The triangles show where lick responses were made on the food reward (R) trials.

6.4.3.2 Tail of the caudate nucleus, and posteroventral putamen

The projections from the inferior temporal cortex and the prestriate cortex to the striatum arrive mainly, although not exclusively, in the tail (and genu) of the caudate nucleus and in the posteroventral portions of the putamen (Kemp and Powell 1970; Saint-Cyr *et al.* 1990). The activity of single neurons was analysed in the tail of the caudate nucleus and adjoining part of the ventral putamen by Caan, Perrett and Rolls (1984). Of 195 neurons analysed in two macaque monkeys, 109 (56%) responded to visual stimuli, with latencies of 90–150 ms for the majority of the neurons. The neurons responded to a limited range of complex visual stimuli, and in some cases responded to simpler stimuli such as bars and edges. Typically (for 75% of neurons tested) the neurons habituated rapidly, within 1–8 exposures, to each visual stimulus, but remained responsive to other visual stimuli with a different pattern. This habituation was orientation-specific, in that the neurons responded to the same pattern shown at an orthogonal orientation. The habituation was also relatively short-term, in that at least partial dishabituation to one stimulus could be produced by a single intervening presentation of a different visual stimulus. These neurons were relatively unresponsive in a visual discrimination task, having habituated to the stimuli which had been presented in the task on many previous trials. Given these responses, it may be suggested that these neurons are involved in short-term pattern-specific habituation to visual stimuli. This system would be distinguishable from other habituation systems (involved, for example, in habituation to spots of light) in that it is specialized for patterned visual stimuli which have been highly processed through visual cortical analysis mechanisms, as shown not only by the nature of the neuronal responses, but also by the fact that this system receives inputs from the inferior temporal visual cortex. It may also be suggested that this sensitivity to visual pattern change may have a role in alerting the monkey's attention to new stimuli. This suggestion is consistent with the changes in attention and orientation to stimuli produced by damage to the striatum. In view of these neurophysiological findings, and the finding that in a visual discrimination task neurons which reflected the reinforcement contingencies of the stimuli were not found, we (Caan, Perrett and Rolls 1984) suggested that the tail of the caudate nucleus is not directly involved in the development and maintenance of reward or punishment associations to stimuli (and therefore is not closely involved in emotion-related processing), but may aid visual discrimination performance by its sensitivity to change in visual stimuli. Neurons in some other parts of the striatum may, however, be involved in connecting visual stimuli to appropriate motor responses. For example, in the putamen some neurons have early movement-related firing during the performance of a visual discrimination task (Rolls, Thorpe *et al.* 1984); and some neurons in the head of the caudate nucleus respond to environmental cues which signal that reward may be obtained (Rolls, Thorpe and Maddison 1983b).

6.4.3.3 Postero-ventral putamen

Following these investigations on the caudal striatum which implicated it in visual functions related to a short-term habituation or memory process, a further study was performed to investigate the role of the posterior putamen in visual short-term memory tasks (Johnstone and Rolls 1990; Rolls and Johnstone 1992). Both the inferior temporal visual cortex and the prefrontal cortex project to the posterior ventral parts of the putamen (e.g. Goldman and Nauta 1977; Van Hoesen *et al.* 1981) and these cortical areas are known to subserve a variety of complex functions, including functions related to memory. For example, cells in both areas respond in a variety of short-term memory tasks (Fuster 1973, 1996; Fuster and Jervey 1982; Baylis and Rolls 1987; Miyashita and Chang 1988). Two main groups of neuron with memory-related activity were found in delayed match to sample (DMS) tasks, in which the monkey was shown a sample stimulus, and had to remember it during a 2–5 s delay period, after which if a matching stimulus was shown he could make one response, but if a non-matching stimulus was shown he had to make no response (Johnstone and Rolls 1990; Rolls and Johnstone 1992). First, 11% of the 621 neurons studied responded to the test stimulus which followed the sample stimulus, but did not respond to the sample stimulus. Of these neurons, 43% responded only on non-match trials (test different from sample), 16% only on match trials (test same as the sample), and 41% to the test stimulus irrespective of whether it was the same or different from the sample. These neuronal responses were not related to the licking since (i) the units did not respond in other tasks in which a lick response was required (for example, in an auditory delayed match-to-sample task which was identical to the visual delayed match-to-sample task except that auditory short-term memory rather than visual short-term memory was required, in a serial recognition task, or in a visual discrimination task), and

Table 6.1
Types of neuronal response found in the macaque ventral striatum
(after Williams, Rolls, Leonard and Stern 1993)

		Ventral Striatum	
		No./1013	%
1	Visual, recognition-related		
	−novel	39	3.5
	−familiar	11	1.1
2	Visual, association with reinforcement		
	−aversive	14	1.4
	−food	44	4.3
	−food and S+	18/1004	1.8
	−food, context dependent	13	1.3
	−opposite to food/aversive	11	1.1
	−differential to S+ or S− only	44/1112	4.0
3	Visual		
	−general interest	51	5.0
	−non-specific	78/1112	7.0
	−face	17	1.7
4	Movement-related, conditional	50/1112	4.5
5	Somatosensory	76/1112	6.8
6	Cue related	177/1112	15.9
7	Responses to all arousing stimuli	9/1112	0.8
8	Task-related (non-discriminating)	17/1112	1.5
9	During feeding	52/1112	4.7
10	Peripheral visual and auditory stimuli	72/538	13.4
11	Unresponsive	608/1112	54.7

The sample size was 1013 neurons except where indicated. The categories are non-exclusive.

(ii) a periresponse time spike-density function indicated that the stimulus onset better predicted neuronal activity. Second, 9.5% of the neurons responded in the delay period after the sample stimulus, during which the sample was being remembered. These neurons did not respond in the auditory version of the task, indicating that the responses were visual modality-specific (as were the responses of all other neurons in this part of the putamen with activity related to the delayed match to sample task). Given that the visual and auditory tasks were very similar apart from the modality of the input stimuli, this suggests that the activity of the neurons was not related to movements, or to rewards or punishments obtained in the tasks (and is thus not closely linked to emotion-related processing), but instead to modality-specific short-term memory-related processing.

In recordings made from pallidal neurons it was found that some responded in both visual and auditory versions of the task (Johnstone and Rolls 1990; Rolls and Johnstone 1992). Of 37 units responsive in the visual DMS task which were also tested in the auditory version, seven (19%) responded also in the auditory DMS task. The finding that some of the pallidal neurons active in the DMS task were not modality-specific, whereas only visual modality-specific DMS units were located in the posterior part of the striatum, suggests that the pallidum may represent a further stage in information processing in which information from different parts of the striatum can converge.

6.4.3.4 Head of the caudate nucleus

The activity of 394 neurons in the head of the caudate nucleus and most anterior part of the putamen was analysed in three behaving rhesus monkeys (Rolls, Thorpe and Maddison 1983b). 64.2% of these neurons had responses related to environmental stimuli, movements, the performance of a visual discrimination task, or eating. However, only relatively small proportions of these neurons had responses that were unconditionally related to visual (9.6%), auditory (3.5%), or gustatory (0.5%) stimuli, or to movements (4.1%). Instead, the majority of the neurons had responses that occurred conditionally in relation to stimuli or movements, in that the responses occurred in only some test situations, and were often dependent on the performance of a task by the monkeys. Thus, it was found that in a visual discrimination task 14.5% of the neurons responded during a 0.5 s tone/light cue which signalled the start of each trial; 31.1% responded in the period in which the discriminative visual stimuli were shown, with 24.3% of these responding more either to the visual stimulus which signified food reward or to that which signified punishment; and 6.2% responded in relation to lick responses. Yet these neurons typically did not respond in relation to the cue stimuli, to the visual stimuli, or to movements, when these occurred independently of the task, or performance of the task was prevented. Similarly, although of the neurons tested during feeding, 25.8% responded when the food was seen by the monkey, 6.2% when he tasted it, and 22.4% during a cue given by the experimenter that a food or non-food object was about to be presented, only few of these neurons had responses to the same stimuli presented in different situations. Further evidence on the nature of these neuronal responses was that many of the neurons with cue-related responses only responded to the tone/light cue stimuli when they were cues for the performance of the task or the presentation of food, and some responded to the different cues used in these two situations.

The finding that such neurons may respond to environmental stimuli only when they are significant (Rolls, Thorpe *et al.* 1979c; Rolls, Thorpe and Maddison 1983b) was confirmed by Evarts and his colleagues. They showed that some neurons in the putamen only responded to the click of a solenoid when it indicated that a fruit juice reward could be obtained (see Evarts and Wise 1984). We have found that this decoding of the significance of environmental events which are signals for the preparation for or initiation of a response is represented in the firing of a population of neurons in the dorsolateral prefrontal cortex, which projects into the head of the caudate nucleus (E. T. Rolls and G. C. Baylis, unpublished observations 1984). These neurons respond to the tone cue only if it signals the start of a trial of the visual discrimination task, just as do the corresponding population of neurons in the head of the caudate nucleus. The indication that the decoding of significance is performed by the cortex, and that the striatum receives only the result of the cortical computation, is considered below and elsewhere (Rolls and Williams 1987a).

These findings indicate that the head of the caudate nucleus and most anterior part of the putamen contain populations of neurons which respond to cues which enable preparation for the performance of tasks such as feeding and tasks in which movements must be initiated, and others which respond during the performance of such tasks in relation to the stimuli used and the responses made, yet that the majority of these neurons has no unconditional sensory or motor responses. It has therefore been suggested (Rolls, Thorpe *et al.* 1979c; Rolls, Thorpe and Maddison 1983b) that the anterior neostriatum contains neurons which are important for the utilization of environmental cues for the preparation

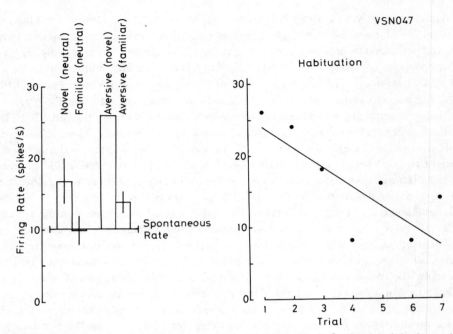

Fig. 6.8 Responses of a ventral striatal neuron to novel visual stimuli. On the right it is shown that the response to novel stimuli, an increase in firing rate to 25 spikes s^{-1} from the spontaneous rate of 10 spikes s^{-1}, habituated over repeated presentations of the stimulus. The lack of response shown in the left panel to the familiar stimulus was thus only achieved after habituation produced by 4–7 presentations of the stimulus. It is also shown that the neuron responded to aversive stimuli when they had not been seen for more than one day (Aversive (novel)), but did not respond to aversive visual stimuli (such as the sight of a syringe from which the monkey was fed saline, Aversive (familiar)), even though the latter produced arousal. (From Williams, Rolls, Leonard and Stern 1993.)

for behavioural responses, and for particular behavioural responses made in particular situations to particular environmental stimuli, that is in stimulus–motor response habit formation. Different neurons in the cue-related group often respond to different subsets of environmentally significant events, and thus convey some information which would be useful in switching behaviour, in preparing to make responses, and in connecting inputs to particular responses (Rolls, Thorpe *et al.* 1979c; Rolls, Thorpe and Maddison 1983b; Rolls 1984a). Striatal neurons with similar types of response have also been recorded by Schultz and colleagues (see for example Schultz *et al.* 1995a), and striatal (tonically active) interneurons whose activity probably reflects the responses of such neurons have been described by Graybiel and Kimura (1995).

6.4.3.5 Anterior putamen

It is clear that the activity of many neurons in the putamen is related to movements (Anderson 1978; Crutcher and DeLong 1984a,b; DeLong *et al.* 1984). There is a somatotopic organization of neurons in the putamen, with separate areas containing neurons responding to arm, leg, or orofacial movements. Some of these neurons respond only to active movements, and others to active and to passive movements. Some of these neurons respond to somatosensory stimulation, with multiple clusters of neurons responding, for example, to the movement of each joint (see Crutcher and DeLong 1984a; DeLong *et al.* 1984). Some neurons in the putamen have been shown in experiments in which the arm has been given assisting and opposing loads to respond in relation to the direction of an intended movement, rather than in relation to the muscle forces required to execute the movement (Crutcher and DeLong 1984b). Also, the firing rate of neurons in the putamen tends to be linearly related to the amplitude of movements (Crutcher and DeLong 1984b), and this is of potential clinical relevance, since patients with basal ganglia disease frequently have difficulty in controlling the amplitude of their limb movements.

In order to obtain further evidence on specialization of function within the striatum, the activity of neurons in the putamen has been compared with the activity of neurons recorded in different parts of the striatum in the same tasks (Rolls, Thorpe, Boytim, Szabo and Perrett 1984). Of 234 neurons recorded in the putamen of two macaque monkeys during the performance of a visual discrimination task and the other tests in which other striatal neurons have been shown to respond (Rolls, Thorpe and Maddison 1983b; Caan, Perrett and Rolls 1984), 68 (29%) had activity that was phasically related to movements (Rolls, Thorpe *et al.* 1984). Many of these responded in relation to mouth movements such as licking. Similar neurons were found in the substantia nigra, pars reticulata, to which the putamen projects (Mora, Mogenson and Rolls 1977). The neurons did not have activity related to taste, in that they responded, for example, during tongue protrusion made to a food or non-food object. Some of these neurons responded in relation to the licking mouth movements made in the visual discrimination task, and always also responded when mouth movements were made during clinical testing when a food or non-food object was brought close to the mouth. Their responses were thus unconditionally related to movements, in that they responded in whichever testing situation was used, and were therefore different from the responses of neurons in the head of the caudate nucleus (Rolls, Thorpe and Maddison 1983b). Of the 68 neurons in the putamen with movement-related activity in these tests, 61 had activity related to mouth movements, and seven had activity related to movements of the body. Of the remaining neurons, 24 (10%) had activity which was task-related in that some change of firing rate associated with the presentation of the tone cue or the opening of the shutter occurred on each trial (see Rolls, Thorpe *et al.* 1984), four had auditory responses, one responded to environmental stimuli (see Rolls, Thorpe and Maddison 1983b), and 137 were not responsive in these test situations.

These findings (Rolls, Thorpe *et al.* 1984) provide further evidence that differences between neuronal activity in different regions of the striatum are found even in the same testing situations, and also that the inputs which activate these neurons are derived functionally from the cortex which projects into a particular region of the striatum (in this case sensori-motor cortex, areas 3, 1, 2, 4, and 6).

6.4.4   What computations are performed by the basal ganglia?

The neurophysiological investigations described in Section 6.4.3 indicate that reinforcement-related signals do affect neuronal activity in some parts of the striatum, particularly in the ventral striatum. This finding suggests that pharmacological agents such as dopaminergic drugs that produce reward by acting on the ventral striatum may do so because they are tapping into a system normally involved in providing a route to behavioural output for signals carrying information about learned incentives. Some questions arise. Does the ventral striatum process the inputs in any way before passing them on? Can the ventral striatum be considered as one part of a larger computational system that includes all parts of the basal ganglia, and which operates as a single system with inputs from all parts of the cerebral cortex, allowing selection by competition between all the inputs as well as convergence between them to produce a single behavioural output stream? How do the outputs of the basal ganglia lead to or influence action?

One way to obtain evidence on the information processing being performed by the striatum is to compare neuronal activity in the striatum with that in its corresponding input and output structures. For example, the taste and visual information necessary for the computation that a visual stimulus is no longer associated with taste reward reaches the orbitofrontal cortex, and the putative output of such a computation, namely neurons which respond in this non-reward situation, are found in the orbitofrontal cortex (Thorpe, Rolls and Maddison 1983; Rolls 1989a, 1996b). However, such neurons which represent the necessary sensory information for this computation, and neurons which respond to the non-reward, were not found in the head of the caudate nucleus or the ventral striatum (Rolls, Thorpe and Maddison 1983b; Williams, Rolls, Leonard and Stern 1993). Instead, in the head of the caudate nucleus, neurons in the same test situation responded in relation to whether the monkey had to make a response on a particular trial, that is many of them responded more on go than on no-go trials. This could reflect the *output* of a cognitive computation performed by the orbitofrontal cortex, indicating whether on the basis of the available sensory information, the current trial should be a go trial, or a no-go trial because a visual stimulus previously associated with punishment had been shown. Similarly, neurons were not found in the ventral striatum that are tuned to all the visual reward, taste reward, olfactory reward, and visual non-reward functions about which macaque orbitofrontal cortex neurons carry information (see Chapters 2 and 4). Instead the ventral striatal neurons were usually less easy to classify in these sensory ways, and were especially engaged when tasks were being performed. For example, many of the ventral striatal neurons that respond to visual inputs do so preferentially on the basis of whether the stimuli are recognized, or are associated with reinforcement (Williams, Rolls, Leonard and Stern 1993). Much of the sensory and memory-related processing required to determine whether a stimulus is a face, is recognized, or is associated with reinforcement has been performed in and is evident in neuronal responses in structures such as the amygdala (Leonard, Rolls, Wilson and Baylis 1985; Rolls 1992a,b), orbitofrontal cortex (Thorpe, Rolls and Maddison 1983; Rolls 1996b) and hippocampal system.

Similar comparisons can be made for the head and tail of the caudate nucleus, and the posterior putamen (see Rolls and Johnstone 1992; Rolls and Treves 1998). In these four parts of the striatum in which a comparison can be made of processing in the striatum with that in the cortical area which projects to that part of the striatum, it appears that the full information represented in the cortex does not reach the striatum, but that rather the striatum receives the output of the computation being performed by a cortical area, and could use this to switch or alter behaviour.

The hypothesis arises from these findings that some parts of the striatum, particularly the caudate nucleus, ventral striatum, and posterior putamen, receive the output of these memory-related and cognitive computations, but do not themselves perform them. Instead, on receiving the cortical and limbic outputs, the striatum may be involved in switching behaviour as appropriate as determined by the different, sometimes conflicting, information received from these cortical and limbic areas. On this view, the striatum would be particularly involved in the selection of behavioural responses, and in producing one coherent stream of behavioural output, with the possibility to switch if a higher priority input was received. This process may be achieved by a laterally spreading competitive interaction between striatal or pallidal neurons, which might be implemented by direct connections between nearby neurons in the striatum and globus pallidus. In addition, the inhibitory interneurons within the striatum, the dendrites of which in the striatum may cross the boundary between the matrix and striosomes, may play a part in this interaction between striatal processing streams (Groves 1983; Graybiel and Kimura 1995; Groves *et al.* 1995). Dopamine could play an important role in setting the sensitivity of this response selection function, as suggested by direct iontophoresis of dopamine on to single striatal neurons, which produces a similar decrease in the response of the neuron and in its spontaneous activity in the behaving macaque (Rolls, Thorpe *et al.* 1984; Rolls and Williams 1987a). In addition to this response selection function by competition, the basal ganglia may, by the convergence discussed, enable signals originating from non-motor parts of the cerebral cortex to be mapped into motor signals to produce behavioural output. The ways in which these computations might be performed are considered next.

6.4.5 How do the basal ganglia perform their computations?

On the hypothesis just raised, different regions of the striatum, or at least the outputs of such regions, would need to interact. Is there within the striatum the possibility for different regions to interact, and is the partial functional segregation seen within the striatum maintained in processing beyond the striatum? For example, is the segregation maintained throughout the globus pallidus and thalamus with projections to different premotor and even prefrontal regions reached by different regions of the striatum, or is there convergence or the possibility for interaction at some stage during this post-striatal processing?

Given the anatomy of the basal ganglia, interactions between signals reaching the basal ganglia could happen in a number of different ways. One would be for each part of the striatum to receive at least some input from a number of different cortical regions. As discussed above, there is evidence for patches of input from different sources to be brought adjacent to each other in the striatum (Van Hoesen *et al.* 1981; Seleman and Goldman-Rakic 1985; Graybiel and Kimura 1995). For example, in the caudate nucleus, different regions of association cortex project to adjacent longitudinal strips (Seleman and Goldman-Rakic 1985). Now, the dendrites of striatal neurons have the shape of large plates which lie at right angles to the incoming cortico-striate fibres (Percheron *et al.* 1984a,b, 1994) (see Figs. 6.9 and 6.10). Thus one way in which interaction may start in the basal ganglia is by virtue of the same striatal neuron receiving inputs on its dendrites from more than just a limited area of the cerebral cortex. This convergence may provide a first

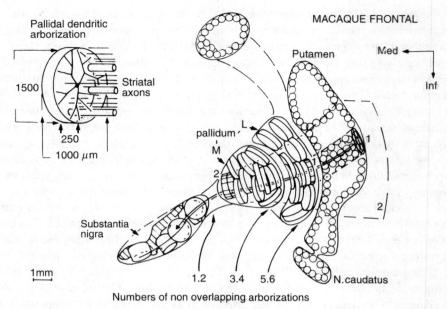

Fig. 6.9 Semi-schematic spatial diagram of the striato-pallido-nigral system (see text). The numbers represent the numbers of non-overlapping arborizations of dendrites in the plane shown. L, lateral or external segment of the globus pallidus; M, medial or internal segment of the globus pallidus. The inserted diagram in the upper left shows the geometry of the dendrites of a typical pallidal neuron, and how the flat dendritic arborization is pierced at right angles by the striatal axons, which make occasional synapses en passage. (Reprinted with permission from Percheron et al. 1984b.)

level of integration over limited sets of cortico–striatal fibres. The large number of cortical inputs received by each striatal neuron, in the order of 10 000 (Wilson 1995), is consistent with the hypothesis that convergence of inputs carrying different signals is an important aspect of the function of the basal ganglia. The computation which could be performed by this architecture is discussed below for the inputs to the globus pallidus, where the connectivity pattern is comparable (Percheron *et al.* 1984a,b, 1994).

6.4.5.1   Interaction between neurons and selection of output

The regional segregation of neuronal response types in the striatum described above is consistent with mainly local integration over limited, adjacent sets of cortico–striatal inputs, as suggested by this anatomy. Short-range integration or interactions within the striatum may also be produced by the short length (for example 0.5 mm) of the intrastriatal axons of striatal neurons. These could produce a more widespread influence if the effect of a strong input to one part of the striatum spread like a lateral competition signal (cf. Groves 1983; Groves *et al.* 1995). Such a mechanism could contribute to behavioural response selection in the face of different competing input signals to the striatum. The lateral inhibition could operate, for example, between the striatal principal (that is spiny) neurons by direct connections (they receive excitatory connections from the cortex, respond by increasing their firing rates, and could inhibit each other by their local axonal arborizations, which spread in an area as large as their dendritic trees, and which utilize GABA as their inhibitory transmitter). Further lateral inhibition could operate in the pallidum and substantia nigra (see Fig. 6.10). Here again there are local axon collaterals, as extensive as the very large pallidal and nigral dendritic fields. The lateral competition could again operate by direct connections between the cells. (Note that pallidal and nigral cells have high spontaneous firing rates (often 25–50 spikes s^{-1}), and respond (to their inhibitory striatal inputs) by reducing their firing rates below this high spontaneous rate. Such a decrease in the firing rate of one neuron would release inhibition on nearby neurons, causing them to increase their firing rates, equivalent to responding less.) A selection function of this type between processing streams in the basal ganglia, even without any convergence anatomically between the processing streams, might provide an important computational *raison d'être* for the basal ganglia. The direct inhibitory local connectivity between the principal neurons within the striatum and globus pallidus would seem to provide a simple, and perhaps evolutionarily old, way in which to implement competition between neurons and processing streams. This might even be a primitive design principle that characterizes the basal ganglia. A system such as the basal ganglia with direct inhibitory recurrent collaterals may have evolved easily because it is easier to make stable than architectures such as the cerebral cortex with recurrent excitatory connections. The basal ganglia architecture may have been especially appropriate in motor systems in which instability could produce movement and co-ordination difficulties (see Rolls and Treves 1998).

This hypothesis of lateral competition between the neurons of the basal ganglia can be sketched simply (see also Fig. 6.10 and Rolls and Treves 1998, Chapter 9, where a more detailed neuronal network theory of the operation of the basal ganglia is presented). The inputs from the cortex to the striatum are excitatory, and competition between striatal neurons is implemented by the use of an inhibitory transmitter (GABA), and direct connections between striatal neurons, within an area which is approximately co-extensive with the dendritic arborization. Given that the lateral connections between the striatal neurons are collaterals of the output axons, the output must be inhibitory on to pallidal and nigral neurons. This means that to transmit signals usefully, and in contrast with striatal neurons, the neurons in the globus pallidus and substantia nigra (pars reticulata) must have high spontaneous firing rates, and respond by reducing their firing rates. These pallidal and nigral neurons then repeat the simple scheme for lateral competition between output neurons by having direct lateral inhibitory connections to the other pallidal and nigral neurons. When nigral and pallidal neurons respond by reducing their firing rates, the reduced inhibition through the recurrent collaterals allows the connected pallidal and nigral neurons to fire faster, and also at the same time the main output of the pallidal and nigral neurons allows the thalamic neurons to fire faster. The thalamic neurons then have the standard excitatory influence on their cortical targets. The simple, and perhaps evolutionarily early, aspect of this basal ganglia architecture is that the striatal, pallidal, and nigral neurons implement competition (for selection) by direct inhibitory recurrent lateral connections of the main output neurons on to other output neurons, with the inputs to a stage synapsing directly on to the output neurons (see Fig. 6.10).

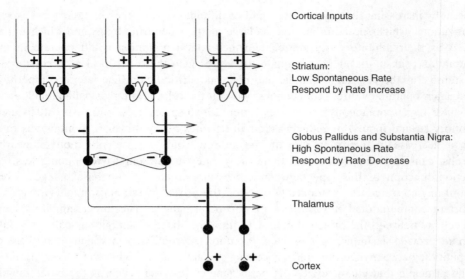

Cortical Inputs

Striatum:
Low Spontaneous Rate
Respond by Rate Increase

Globus Pallidus and Substantia Nigra:
High Spontaneous Rate
Respond by Rate Decrease

Thalamus

Cortex

Fig. 6.10 Simple hypothesis of basal ganglia network architecture. A key aspect is that in both the striatum and globus pallidus there are direct inhibitory connections (−) between the principal neurons, as shown. These synapses use GABA as a transmitter. Excitatory inputs to the striatum are shown as +. (From Rolls and Treves 1998.)

Another possible mechanism for interaction within the striatum is provided by the dopaminergic pathway, through which a signal which has descended from, for example, the ventral striatum might influence other parts of the striatum (Nauta and Domesick 1978). Because of the slow conduction speed of the dopaminergic neurons, this latter system would probably not be suitable for rapid switching of behaviour, but only for more tonic, long-term adjustments of sensitivity.

Further levels for integration within the basal ganglia are provided by the striato–pallidal and striato–nigral projections (Percheron *et al.* 1984a,b, 1994). The afferent fibres from the striatum again cross at right angles a flat plate or disc formed by the dendrites of the pallidal or nigral neurons (see Fig. 6.9). The discs are approximately 1.5 mm in diameter, and are stacked up one upon the next at right angles to the incoming striatal fibres. The dendritic discs are so large that in the monkey there is room for only perhaps 50 such discs not to overlap in the external pallidal segment, for 10 non-overlapping discs in the medial pallidal segment, and for one overlapping disc in the most medial part of the medial segment of the globus pallidus and in the substantia nigra.

One result of this convergence achieved by this stage of the medial pallidum/substantia nigra is that even if inputs from different cortical regions were kept segregated by specific wiring rules on to different neurons, there might nevertheless well be the possibility for mutual competition between different pallidal neurons, implemented by interneurons. Given the relatively small number of neurons into which the cortical signals had now been compressed, it would be feasible to have competition (the same effect as lateral inhibition would achieve elsewhere) implemented between the relatively small population of neurons, now all collected into a relatively restricted space, so that the competition could spread widely within these nuclei. This could allow selection by competition between these pathways, that is effectively between information processing in different cortical areas. This could be important in allowing each cortical area to control output when appropriate (depending on the task being performed). Even if full segregation were maintained in the return paths to the cerebral cortex, the return paths could influence each cortical area, allowing it to continue processing if it had the strongest 'call'. Each cortical area on a fully segregated hypothesis might thus have its own non-basal ganglia output routes, but might according to the current suggestion utilize the basal ganglia as a system to select a cortical area or set of areas, depending on how strongly each cortical area is calling for output. The thalamic outputs from the basal ganglia (areas VA and VLo of the thalamus) might according to this hypothesis have to some extent an activity or gain-controlling function on an area (such as might be mediated by diffuse terminals in superficial cortical layers), rather than the strong and selective inputs implemented by a specific thalamic nucleus such as the lateral geniculate.

The way in which selection of behavioural output to produce feeding could take place within the basal ganglia is considered further in Section 2.4.8.

6.4.5.2 Convergent mapping within the basal ganglia

In addition to this selection function, it is also attractive to at least consider the further hypothesis that there is some convergent mapping achieved by the basal ganglia. This hypothesis is now considered in more detail. The anatomical arrangement just described does provide a possibility for some convergence on to single striatal neurons of cortical input, and on to single pallidal and nigral neurons of signals from relatively different parts of the striatum. For what computation might such anatomy provide a structural basis? Within the pallidum, each dendritic disc is flat, is orthogonal to the input fibres which pierce it, but is not filled with dendritic arborizations. Instead, each dendrite typically consists of 4–5 branches which are spread out to occupy only a small part of the surface area of the dendritic disc (see Fig. 6.9). There are thousands of such sparsely populated plates stacked on top of one another. Each pallidal neuron is contacted by a number of the mass of fibres from the striatum which pass it, and given the relatively small collecting area of each pallidal or nigral neuron (4 or 5 dendritic branches in a plane), each such neuron is thus likely to receive a random combination of inputs from different striatal neurons within its collection field. The thinness of the dendritic sheet may help to ensure that each axon does not make more than a few synapses with each dendrite, and that the combinations of inputs received by each dendrite are approximately random. This architecture thus appears to be appropriate for bringing together at random on to single pallidal and nigral neurons inputs which originate from quite diverse parts of the cerebral cortex. (This is a two-stage process, cortex to striatum, and striatum to pallidum and substantia nigra). By the stage of the medial pallidum and substantia nigra, there is the opportunity for the input field of a single neuron to effectively become very wide, although whether in practice this covers very different cortical areas, or is instead limited to a rather segregated cortex–basal ganglia–cortex loop, remains to be confirmed.

Given then that this architecture could allow individual pallidal and nigral neurons to receive random combinations of inputs from different striatal neurons, the following functional implications arise. Simple Hebbian learning in the striatum would enable strongly firing striatal neurons to increase the strength of the synapses from the active cortical inputs. In the pallidum, such conjunctive learning of coactive inputs would be more complex, requiring, for example, a strongly inhibited pallidal neuron to show synaptic strengthening from strongly firing but inhibitory inputs from the striatum. Then, if a particular pallidal or nigral neuron received inputs by chance from striatal neurons which responded to an environmental cue signal that something significant was about to happen, and from striatal neurons which fired because the monkey was making a postural adjustment, this conjunction of events might make that pallidal or nigral neuron become inhibited (that is respond to) either input alone. Then, in the future, the occurrence of only one of the inputs, for example only the environmental cue, would result in a decrease of firing of that pallidal or nigral neuron, and thus in the appropriate postural adjustment being made by virtue of the output connections of that pallidal or nigral neuron.

This is a proposal that the basal ganglia are able to detect combinations of conjunctively active inputs from quite widespread regions of the cerebral cortex using their combinatorial architecture and a property of synaptic modifiability. In this way it would be possible to trigger any complex pattern of behavioural responses by any complex pattern of environmental inputs, using what is effectively a pattern associator. According to this possibility the unconditioned input would be the motor input, and the to-be-associated inputs the other inputs to the basal ganglia.

It may be noted that the input events need not include only those from environmental stimuli represented in the caudate nucleus and ventral striatum, but also, if the overlapping properties of the dendrites described above provide sufficient opportunity for convergence, of the context of the movement, provided by inputs via the putamen from sensorimotor cortex. This would then make a system appropriate for triggering an appropriate motor response (learned by trial and error, with the final solution becoming associated with the triggering input events) to any environmental input state. As such, this hypothesis provides a suggested neural basis for 'habit' learning in which the basal ganglia have been implicated (R. Phillips *et al.* 1988; Petri and Mishkin 1994). The hypothesis could be said to provide a basis for the storage of motor plans in the basal ganglia, which would be instantiated as a series of look-ups of the appropriate motor output pattern to an evolving sequence of input information. An interesting aspect of this hypothesis is that other parts of the motor system, such as the cortico–cortical pathways, may mediate the control of action in a voluntary, often slow way in the early stages of learning. The input context for the movement and the appropriate motor signals (originating during learning from motor cortical areas) could then be learned by the basal ganglia, until after many trials the basal ganglia can perform the required look-up of the correct motor output in an automated, 'habit', mode. In this sense, the cortico–cortical pathways would set up the conditions, which because of their continuing repetition would be learned by the basal ganglia. The hypothesis introduced above also may provide a basis for the switching between different types of behaviour proposed as a function of the basal ganglia, for if a strong new pattern of inputs was received by the basal ganglia, this would result in a different pattern of outputs being 'looked up' than that currently in progress.

The way in which reinforcement signals present in the ventral striatum could contribute to these functions is that whether reinforcement availability is being indicated by the firing of ventral striatal neurons could be part of the output context being provided by the basal ganglia. If positive reinforcement was being signalled, the implication of the striatal output would be that the animal should make behavioural responses that would lead to approach to the conditioned positive reinforcers, and thus to obtaining primary reinforcement.

6.4.5.3   Learning within the basal ganglia, and the role of dopamine

The outputs of the globus pallidus and substantia nigra directed via the thalamus to motor regions such as the supplementary motor cortex and the premotor cortex potentially provide important output routes for the basal ganglia to produce actions (see Figs. 6.5 and 6.6). However, there are also outputs of the basal ganglia to structures which may not be primarily motor, such as the dorsolateral prefrontal cortex of primates (Middleton and Strick 1994, 1996b), and the inferior temporal visual cortex (Middleton and Strick 1996a). The outputs to the dorsolateral prefrontal cortex might be to enable that region to know what response had recently been selected, and thus to remember the response over a delay period (see Rolls and Treves 1998).

The hypothesis of basal ganglia function just described incorporates associative learning of coactive inputs on to neurons, at both the cortico–striatal stages, and the striato–pallidal and nigral stages. Consistent with this hypothesis (Rolls 1979, 1987, 1984b, 1994d; Rolls and Johnstone 1992), it has now been possible to demonstrate long-term potentiation (LTP) in at least some parts of the basal ganglia. For example, Pennartz et al. (1993) demonstrated LTP of limbic inputs to the nucleus accumbens, and were able to show that such LTP is facilitated by dopamine (see also Calabresi et al. 1992; Wickens and Kotter 1995; Wickens et al. 1996).

Thus one function of dopamine in the basal ganglia may be to set the threshold for learning within the basal ganglia. In what further ways might dopamine come to be so important in reward, as indicated by the evidence described in Section 6.3? Given that there are relatively few dopaminergic neurons, it is likely that the information conveyed by the dopamine pathway is relatively general or modulatory, rather than conveying the specific information that must be learned and mapped to the output of the basal ganglia, or the full details of the primary reinforcer obtained (for example which taste, which touch, etc.). A second possible function, noted above, is that dopamine may play an important role in setting the thresholds of striatal neurons, as suggested by direct iontophoresis of dopamine on to single striatal neurons, which produces a similar decrease in the response of the neuron and in its spontaneous activity in the behaving macaque (Rolls and Williams 1987a; Rolls, Thorpe et al. 1984). In this way, or perhaps by a different mechanism, the dopamine might also modulate learning in the basal ganglia. A very simple hypothesis is that the modulation of learning is likely to be quite general, making it more likely that information will be stored, that is that conjunctive activity at the inputs to the basal ganglia will become associated. An alternative possibility is that activity in the dopamine pathways carries a teaching signal, which might operate as a reinforcer in the type of reinforcement learning network described in the Appendix (Section A.3) and by

Rolls and Treves (1998, Chapter 5). Schultz *et al.* (1995b) have argued from their recordings from dopamine neurons that this may be the case. For example, dopamine neurons can respond to the taste of a liquid reward in an operant task. However, these neurons may stop responding to such a primary (unlearned) reinforcer quite rapidly as the task is learned, and instead respond only to the earliest indication that a trial of the task is about to begin (Schultz *et al.* 1995b). Thus they could not convey information about a primary reward obtained if the trial is successful, but instead appear to convey information which would be much better suited to a preparation or 'Go' role for dopamine release in the striatum. Further evidence that the dopamine projection does not convey a specific 'reward' signal is that dopamine release occurs not only to rewards (such as food or brain-stimulation reward, or later in training to an indication that a reward might be given later), but also to aversive stimuli such as aversive stimulation of the medial hypothalamus (see Hoebel *et al.* 1996; Hoebel, personal communication 1996; Gray, Young and Joseph 1997). These findings are much more consistent with the hypothesis that instead of acting as the reinforce or error signal in a reinforcement learning system, as suggested by Houk *et al.* (1995), the dopamine projection to the striatum may act as a 'Go' or 'preparation' signal to set the thresholds of neurons in the striatum, and/or as a general modulatory signal that could help to strengthen synapses of conjunctively active pre- and postsynaptic neurons. In such a system, what is learned would be dependent on the presynaptic and postsynaptic terms, and would not be explicitly guided by a reinforce/teacher signal that would provide feedback *after* each trial on the degree of success of each trial as in the reinforcement learning algorithm (see Section A.3).

An alternative view of striatal function is that the striatum might be organized as a set of segregated and independent transmission routes, each one of which would receive from a given region of the cortex, and project finally to separate premotor or prefrontal regions (Strick *et al.* 1995; Middleton and Strick 1996a,b) (see Figs. 6.5 and 6.6). Even if this is correct, the detection of combinations of conjunctively active inputs, but in this case from limited populations of input axons to the basal ganglia, might still be an important aspect of the function of the basal ganglia.

On both views of basal ganglia function, the ventral striatum would still be an area allowing convergence from signals from the amygdala, orbitofrontal cortex, and hippocampus. Transmission in this system would be modulated by dopamine. This modulation could influence how much effect reinforcing inputs to the striatum produce on their outputs. *Increasing the gain or reducing the threshold could enhance positive reinforcing output if the inputs to the ventral striatum were predominantly indicating positive reinforcement. In a positively reinforcing context, facilitating dopamine transmission in the ventral striatum could lead to a net increase in reward output, and this could be at least part of the mechanism by which dopamine release in the ventral striatum could be rewarding.*

6.5 Conclusions on the role of dopamine in reward and addiction

Dopamine does appear to be involved in the reward produced by stimulation of some brain-stimulation reward sites, notably the ventral tegmental area where the dopamine cell bodies are located. This self-stimulation depends on dopamine release in the nucleus accumbens. Self-stimulation at other sites does not depend on dopamine.

The self-administration of the psychomotor stimulants such as amphetamine and cocaine depends on activation of a dopaminergic system in the nucleus accumbens.

The dopamine release produced by these behaviours may be rewarding because it is influencing the activity of an amygdalo–striatal (and in primates also possibly orbitofrontal–striatal) system involved in linking the amygdala and orbitofrontal cortex, which can learn stimulus–reinforcement associations, to output systems. Effectively, activation of neurons in this system has to be reinforcing if secondary reinforcers are to influence behaviour. Put very directly, animals must be built to want to activate the neurons in this system which can be activated by stimuli learned to be reinforcers in the amygdala and orbitofrontal cortex. In this system, dopamine release, and the firing of dopamine neurons, may only produce reward if the net input to the ventral striatum from the amygdala and orbitofrontal cortex is positive. The dopamine in this system may just be acting as an input which tends to facilitate transmission through this system, and effectively to help the transmission to produce a 'Go' signal. A particular way to show that the dopamine in this system means 'Go' rather than 'reward' would be to test whether the dopamine neurons fire, and dopamine release occurs and is necessary for, behaviour such as active avoidance to a strong punishing, arousing, stimulus. There is indeed evidence that dopamine is released in the nucleus accumbens by aversive as well as by rewarding stimuli (see Section 6.3.3).

The pathway from the amygdala to the ventral striatum may, as discussed above, be especially involved in linking conditioned incentives (secondary reinforcers) to behavioural output. Consistent with this, and in the context of drug seeking behaviour and the role of stimuli associated by stimulus-reinforcement learning with the reinforcement produced by psychomotor stimulants, Whitelaw, Markou, Robbins and Everitt (1996) showed that excitotoxic lesions of the basolateral amygdala in rats impaired behavioural responses to a light associated with intravenous administration of cocaine, but not to the primary reinforcer of the cocaine itself (see Section 4.4.2).

If the psychomotor stimulant drugs produce their rewarding and addictive effects by influencing this amygdalo–striatal transmission, and effectively producing reward by tapping into a system normally involved in secondary as opposed to primary reinforcement, it might be asked why the reward produced by the drug does not extinguish. When no primary reinforcement is being received, the effects that secondary reinforcers have on behaviour normally do decline considerably. Why is the reward apparently in contrast so persistent with the dopaminergic stimulant drugs? Perhaps the following is at least part of the explanation. If the amygdala and orbitofrontal cortex are parts of the brain involved in stimulus–reward association learning and extinction, then the extinction would be expected to be implemented by a reduction in the neuronal responses to a secondary reinforcer during extinction. If the mechanism for extinction (as well as learning) is in the amygdala and orbitofrontal cortex, then tapping into the circuitry *after* the amygdala would not be expected to be subject to the learning and extinction. That is, the firing at the entry into the ventral striatum would have to be interpreted by the system as meaning reward (i.e. that actions should be performed to make these neurons fire), as the stimulus–reward learning system precedes this stage of the amygdalo–striatal circuitry (see Fig. 9.4). Thus, in so far as the psychomotor dopaminergic stimulant drugs of addiction are tapping into a part of the circuitry after stimulus–reward learning and unlearning has been implemented, we would not expect the reward introduced into that part of the system to extinguish.

Given that the ventral striatum has inputs from the orbitofrontal cortex as well as the amygdala, and that some primary rewards are represented in the orbitofrontal cortex, the dopaminergic effects of psychomotor stimulant drugs may produce their effects also in part because they are tapping into a primary reward-to-action pathway. However, at least part of the reason that drugs are addictive may indeed be that they activate the brain at the stage of processing after that at which reward or punishment associations have been learned, where the signal is normally interpreted by the system as indicating 'select actions to achieve the goal of making these striatal neurons fire' (see Fig. 9.4).

6.6 The pharmacology of other reward systems, of depression, and of anxiety

6.6.1 Opiate reward systems, and analgesia

Electrical stimulation of some regions of the brain can lead to analgesia in animals ranging from rats to humans and can be equivalent in its pain-reducing properties to large doses of morphine (Liebeskind and Paul 1977). These analgesic effects can last for hours after only seconds of stimulation. The analgesia is often for only part of the body, so that a strong pinch to one side but not to the other might be ignored. This shows that the stimulation-produced analgesia is not simply some general interference with the animal's ability to respond to stimulation. The effective stimulation sites are in the medial brainstem, and extend from the rostral medulla (nucleus raphe magnus), through the midbrain central grey matter, towards the hypothalamus. As described in Section 5.5.5, at some sites both analgesia and self-stimulation are found, and at other sites the stimulation is aversive but is followed by analgesia. It has been shown that naloxone, a specific morphine antagonist, reverses, at least partly, stimulation-produced analgesia in both the rat and in humans (Adams 1976; Akil et al. 1976). The endogenous morphine-like peptide enkephalin (Hughes 1975; Hughes et al. 1975) injected intraventricularly yields analgesia (Beluzzi et al. 1976), and central grey matter stimulation releases this substance or a peptide similar to it (Stein et al., unpublished results; Liebeskind et al. 1976). Further, there are stereospecific opiate-binding sites in the central grey matter, and elsewhere in the brain (Kuhar et al. 1973). These findings raise the possibility that stimulation-produced analgesia is effective because it causes the release of a naturally occurring morphine-like substance which acts on opiate receptors in the central grey matter and elsewhere to provide analgesia. The function of this pain-reduction may be, after injury and the initial behavioural reaction to it to prevent further injury, to reduce the on-going effects of continuing severe pain, which could otherwise impair the animal's ability to cope well behaviourally with other needs.

At some of these analgesia-producing sites the electrical stimulation can produce reward (see Koob and LeMoal 1997). The reward at these sites might be related to the pain-reducing effect of the release of opiates, which can itself be pleasurable and positively reinforcing. However, it is also known that endogenous opiates can be released by behaviours such as grooming (see Dunbar 1996), and this may be part of the mechanism by which grooming produces pleasure and relaxation, for blockade of opiate receptors with naloxone greatly reduces grooming interactions.

6.6.2 Pharmacology of depression in relation to brain systems involved in emotion

One class of antidepressant drug, the tricyclic antidepressants, of which imipramine is an example, block the reuptake of 5-HT, NA, and DA, in that order of potency. (They inhibit the presynaptic transporters with that order of efficacy.) Another class of drug that has antidepressant properties, the monoamine oxidase inhibitors, blocks the reuptake of all three of these monoamines. Both types of drug increase the concentration of the catecholamines NA and DA in the synaptic cleft of catecholaminergic neurons, and the catecholamine hypothesis of affective disorders was based on this type of evidence, and also on the concentrations of these monoamines and their metabolites in the brains of depressed patients. The catecholamine hypothesis was that low concentrations of the catecholamines produced depression, and that the antidepressant drugs worked by increasing the concentrations again. However, this hypothesis is too simple as it stands, for at least two reasons. First, most of the treatments affect 5-HT (serotonin), and indeed some newer drugs such as fluoxetine (Prozac) are relatively selective serotonin uptake inhibitors. (Serotonin, which chemically is 5-hydroxytryptamine, 5-HT, is an indoleamine, not a catecholamine like NA and DA.) Second, when antidepressant drugs are given, the pharmacological effects described take place within hours, whereas the antidepressant effects may take $10-14$ days to become apparent. In the search for biochemical processes that take $10-14$ days to develop with the administration of antidepressant drugs, it has been observed that with a time course more like this (1) 5-HT receptors become upregulated (more sensitive); (2) in relation to NA, there is an increase in the sensitivity of central α-adrenoceptors (and a decrease in the sensitivity of central β-adrenoceptors). Overall, the evidence tends to support the hypothesis that central 5-HT is involved in depression, with probably some involvement of NA but much less evidence that DA is involved (see further Cooper, Bloom and Roth 1996). The traditional way forward for pharmacological research in this area involves screening a large number of new drugs for potential antidepressant effects. This research has not been closely linked to understanding of the brain systems involved in emotion. It may be hoped that in the future there will be closer links now that progress is being made in understanding the brain mechanisms of emotion. One potentially fruitful link would be to develop drugs that have potency particularly for some of the brain areas now known to be involved in emotion, such as the amygdala, orbitofrontal cortex, and cingulate cortex. Another potentially fruitful link is to investigate with neuroimaging the brain changes that occur in depression and in its treatment with antidepressants (see, e.g., Fig. 4.26), to gain further evidence in humans about the brain systems involved in depression, and potentially, with the use of transmitter-specific techniques available with PET, to continue to investigate neuro-pharmacological and neurochemical aspects of depression in humans (see Section 4.5.5).

6.6.3 Pharmacology of anxiety in relation to brain systems involved in emotion

One class of antianxiety drug, the benzodiazepines, bind to 'benzodiazepine receptors' in the brain, increasing the frequency of opening of the $GABA_A$ (γ-aminobutyric acid) receptor-activated chloride channels. The influx of chloride through these channels produces hyperpolarization of cells, and thus a decrease in firing (see Cooper, Bloom and Roth 1996). Barbiturates, which have antianxiety properties, prolong the opening of the same chloride channels. Given that GABA is the most widespread inhibitory transmitter in the brain, these findings leave open, of course, where the antianxiety drugs work. One early suggestion is that they influence the hippocampus (see J. Gray 1987). However, there is almost no evidence linking the hippocampus to emotion, and instead the evidence indicates that it is involved in memory, often when this has a spatial aspect (including a spatial context), or is episodic, about a particular past event or episode (see Rolls and Treves 1998). Indeed, fornix section, which produces many of the effects of hippocampal and related damage on memory, has no effects on stimulus–reinforcement association learning or reversal (see D. Gaffan *et al.* 1984; see also Jones and Mishkin 1972). Further, Rawlins, Winocur and Gray (1983) showed that damage to the hippocampus of rats did not abolish the antianxiety effects of the antianxiety drug chlordiazepoxide in an animal model of anxiety. As in the case of antidepressant drugs, it may be hoped that future studies will be able to link the effects of antianxiety drugs more closely to areas of the brain known to be involved in emotion, as this may help in the development of better treatments for anxiety, whether by drugs (e.g. File 1987) or by other forms of treatment.

6.7 Overview of behavioural selection and output systems involved in reward, punishment, emotion, and motivation

Some of the output systems involved in emotion are outlined in Section 4.6. There, output systems from the orbitofrontal cortex and amygdala that project through the hypothalamus and directly to the dorsal nucleus of the vagus are described for learned autonomic responses. Output systems involving the striatum and rest of the basal ganglia are implicated in implicit behavioural responses to at least conditioned incentives. In addition, there are systems for producing explicit emotional responses (Section 4.6.3). In Chapter 10 I consider the fact that a cost–benefit analysis must be performed in order to select an appropriate response. Here I draw out how reward systems in the brain may act as a suitable interface between sensory and motor systems, and some of the ways in which such interfacing may be implemented in the brain.

In terms of sensory analysis, we have seen in Chapters 2 and 4 how sensory systems set up representations of objects in the world that are without reward/punishment valence, but are suitable as inputs to succeeding stages of processing such as the orbitofrontal cortex and amygdala where the valence can be learned by pattern association with primary reinforcers such as taste and touch. We have seen how the representations are highly appropriate as inputs to pattern-association mechanisms, in that they can be read with a dot product type of decoding that is very neurophysiologically plausible, implemented in the brain by adding in the post-synaptic neuron the contributions of many thousands of inputs each weighted by its synaptic connection strength (see Appendix), and in that each input carries information that is essentially independent (within the limits enforced by the number of stimuli being processed). After this pattern association, we have a representation that is coded in terms of its reward/punishment valence. We also have other sensory stimuli which are decoded by the brain as being primary, that is unlearned, reinforcers, such as the taste of food (Chapter 2), or pleasant touch or pain (Chapter 4), or many others (Chapter 10, Table 10.1). We should think of these representations coded in terms of reward and punishment as potential goals for action. Although Milner and Goodale (1995) have characterized the dorsal visual system as being appropriate for the control of action, and the ventral visual system projecting to the primate temporal lobe as being appropriate for perception, the view taken here is that the ventral visual system is also involved in action, indeed is at the heart of action, by providing the representations that are the goals for action. It is precisely because the goals for action are typically objects in the world that the ventral visual system, which is involved in the representation of objects, is an important component for the action system (see further Rolls and Treves 1998).

We have seen then that reward and punishment decoding systems require certain types of sensory system, so that an important way of understanding much sensory information processing is to realize that it is involved in producing representations suitable as goals for action. The reasons for brain design that have resulted in it using rewards and punishers (including expected rewards and punishers) as goals for actions are considered in Chapter 10. The issue considered here is how, in the brain, reward and punishment systems, which represent goals, are connected to output systems. One feature of the output systems is that they must be built to try to obtain activation of the reward representations in the brain, and to avoid or escape from activation of punishment-related representations in the brain. A second feature is that of response selection, and a third is that of cost–benefit 'analysis' (see Chapter 10).

In Section 6.4, we considered the operation of the basal ganglia in terms of receiving inputs from many reward systems. We showed how they could implement a selection based on competition between inputs, the strongest current reward or punishment (in the common currency, see Chapter 10) winning. Some of the mechanisms for ensuring that one reward does not dominate behaviour for too long include satiety mechanisms, sensory-specific satiety, etc. (see Chapters 2, 4, 8, and 10). We showed how the basal ganglia could perhaps also map (by association) the selected reward on to the other systems that also project into the basal ganglia. These other inputs, from the cerebral cortex, include motor and somatosensory systems so that the rewards could produce responses with which they had been associated in the past. This would implement response–reinforcer learning. The other cortical inputs though come from all areas of cerebral cortex, so effectively the reinforcers could be associated to much more complex actions than just 'responses' of the type represented in primary motor and somatosensory areas (see Rolls and Treves 1998). The basal ganglia could thus in principle provide one way in which the rewards and punishment representations in the brain could be interfaced to response and action systems. This is an implicit route to action (see Chapter 9), and in line with this, the basal ganglia do not have backprojections to the cortical areas that project into them. This is in contrast with memory systems such as the hippocampus, orbitofrontal cortex, and amygdala, which do have backprojections to the cortical areas from which they receive, potentially allowing retrieval of information from those systems about memories and emotional states (see Rolls and Treves 1998). In contrast, the basal ganglia, with no such backprojections, may not allow such explicit retrieval, and indeed we are not aware of how our motor systems solve and are processing well-learned problems. These suggestions on basal ganglia function, and their possible role in action–reinforcer learning and connecting reinforcers to actions, are complemented by a neuronal network computational model of how the basal ganglia could actually operate (Rolls and Treves 1998, Chapter 9). However, at the same time it must be stated that our understanding of basal ganglia function, and of how actions are selected and learned in terms of their anticipated reinforcer outcomes, is far from well developed, and we should regard the points made here as hypotheses which may help to guide future research (see also Rolls and Treves 1998, Chapter 9). What is strongly suggested here is that rewards and punishers, and anticipated rewards and punishers, decoded and represented as described in this book, provide the inputs to the behaviour selection processes.

In addition to the basal ganglia route, and the route for explicit reasoning about courses of action to take concerning rewards and punishments (see Section 4.6.3, and Chapters 9 and 10), there are some other possible routes for stimuli that are reinforcers to influence behaviour. There may for example be many brainstem connections between aversive sensory inputs such as the pain-related inputs coming from the C and $A\delta$ fibres, and brainstem response systems. Such systems operate at the reflex level, enabling for example a limb to be pulled away from a noxious stimulus. However, in terms of the definition given in Chapter 1 for reinforcers, which require operant, that is arbitrary, acts to be learnable to the stimuli, such brainstem reflexes would not qualify as being involved in behavioural responses to reinforcers. There may be other sensory-motor routes which also operate at a relatively low level, and which may correspondingly not qualify as reward or punishment systems. To qualify, the systems have to provide a representation of the goals for actions, and allow arbitrary (operant) responses to be learned to obtain such rewards or avoid or escape from such punishers. Although the basal ganglia are key brain systems involved in this function, it is possible that there are others. Now that we have clear hypotheses about how and where rewards and punishers are decoded and represented by the brain, it must be an aim of future research to clarify and better understand how the selection is made between the different goals, how the costs of actions are taken into account (perhaps because they are encoded into the common currency as punishers and expected punishers), and how responses for obtaining the selected goal are made.

7 Brain mechanisms for thirst

7.1 Introduction

In this chapter we consider the rewards relevant to thirst and drinking. In the case of thirst there are internal signals which indicate that there is a need for water. The water is a reward, in that the organism will work to obtain the water. The signals that make the water rewarding originate internally. In the case of thirst, the internal signals reflect the volumes of the cellular and extracellular fluid. Thirst and drinking operate to maintain the constancy of the internal milieu. The internal signals operate to alter the reward value which water has for the thirsty organism. The reward signals are conveyed primarily by the taste and sight of water. In this chapter, we will consider where in information processing in these sensory systems the sensory stimulation produced by water is decoded not just as a physical stimulus, but is coded in terms of its reward value. An important aspect of brain organization is that these two aspects of information processing are kept separate, at least in primates including humans. Another important aspect of brain organization for this type of reward is that the learning of which visual stimuli are water, or are associated with water, takes place in specialized parts for the brain for this type of learning, which take place after analysis of what the stimulus is.

For thirst, and hunger, the origin of the drive signal that modulates the reward value of sensory input is internal, and related to homeostasis. For comparison, in Chapter 8 we consider the processing of rewards relevant to sexual behaviour, in which the conditions that initiate the drive are not simply homeostatic to maintain the internal milieu.

Thirst is a sensation normally aroused by a lack of water and associated with a desire to drink water. The mechanisms involved in the control of drinking are useful to study, not only because of their medical relevance, but also because the stimuli that lead to drinking can be identified, measured and manipulated, so allowing the basis of a relatively complex, motivated behaviour to be analysed. The type of control of the reward value produced by the taste of water being modulated by internal thirst signals is analogous to the control of the reward value of the taste of food by internal hunger and satiety signals. However, thirst is a useful case to study because the internal signals that control thirst can be defined and precisely measured.

Body water is contained within two main compartments. The intracellular water accounts for approximately 40% of body weight, and the extracellular water is approximately 20% of body weight, divided between the blood plasma (the blood without the cells) (5% of body weight) and the interstitial fluid (the fluid between/outside the cells of the body and not in the blood vascular system) (15% of body weight) (see Fig. 7.1). After water deprivation, significant depletions of both the cellular and extracellular fluid compartments are found. To discover whether changes in either or both fluid compartments can act as stimuli for drinking, effects of selective depletion of one of the compartments on drinking, and the mechanisms activated, have been investigated as described below.

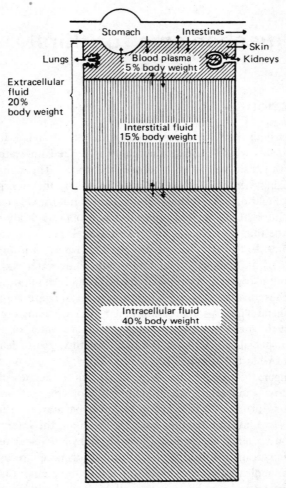

Fig. 7.1 Body water compartments. Arrows represent fluid movement. (After B. Rolls and Rolls 1982.)

References to original sources are contained in B. Rolls and Rolls (1982), B. Rolls, Wood and Rolls (1980a), Grossman (1990), and Fitzsimons (1992).

7.2 Cellular stimuli for drinking

The drinking that occurs when the body fluids become concentrated due to net water loss or the ingestion of foods rich in salts such as meat appears to be initiated by cellular dehydration, leading to cell shrinkage. Evidence for this is that the administration of concentrated sodium chloride solution leads to withdrawal of water from the cells by osmosis and produces drinking. (Osmosis is the process by which water may be withdrawn through the semipermeable membrane of cells if the concentration of salts and other osmotically active substances outside the cells is increased.) The effective change appears to be cellular dehydration and not an increase in absolute osmotic pressure (i.e. osmolality, as measured by freezing-point depression), in that administration of hypertonic substances such as sodium chloride and sucrose, which remain outside the cells and therefore cause cellular dehydration by osmosis, stimulates drinking. In contrast, similar concentrations of substances such as glucose, urea, and methylglucose, which cross the cell membrane and therefore do not lead to cellular dehydration, stimulate little or no drinking. Increases in sodium concentration rather than cellular dehydration might be thought to be the thirst stimulus, but this seems unlikely since drinking is stimulated by the application of sucrose (which withdraws water from cells but does not raise sodium concentration) either directly to brain tissue (Blass and Epstein 1971; Peck and Novin 1971) or into the cerebral ventricles. The degree of cellular dehydration must be monitored accurately, because sufficient water is consumed to dilute administered hypertonic sodium chloride solutions to the same concentration as the body fluids, that is to the same effective osmotic pressure (isotonicity).

Cellular dehydration as a stimulus for drinking is sensed centrally, in the brain, rather than peripherally, in the body, because low doses of hypertonic sodium chloride (or sucrose) infused into the carotid arteries, which supply the brain, produced drinking in the dog. Similar peripheral infusions had no effect on drinking (Wood, Rolls and Ramsay 1977). The brain regions in which cellular dehydration is sensed and leads to drinking appear to be near or lie in a region extending from the preoptic area through the hypothalamus, and including tissue surrounding the anteroventral part of the third ventricle, to the zona incerta posteriorly (Fig. 7.2). In these regions (but not in other brain regions) injections of small volumes of mildly hypertonic sodium chloride or sucrose lead to drinking, which at least at some sites is motivationally specific, as drinking, but not eating, is elicited (Blass and Epstein 1971; Peck and Novin 1971). Consistent with the hypothesis that these brain regions are involved in drinking in response to cellular dehydration, small lesions here can specifically impair drinking in response to cellular thirst stimuli yet leave drinking in response to other thirst stimuli intact, although more non-specific effects of the lesions are common (see B. Rolls and Rolls 1982).

7.3 Extracellular thirst stimuli

7.3.1 Extracellular stimuli for thirst

Thus far we have considered only the effect of loss of fluid from inside cells on thirst. Although the amount of fluid in the extracellular fluid (ECF) compartment is less than that in the cells, it is vital for the organism that the ECF be conserved to avoid debilitating changes in vascular fluid volume and pressure. The effects of loss of extracellular fluid include fainting, caused by insufficient blood reaching the brain. In addition to the physiological and hormonal mechanisms that contribute to the maintenance of the ECF volume (e.g. baroreceptor reflexes stimulated by a fall in blood pressure, antidiuretic hormone (ADH) (which reduces the excretion of water in the urine), and aldosterone

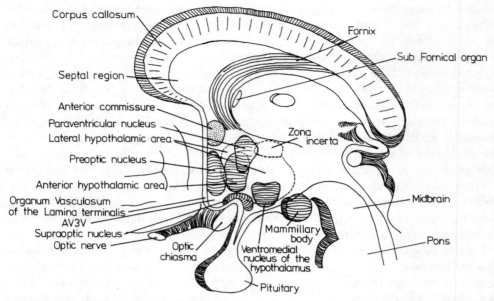

Fig. 7.2 Sagittal three-dimensional representation of the brain to illustrate some brain regions implicated in the control of drinking. AV3V: anteroventral region of the third ventricle. (After B. Rolls and Rolls 1982.)

(which reduces the excretion of sodium ion in the urine)), the behavioural response of drinking ensures that plasma volume does not fall to dangerously low levels.

The extracellular compartment has two components: the intravascular which contains the plasma, and the extravascular or interstitial fluid. These two components are in equilibrium and the receptors for controlling the ECF volume are located within the vasculature. ECF volume can become depleted in a variety of clinical conditions, which are accompanied by the loss of isotonic fluid as a result of vomiting, diarrhoea, or blood loss. (Isotonic fluid is fluid that is at the same 'strength' or effective osmotic pressure as the body fluids.) Significant ECF volume depletion will cause the release of ADH, which will reduce renal fluid loss. There might also be a need to replenish lost fluid, and it is advantageous that thirst often follows the ECF depletion in these clinical conditions.

There are several ways that ECF volume can be depleted experimentally in order to study the role of ECF volume in thirst. Obvious methods include haemorrhage, lowering the sodium content of the diet, and encouraging excessive sweating, urine production, or salivation, depending on the species being tested. However, ECF can be removed quickly and simply by injecting high concentrations of colloids (gum acacia or polyethylene glycol) either into the peritoneal cavity or subcutaneously. Isotonic fluid accumulates around the colloid, thereby depleting the ECF. Such depletion leads to a reduction in urine flow and an increase in water intake which is related to the magnitude of the depletion. Some hours after the onset of thirst, a marked appetite for sodium develops and the ingestion of sodium restores the volume and composition of the ECF to normal.

The drinking that follows ECF depletion could be mediated by receptors in the vasculature. The role of such putative receptors in thirst can be studied by either constricting or expanding blood vessels in regions where such manipulations would be interpreted as under- or over-filling. Such studies have indicated that the receptors for extracellular thirst are located in two main regions of the vasculature, in and around the kidneys and the heart (see Fig. 7.3), as shown by the following evidence.

7.3.2 Role of the kidney in extracellular thirst: the renin–angiotensin system

In the rat ligation of the inferior vena cava, which reduces venous return to the heart and reduces arterial blood pressure, leads to a marked increase in water intake and a positive fluid balance due to decreased urine flow. If both kidneys are removed before ligation, water intake is significantly reduced, which suggests that an essential thirst stimulus following caval ligation could be a reduction in blood pressure to the kidneys. In order to test this hypothesis, Fitzsimons reduced the pressure to the kidneys by partially constricting the renal arteries, and found that water intake increased. When reductions in blood pressure or volume are sensed by the juxtaglomerular apparatus in the kidneys, the enzyme renin is released. Renin acts on substrate in the plasma to form angiotensin I, which is converted to angiotensin II, a vasoactive octapeptide (see Fig. 7.4). Angiotensin II is an active dipsogen in that intravenous infusions stimulate copious drinking (Fitzsimons and Simons 1969). The receptors for angiotensin-induced drinking are located in the central nervous system, since injections into localized brain regions of doses of angiotensin at least 1000 times smaller than those required peripherally stimulate rats in fluid balance to drink large quantities of water (Epstein, Fitzsimons and Rolls 1970). Not only is angiotensin very potent, it is also very specific. Drinking is the only behavioural response which follows its administration and this drinking is highly motivated. A wide variety of species (including mammals, birds, and reptiles) have been shown to drink after administration of angiotensin (see B. Rolls and Rolls 1982).

Since the initial discovery that intracranial angiotensin stimulates drinking, much work has been aimed at locating precisely the receptive site(s) in the brain. Angiotensin does not cross the blood–brain barrier, but the circumventricular organs, which are located on the surface of the cerebral ventricles, are outside the blood–brain barrier. Several circumventricular organs have now been suggested as receptive sites for angiotensin and one of these is the subfornical organ (SFO) (see Fig. 7.4). Local application of angiotensin to the SFO in very low doses (1.0 pg) can stimulate drinking, and lesions of the SFO or application to it of a competitive, angiotensin receptor-blocking agent, at least in the rat, can abolish drinking in response to intravenous angiotensin without affecting drinking in response to cellular thirst stimuli (Simpson et al. 1977). The SFO has been shown electrophysiologically to contain angiotensin-sensitive neurons (M. Phillips and Felix 1976), and anatomically to send projections to the medial preoptic area, the supraoptic nucleus, and the brain close to the anteroventral part of the third ventricle (AV3V) (Miselis et al. 1979). Injections of low doses of angiotensin in the region of another circumventricular organ, the organum vasculosum of the lamina terminalis (OVLT) in the anteroventral part of the third ventricle (see Fig. 7.3), also elicit drinking (M. Phillips 1978). Relatively large lesions in this region, which included damage to fibres from the SFO, reduced drinking in response to angiotensin (and to hypertonic sodium chloride)

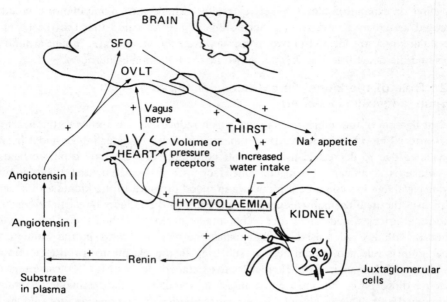

Fig. 7.3 A summary of the mechanisms involved in extracellular thirst. SFO, subfornical organ; OVLT, organum vasculosum of the lamina terminalis. (After B. Rolls and Rolls 1982.)

(Buggy and Johnson 1977a,b; Thrasher *et al.* 1980a,b). Thus there is reasonable evidence that there are specialized and localized regions of neural tissue in or near the SFO and the OVLT involved in drinking produced by angiotensin (see B. Rolls and Rolls 1982).

7.3.3 Cardiac receptors for thirst

Local changes in volume and pressure in and around the heart are involved in extracellular thirst. Reducing the blood flow to the heart by partially constricting the thoracic inferior vena cava in the dog (a method used to produce low-output experimental cardiac failure) markedly increased water intake, which led to excessive oedema (Ramsay, Rolls and Wood 1975). Inflation of a balloon in the abdominal inferior vena cava also led to drinking which was correlated with the maximal fall in central venous pressure, but some drinking still occurred after administration of an angiotensin receptor-blocking agent and presumably was mediated by cardiac receptors (Fitzsimons and Moore-Gillon 1980). It is still not clear precisely where such cardiac receptors are located, but it seems most likely that they are in the low-pressure (venous) circulation around the heart (see Fig. 7.3), since the compliance of these vessels is high, making them responsive to changes in blood volume. It is thought that the information from these receptors is carried to the central nervous system via the vagosympathetic nerves, which normally exert an inhibitory effect on thirst.

7.4 Control of normal drinking

It has been shown above that there are mechanisms by which depletion of the cellular or the extracellular fluid compartments can stimulate drinking. An important question is to what extent these mechanisms are normally activated during thirst and drinking, whether produced by water deprivation or occurring when there is free access to water. Perhaps habit is one factor normally important in the initiation of drinking, but are deficits in the body fluid compartments normally involved in the initiation of drinking?

To gain evidence on this, it is first important to know whether deficits in the body fluid compartments are produced, for example, by water deprivation. There are deficits in both fluid compartments produced by water deprivation (see B. Rolls, Wood and Rolls 1980a; B. Rolls and Rolls 1982). This is the case not only in the rat, dog, and monkey, but also in humans (B. Rolls and Rolls, 1982; Rolls, Wood, Rolls, Lind, Lind and Ledingham, 1980b). Next, it is found that the deficit in the cellular fluid compartment is large enough to lead to drinking, as shown by threshold measurements determined for the initiation of drinking in response to cellular dehydration. For example, following infusions of sodium chloride in the monkey, the threshold increase in plasma concentration necessary to evoke drinking was found to be 7 mOsmol kg^{-1} H_2O, which was less than the increase produced by water deprivation for 24 h (Wood, Maddison, Rolls, Rolls and Gibbs 1980). Other evidence comes from repletion experiments. When, after water deprivation, intravenous water preloads were given which effectively abolished the cellular fluid deficit, drinking was reduced by 65% in the rat and by 85% in the monkey (Wood, Maddison, Rolls, Rolls and Gibbs 1980; Wood, Rolls and Rolls 1982). If the ECF deficit is corrected by intravenous infusions of isotonic sodium chloride, then drinking is reduced by 20% and 5% in the rat and monkey, respectively (see B. Rolls, Wood and Rolls, 1980a). Thus depletion of the fluid compartments is an important determinant of drinking after water deprivation, with the depletion in the cellular compartment being more important, particularly in the primate (see further B. Rolls, Wood and Rolls, 1980a; B. Rolls and Rolls 1982).

In humans, it was found that with free access to water, the osmotic and extracellular thresholds for the elicitation of thirst were not normally reached before the humans had water to drink (P. Phillips, Rolls, Ledingham and Morton 1984). Thus in humans, at least when working in an air-conditioned temperature-controlled environment, drinking may anticipate needs. This anticipation is likely to be at least partly based on learning, so that after some time, actual body fluid deficits would be avoided. The humans would learn to initiate drinking based on any stimuli that are associated later with thirst signalled by cellular or extracellular body fluid deficits. In this way, drinking might become conditioned to stimuli such as large meals, salty food, or hot temperatures and dry conditions, or even to time of day. Of course, the primary thirst signals would be important for setting up this learning, but after the learning, the drinking would occur to the conditioned stimuli, and the primary thirst signals would not be activated. One would expect the primary thirst signals to become activated again if conditions changed, an example of which might be moving from sedentary work in an air-conditioned environment to physical work outdoors in a hot country. As a result of the activation of primary thirst signals, new learning would produce appropriate conditioned drinking for the new conditions. Another factor in humans that may lead to primary body fluid deficit signals being unusual is that there is frequently available a large set of attractive drinks, including soft drinks, tea, and coffee.

Another interesting aspect of thirst is that in humans it was found that infusions of angiotensin did not always elicit drinking (P. Phillips, Rolls, Ledingham *et al.* 1985).

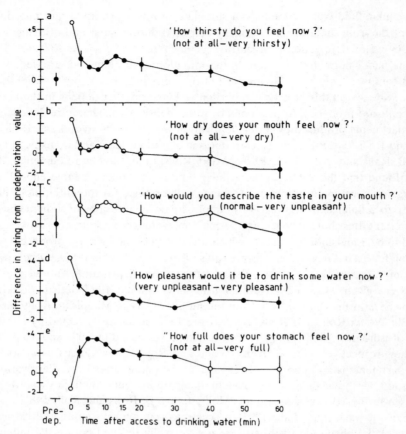

Difference in rating from predeprivation value

a 'How thirsty do you feel now ?' (not at all—very thirsty)

b 'How dry does your mouth feel now ?' (not at all—very dry)

c 'How would you describe the taste in your mouth ?' (normal—very unpleasant)

d 'How pleasant would it be to drink some water now ?' (very unpleasant—very pleasant)

e "How full does your stomach feel now ?' (not at all—very full)

Pre-dep.   0   5   10   15   20   30   40   50   60
Time after access to drinking water (min)

Fig. 7.4 The pleasantness of the taste of water is increased by water deprivation in humans, and decreases rapidly during drinking to satiety, before the water depletion of the body fluids has been completed. This is shown in the fourth graph from the top. In this diagram the effects of 24 h water deprivation on human subjective ratings of thirst and other sensations are shown by the difference between the predeprivation rating (pre-dep.) and the rating at time 0, taken 24 h later just before access to the water was given. The way in which the ratings changed after drinking started at time 0 is also shown. The significance of the changes relative to the value after 24 h water deprivation, at time 0, is indicated by closed circles ($P < 0.01$), half-filled circles ($P < 0.05$), or open circles (not significant). (After B. Rolls, Wood, Rolls, Lind, Lind and Ledingham 1980b and B. Rolls and Rolls 1982.)

Moreover, large variations of angiotensin concentrations are found in humans when the human moves for example from lying down to standing up. The reason for this is that the change of posture in humans to standing upright on two legs produces a sudden drop in pressure in the renal arteries (as blood accumulates initially in the lower half of the standing body), and the release of angiotensin (stimulated by the reduced pressure in the renal arteries) produces vasoconstriction, which helps to compensate for the reduced blood pressure. Under these conditions (just standing up), thirst is not necessarily appropriate, and it may therefore be that the renin–angiotensin system is less important in humans than in other animals. It is nevertheless important to know about angiotensin in humans, for under some pathological conditions such as congestive heart failure, much angiotensin may be released as part of the body's attempt to compensate for some of the lack of fluid on the arterial side of the circulation (see Fitzsimons 1992). However, to the extent that such pathologically high levels of angiotensin may produce thirst and lead to drinking, this is inappropriate, for it may exacerbate the problem. Under these conditions, appropriate clinical care might include monitoring of water and fluid intake, to ensure that it is not excessive.

7.5   Reward and satiety signals for drinking

Drinking still occurs when ingested water is allowed to drain from a fistula in the oesophagus, stomach or duodenum. This is found in the rat, dog, and monkey (see Rolls, Wood and Rolls, 1980a; B. Rolls and Rolls 1982; Gibbs, Rolls and Rolls, 1986), and indicates that the reward for drinking is provided by oropharyngeal (and other pregastric) sensations such as the taste of water (at least in the first instance; compensatory learning may occur after prolonged experience). In fact, even a small quantity (e.g. 0.1 ml) of water delivered orally is sufficient to reinforce drinking, whereas much more water (e.g. 1–2 ml) must be delivered for the rat to learn a response in order to deliver it intragastrically (Epstein 1960) or intravenously (Nicolaidis and Rowland 1974). This underlines the importance of exteroceptors in detecting and responding correctly to the presence of water, and shows that the presence of water in the gut or the dilution of plasma are not the primary rewards which normally control the animal's drinking. A subjective analysis of the oropharyngeal control of drinking found that humans report (using a quantitative visual analogue rating scale) that the pleasantness of the taste of water is increased when they are thirsty as a result of water deprivation for 24 h, relative to the non-deprived condition (B. Rolls, Wood, Rolls, Lind, Lind and Ledingham 1980b; see Fig. 7.4). It thus appears that oropharyngeal factors such as taste and swallowing maintain drinking and provide the incentive (or reward) for drinking.

There are neurons in the orbitofrontal cortex taste regions that respond to the 'taste' of water. An example of this type of neuron is shown in Fig. 7.5. The neuron responded much more to the taste of water than to other stimuli. There are many such neurons in the orbitofrontal cortex (Rolls, Yaxley and Sienkiewicz 1990). Although there might not be water receptors per se on the tongue, the presence of water in the mouth may be signalled by the presence of non-viscous liquid in the mouth, and the absence of firing of sweet, salt, bitter, sour, and umami neurons. (The saliva in the mouth will be diluted when water is in the mouth.) In any case, the processing that has taken place by the time taste information reaches the orbitofrontal cortex results in a population of neurons which conveys information about the presence of water in the mouth, and which is approximately as large a population as that devoted to the other prototypical tastes sweet, salt, bitter, and sour (Rolls, Yaxley and Sienkiewicz 1990). The coding provided by these populations of taste-responsive neurons in the orbitofrontal cortex can be visualized using multidimensional scaling (MDS), as shown in Fig. 7.6. MDS is based on a distance measure of the representations provided by different neurons. It is based, for example, on the correlations between the response profiles of different neurons to a set of stimuli. If all the different neurons respond similarly to two stimuli, they will be close together in the MDS space. If the different neurons have differences in their responses to the two stimuli, the stimuli will

OFC

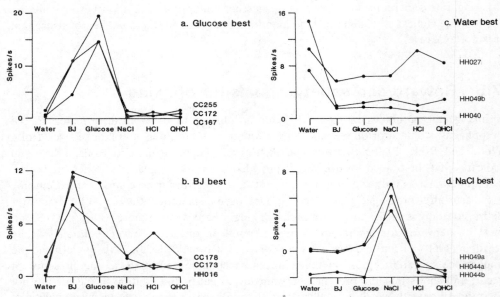

Fig. 7.5 A selection of three orbitofrontal cortex neurons responding best to the taste of water (W) (c, top right). Other neurons responding best to the taste of 1 M glucose are shown in (a), to blackcurrant fruit juice (BJ) in (b), and to 0.1 M sodium chloride (NaCl) in (d). HCl, 0.01 M HCl, sour; QHCl, 0.001 M quinine hydrochloride (bitter). (After Rolls, Yaxley and Sienkiewicz 1990.)

be far apart in the space. The results of MDS on a population of taste neurons in the orbitofrontal cortex is shown in Fig. 7.6. It can be seen that the prototypical taste stimuli are well separated from each other, and that water is well separated from each of the other stimuli, in at least some dimensions of the space. Thus the 'taste' of water is clearly represented as being separate from that of other tastes in the primate orbitofrontal cortex.

The representation of taste in the primate orbitofrontal cortex is probably of the reward value of the taste of water, in that the responses of these neurons to the taste of water is reduced to zero by feeding the monkey to satiety (see Fig. 7.7; Rolls, Sienkiewicz and Yaxley 1989b). After the reward value of the taste of water has been decoded in the orbitofrontal cortex, the output systems that link to action may be analogous to those described in Chapter 2 for hunger. For example, there are neurons in the lateral hypothalamus of the monkey that respond to the taste of water if the monkey is thirsty (Rolls, Burton and Mora 1976; B. Rolls and Rolls 1982; Rolls, Murzi, Yaxley, Thorpe and Simpson 1986; cf. Rolls, Rolls and Rowe 1983a). There are also neurons in the primate lateral hypothalamus that respond in a motivation-selective way to the sight of a visual stimulus associated with the sight of water but not of food when both thirst and hunger are present (see Fig. 2.11).

In the termination of drinking, gastric and post-gastric factors such as gut stimulation by water, and the systemic effects of absorbed water are important, and oropharyngeal factors are of less importance. If, for example, drinking is measured with an oesophageal,

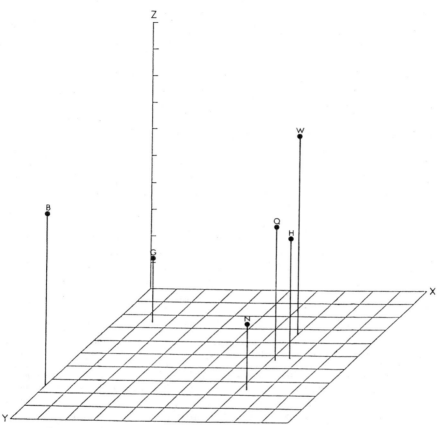

Fig. 7.6 The space produced by multidimensional scaling (MDS) of the responses of primate orbitofrontal cortex neurons to different tastes. The representation of water (W) is well separated from that of the prototypical tastes glucose (G), salt (N), bitter (Q, quinine) and sour (H, HCl). B, Blackcurrant juice. (After Rolls, Yaxley and Sienkiewicz 1990.)

gastric or duodenal fistula open, then much more water (e.g. 1.5–10 times) is consumed than normally or when the fistula is closed (Maddison, Wood, Rolls, Rolls and Gibbs 1980; B. Rolls, Wood and Rolls 1980a). Gastric distension appears to be one factor in satiety, for if drinking is allowed to terminate normally in the monkey, and then a gastric cannula is opened to allow water in the stomach to drain out, drinking starts again very promptly (Maddison *et al,* 1980). Gastric distension can only operate normally if ingested water reaches the intestine to inhibit gastric emptying, because excessive drinking occurs with a duodenal fistula open (Maddison *et al.* 1980). Gut stimulation by water, and possibly activation of immediately post-absorptive hepatic–portal mechanisms, may also contribute to satiety, because intraduodenal infusions of water are relatively more effective in terminating drinking than intravenous infusions (Wood, Maddison, Rolls, Rolls and Gibbs 1980). In the monkey and other relatively rapid drinkers such as the dog and human, systemic dilution produced by ingested water is not rapid enough to account for the termination of drinking, although, within 15–20 minutes after access to water, dilution of

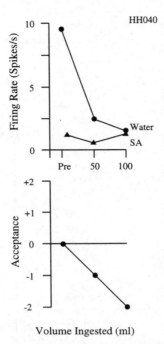

Fig. 7.7 An orbitofrontal cortex neuron in the monkey responding to the taste of water when thirsty, and gradually responding less to the taste of water during drinking to satiety. SA, spontaneous activity of the neuron; Pre, the firing rate before satiety was produced, by allowing the monkey to drink 100 ml water. The acceptability of the water is shown in the lower graph, on a scale from +2 indicating strong acceptance to −2 indicating strong rejection when satiety has been reached. (After Rolls, Sienkiewicz and Yaxley 1989b.)

the body fluids is occurring (B. Rolls, Wood, Rolls, Lind, Lind and Ledingham 1980a; B. Rolls and Rolls, 1982). This dilution does at least contribute to satiety, since equivalent dilution produced by intravenous infusions of water reduces drinking (Wood, Maddison, Rolls, Rolls and Gibbs 1980). The termination of drinking is best considered as the sequential activation of a number of contributing factors, starting with oropharyngeal stimulation by water (which appears to make a partial contribution to satiety as shown by observations that drinking with an oesophageal fistula open does usually stop in very rapid drinkers such as the dog—Towbin 1949), gastric distension (which humans report subjectively to occur rapidly as satiety develops—B. Rolls et al. 1980a), gut and hepatic–portal stimulation by water, and finally systemic dilution and expansion (see B. Rolls et al. 1980a; B. Rolls and Rolls 1982). Thus the reward value of the taste of water can be reduced by preabsorptive factors such as gastric distension, and later systemic dilution can contribute to satiety.

7.6 Summary (see Fig. 7.8)

Drinking can be initiated by depletion of either the cellular or extracellular fluid compartments.

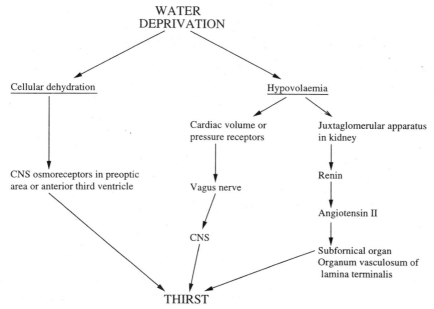

Fig. 7.8 A summary of the factors that can lead to drinking after water deprivation. (After B. Rolls and Rolls 1982.)

Both cellular and extracellular thirst stimuli (i.e. cellular dehydration and hypovolaemia) are produced by water deprivation in a variety of mammalian species, including humans. Experiments in which the deficits in the fluid compartments are selectively repleted indicate that changes in both compartments contribute to drinking following water deprivation, but that changes in the cellular compartment are the more important.

Cellular dehydration as a thirst stimulus is indicated by the shrinkage of cells in or near the preoptic area of the brain.

Extracellular depletion as a thirst stimulus is indicated by activation of the renin–angiotensin system, and by signals from volume receptors in the low-pressure circulation on the venous side of the heart. Angiotensin is sensed by neurons in the subfornical organ, which have connections to a brain region close to the preoptic area.

Drinking is maintained or reinforced by oropharyngeal factors such as the taste of water, and it appears that the pleasantness of the taste of water in humans is influenced by the degree of thirst.

When water is consumed, the following changes occur in sequence and all contribute to the termination of drinking: oropharyngeal stimulation by water, gastric distension and gut stimulation by water, and finally systemic dilution.

The 'taste' of water is represented in the cortical taste areas. The reward value of the taste of water is represented in the primate orbitofrontal cortex taste areas and in the lateral hypothalamus.

Some neurons in the primate orbitofrontal cortex and the lateral hypothalamus respond to the sight of water.

8 Sexual behaviour, reward, and brain function

8.1 Introduction

The theme of this chapter is the brain control of sexual behaviour, and especially how the brain has evolved to respond to different types of reward to produce sexual behaviour that is adaptive, that is, increases fitness.

The first part of the chapter is therefore concerned with what is known of the brain mechanisms that underlie sexual behaviour. Understanding the actual neural mechanisms is important not only because this helps to clarify the behaviour itself, but also because this is a foundation for understanding medical and other disorders of these systems, and treatments for them.

However, because there have been many advances recently in understanding and theorizing about the different patterns of sexual behaviour and why they have evolved, part of the aim of this chapter is to suggest what reward systems could account for this behaviour, and what the properties are of these reward systems. Specific hypotheses are presented about the operation of the neural systems that could implement these reward-related processes. This is intended to be an approach to how the different types of behaviour observed could be produced by particular reward systems designed by natural selection during evolution, and to provide a basis for investigations of the actual neural mechanisms that implement these processes. The aim thus is to link much recent research on the sociobiology and adaptive value of different types of sexual behaviour to new ideas introduced here about how these behaviours could be produced by the sculpting during evolution of systems that are sensitive to different types of reward. The aim is to provide a better understanding of how natural selection may operate in the course of evolution to produce different types of behavioural adaptation by selecting for different types of reward system. The possibility that during evolution a variety of different reward systems could have their sensitivity set differently in different individuals, leading to tendencies towards different types of behaviour in different individuals, each with its own way of being adaptive, is introduced. These new ideas are intended to provide a foundation for future studies of the actual reward systems in the brain that implement these different aspects of sexual behaviour each with its underlying evolutionary 'strategy'[1].

The intentional stance is adopted in much writing about sociobiology, and is sometimes used here, but should not be taken literally. It is used just as a shorthand. An example is that it might be said that genes are selfish. But this does not mean at all that genes think about whether to be selfish, and then take the decision. Instead it is just shorthand for a statement along the lines 'genes produce behaviour which operates in the context of natural selection to maximize the number of copies of the gene in the next generations'. Much of the behaviour produced is implicit or unconscious, and when the intentional stance is used as a descriptive tool, it should not be taken to mean that there is usually any explicit or conscious processing involved in the behavioural outcome.

Some of the points may seem 'obvious' once they have been made, if the reader is a neo-Darwinian used to the approach taken in evolutionary biology. However, a potential problem of sociobiology is that its stories do seem plausible, given Darwinism—but many stories are plausible. So we must be careful to seek evidence too, not just plausibility; and we need to know how much of the variance of behaviour is accounted for by each sociobiological account of a type of behaviour. In the long-term, once sociobiological hypotheses have been presented, they must be tested.

One of the main themes of this chapter is how the underlying physiology of reward is related to the sexual behaviour shown by different types of women, and different types of men. One of the key ideas is that reward systems become tuned to biological functions which they serve. For this reason, there will be discussion of the biological functions that *could* be implemented by different aspects of sexual behaviour.

Sexual behaviour is an interesting type of motivated behaviour to compare with feeding and drinking. For both feeding and drinking, there are internal signals such as plasma glucose or cellular dehydration related to homeostatic control that set the levels of food or water reward in order to produce the appropriate behaviour. In the case of sexual behaviour, there are no similar short-term homeostatic controls. However, the reward value of sexual behaviour has to be set so that it does occur sufficiently often to lead to successful reproductive behaviour, in terms of passing an individual's genes into the next generation, and helping them to thrive in the offspring. There are several factors that contribute to this, including internal (steroid) hormonal signals that on a seasonal basis, or

---

[1] We should note at the outset that there may be more than one type of evolutionary 'strategy'. One is to have genetically specified polymorphism, with the two types of individual existing in a mixed evolutionarily stable state (ESS). An example is that some individuals might be 'hawks', and others 'doves', in social situations. The behaviours might be set to occur probabilistically by the genes. A second is to have a conditional strategy, in which an individual might change behaviour, based on an assessment of the situation. For example, if one's opponent is large, one might not play a hawk. Conditional strategies can also lead to evolutionarily stable states (Maynard-Smith 1982). Of the examples that are included in this chapter, some might be polymorphic ESSs, e.g. attractiveness (though this can in humans be conditionally modified too!). Others might be conditional ESSs, e.g. the tendency for flirtation. In many of the cases, the type of strategy that is in operation strictly remains to be determined. For further discussion, see M. S. Dawkins (1986).

in relation to the stage of an oestrus cycle, set the relative reward value of sexual behaviour. For example, in rats at the stage of the oestrus cycle when oestrogen is high the appetite for food is suppressed and sexual behaviour is rewarding. The hormonal status can even be set by the environmental stimuli. For example, Lehrman and colleagues (see Lehrman 1965) described a series of events in ring doves in which seasonal factors lead to bow–cooing in the male, the sight of which stimulates the female to become receptive as a result of hormonal changes. External signals can also adjust the reward value of sexual behaviour. For example, female macaques release a pheromone (actually produced by bacteria in the vagina under the influence of androgenic hormones in the female) that acts to promote sexual behaviour in males (Baum, Everitt, Herbert and Keverne 1977). (In this example, a 'male' hormone produced in females 'controls' male sexual behaviour through the effect of the pheromone!) Thus both internal and external stimuli can act to influence the reward value of sexual behaviour.

8.2 Brain regions involved in the control of sexual behaviour, and especially in the rewards produced by sexual behaviour

In males, the preoptic area (see Fig. 8.1) is involved in the control of sexual behaviour. Lesions of this region permanently abolish male sexual behaviour; electrical stimulation can elicit copulatory activity; metabolic activity is induced (as shown by c-fos) in the preoptic area during copulation; and small implants of testosterone into the preoptic area restore sexual behaviour in castrated rats (see Carlson 1994; Everitt *et al*, 1989; Everitt, 1990; Everitt and Robbins, 1992). This region appears to have neurons in it that respond to sex-related rewards in primates, in that Oomura *et al*. (1988) described some preoptic neurons in the male macaque that increased their firing rates when he could see a female

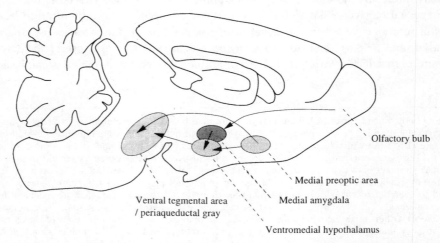

Fig. 8.1 Some of the brain regions implicated in sexual behaviour, shown on a midline view of a rat brain.

macaque seated on a chair which he could pull towards him. The same neurons did not respond to the sight of food (personal communication), and so reflected information about the type of reward available. They also described neuronal activity changes in the medial preoptic area of the male monkey that were related to the commencement of sexual behaviour, penile erection, and the refractory period following ejaculation. Similarly, neuronal activity changes in the female medial preoptic area were related to the commencement of sexual behaviour and presentation. Increased neuronal activity in the dorsomedial hypothalamic nucleus in the male monkey and in the ventromedial hypothalamic nucleus in the female monkey were synchronized to each mating act. These findings, and studies using local electrical stimulation, suggested the involvement of medial preoptic area neurons in sexual arousal, and of male dorsomedial hypothalamic and female ventromedial hypothalamic neurons in copulation (Oomura *et al.* 1988). Further evidence that these brain areas are involved in sex-related rewards is that the hormone testosterone affects brain-stimulation reward at some sites in this general region (e.g. in the posterior hypothalamus), but not at sites in, for example, the lateral hypothalamus (Caggiula 1970), where hunger modulates brain-stimulation reward (see Chapter 5).

In females, the medial preoptic area is involved in the control of reproductive cycles. It is probably also involved in controlling sexual behaviour directly. The ventromedial nucleus of the hypothalamus (VMH) is involved in some aspects of sexual behaviour, including lordosis (standing still in a receptive position) in rodents, and this behaviour can be reinstated in ovariectomized female rats by injections of oestradiol and progesterone into the ventromedial nucleus. Outputs from the VMH project to the periaqueductal gray of the midbrain, which is also necessary for female sexual behaviour such as lordosis in rodents (see Carlson 1994), via descending influences on spinal cord reflexes implemented via the reticular formation neurons and the reticulospinal tracts (Pfaff 1980, 1982; see also Priest and Pfaff 1995) (see Fig. 8.2). The VMH receives inputs from regions such as the medial amygdala.

The preoptic area receives inputs from the amygdala and orbitofrontal cortex, and thus receives information from the inferior temporal visual cortex (including information about face identity and expression), from the superior temporal auditory association cortex, from the olfactory system, and from the somatosensory system. The operation of these circuits has been described in Chapters 2 and 4. In one example described in Section 4.4.2, Everitt *et al.* (1989) showed that excitotoxic lesions of the basolateral amygdala disrupted appetitive sexual responses maintained by a visual conditioned reinforcer, but not the behaviour to the primary reinforcer for the male rats, copulation with a female rat in heat (see further Everitt 1990; Everitt and Robbins 1992). (The details of the study were that the learned reinforcer or conditioned stimulus was a light for which the male rats worked on a FR10 schedule (i.e. 10 responses made to obtain a presentation of the light), with access to the female being allowed for the first FR10 completed after a fixed period of 15 min. This is a second order schedule of reinforcement.) For comparison medial preoptic area lesions eliminated the copulatory behaviour of mounting, intromission and ejaculation to the primary reinforcer, the female rat, but did not affect the learned appetitive responding for the conditioned or secondary reinforcing stimulus, the light. The conclusion from such studies is that the amygdala is involved in stimulus-reinforcement association learning

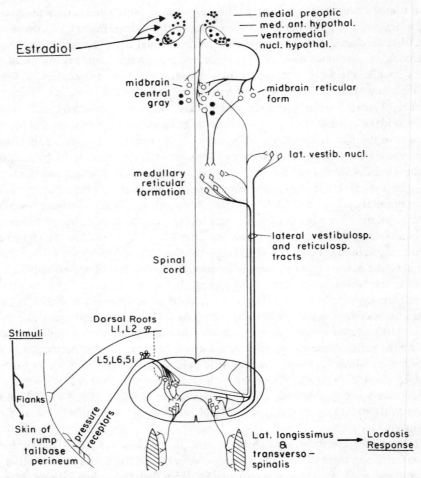

Fig. 8.2 Neural circuitry involved in the lordosis response of the female rat to flank, rump, and perineal stimulation by male rats after she is made sexually receptive by oestrogen (estradiol) in the hypothalamus. (Reproduced with permission from Pfaff 1980.)

when the primary reinforcer is a sexual reward. On the other hand, the preoptic area is not involved in such stimulus-reinforcement association learning, but is involved in the rewarding effects of primary sexual rewards. In an example illustrating part of the importance of the orbitofrontal cortex and of somatosensory reinforcers, evidence from fMRI indicates that the pleasantness of touch is represented especially in the orbitofrontal cortex (see Figs 4.4 and 4.5). Presumably the pleasant effects of sexual touch are also represented in this and connected brain areas (see, e.g., Tiihonen *et al.* 1994). It is presumably by these neural circuits in the orbitofrontal cortex and amygdala that the effects related to the control of sexual behaviour described below in Section 8.5 are implemented, and much of the decoding of the relevant stimuli, and then their interpretation as primary reinforcers, or learning about their reinforcing properties by stimulus–reinforcement association learning, occurs. A number of the effects described in Section 8.5

are related to a diminution over time of the reward value produced by the same stimulus or individual, and the enhancement of behaviour produced by novel stimuli or individuals. It is also presumably in regions such as the orbitofrontal cortex and amygdala that such effects, which require a representation of individuals, and systems that can show a form of learning with stimulus repetition to implement sensory-specific satiety and novelty effects, are implemented.

The outputs of the preoptic area include connections to the lateral tegmental field in the midbrain, and in this region neurons are found that respond in relation to different aspects of male sexual behaviour (Shimura and Shimokochi 1990). However, it is likely that only some outputs of the orbitofrontal cortex and amygdala which control sexual behaviour act through the preoptic area. The preoptic area route may be necessary for computationally simple aspects of sexual behaviour such as copulation in males, but the attractive effect of sexual stimuli may survive damage to the medial preoptic area (see Carlson 1994), suggesting that, as for feeding, outputs of the amygdala and orbitofrontal cortex can influence behaviour through the striatum (see Chapters 2, 4, and 6).

Much research remains to be performed to understand the details of the implementation of the rewards underlying sexual behaviour in brain regions such as the amygdala, orbitofrontal cortex, preoptic area, and hypothalamus. In order to provide an understanding of what reward mechanisms for sexual behaviour are likely to be implemented in these regions, we now turn to an evolutionary and sociobiological approach to sexual behaviour, and from this make suggestions about what the reward mechanisms may be that natural selection has implemented in order to bring about the types of behaviour observed.

8.3   Sperm competition and its consequences for sexual behaviour: a sociobiological approach

Monogamous primates well spread out over territory have small testes, for example the baboon. Polygamous primates living in groups with several males in the group have large testes and frequent copulation, e.g. chimpanzees and monkeys (see Ridley 1993). The reason for this appears to be sperm warfare—in order to pass his genes on to the next population, a male in a polygamous society needs to increase the probability that he will fertilize a female, and the best way to do this is to copulate often, and swamp the female with sperm, so that his sperm have a reasonable chance of getting to the egg to fertilize it. Therefore in polygamous groups with more than one male, males should have large testes, to produce large numbers of sperm and large quantities of seminal fluid. In monogamous societies, with no competition between sperm, the male should just pick a good partner, produce only enough sperm to fertilize an egg and not enough to compete with others' sperm, stay with her to bring up the children, and guard them because they are his genetic investment (Ridley 1993; see further Section 10.5).

What about humans? Despite being apparently mainly monogamous, they are intermediate in testis size and penis size—bigger than expected. Why? Maybe there is some sperm competition? Remember that although humans usually do pair, and are often apparently monogamous, humans do live in groups or colonies. Can we get hints from other animals that are paired, but are also in colonies? A problem with comparing humans with most other primates in this respect is that in most primates (and indeed in most mammals), the main parental investment is by the female (in producing the egg, in carrying the foetus, and in feeding the baby until it can become independent). The male does not have to invest in his children for them to have a reasonable chance of surviving. For this reason, the typical pattern in mammals is that the female is choosy in order to obtain healthy and fit males, and to complement this the males compete for females. However, in humans, because the children must be reared for a number of years before they become independent, there is an advantage to paternal investment in helping to bring up the children, in that the paternal resources (e.g. food, shelter, and protection) can increase the chances of the male's genes surviving into the next generation to reproduce again. Part of the reason why investment by both parents is needed in humans is that because of the large final human brain size, at birth the brain is not fully developed, and for this reason the infant needs to be looked after, fed, protected, and helped for a considerable period while the infant's brain develops, favouring pair bonding between the parents. A more useful comparison can therefore be made with some birds, such as the swallow, which live in colonies but in which the male and the female pair, and both invest in bringing up the offspring, taking it in turns for example to bring food back to the nest. If checks are made in swallows using DNA techniques for determining paternity, it is found that actually approximately one third of a pair's young are not sired by the 'father', the male of the pair (Birkhead and Moller 1992; see Ridley 1993). What happens is that the female mates sometimes with other males—she commits adultery. She probably does not do this just with a random male either—she may choose an 'attractive' male, in which the signals that attract her are signals that indicate health, strength, and fitness. One well known example of such a signal is the gaudy 'tail' of the male peacock. One argument is that, given that the tail is a real handicap in life, any male that can survive with such a large tail must be very healthy or fit. Another argument is that if his tail is very attractive indeed, then the female should choose him, because her sons with him would probably be attractive too, and also chosen by females. (This is an example of the use of the intentional stance in the description, when no real propositional state is likely to occur at all.) In such a social system, such as that of the swallow, the wife needs a reliable husband with whom she mates (so that he thinks the offspring are his, which for the system to be stable they must be sometimes) to help provide resources for 'their' offspring. (Remember that a nest must be built, the eggs must be incubated, and the hungry young must be well fed to help them become fit offspring. Here fit means successfully passing on genes into the next generation —see R. Dawkins 1986 etc.). But the wife (or at least her genes) also benefits by obtaining as fit genes as possible, by sometimes cheating on her husband. To ensure that her husband does not find out and therefore leave her and stop caring for the young, she deceives the husband by committing her adultery as much as possible secretly, perhaps hiding behind a bush to mate with her lover. So the (swallow) wife maximizes care for her children using her husband, and maximizes her genetic potential by finding a lover with fit genes that are likely to be attractive in her sons to other females (see Ridley 1993). (It is interesting that if a male were popular with females, then even if he had genes that were not better in terms of survival etc., it would be advantageous for a female to have offspring with him, as her sons would be more likely to be attractive to other females, and thus maximize her reproductive potential. This is an example of Fisherian selection.)

Could anything like the situation just described for birds such as swallows also apply to humans? It appears that it may apply, at least in part, and that similar evolutionary factors may influence human sexual behaviour, and hence make obtaining particular stimuli in the environment rewarding to humans. We need to understand whether this is the case, in order to understand what rewards drive sexual behaviour in humans. One line of evidence already described is the large testis and penis size of men. (We will get on to the reason for the large penis size soon.) A second line is that studies in humans of paternity using modern DNA tests show that in fact the woman's partner (e.g. husband) is not the father of about 14% of their children. Although possibly surprising, this has been found in a study in Liverpool, and in another in the south of England, and in other studies (Baker and Bellis 1995; see Ridley 1993). So might men produce large amounts of sperm, and have intercourse quite regularly, in order to increase the likelihood that children produced are theirs, whether by their wife or by their mistress? When women choose men as their lovers, do they choose men who are likely to produce children who are fit, that is children good at passing on their genes, half of which originate from the woman? It appears that women may choose like this, as described below, and that this behaviour may even select genetically for certain characteristics in men, because the woman finds these characteristics rewarding during mate selection. Of course, if such a strategy were employed (presumably mainly unconsciously) all the time in women the system would break down (be unstable), because men would not trust their wives, and the men would not invest in making a home and bringing up their children.[2] So we would not expect this to be the only selective pressure on what women find attractive and rewarding as qualities in men. Pursuing this matter further, we might expect women to find reliability, stability, provision of a home, and help with bringing up her children, to be rewarding when selecting a husband; and the likelihood of producing genetically fit children, especially sons who can themselves potentially have many children by a number of women, to be rewarding when selecting a lover. What is even more extraordinary is that women may even have evolved ways of influencing whether it is the woman's lover, as opposed to her husband, who fathers her children. Apparently she may be able to do this even while deceiving her husband, even to the extent of having regular intercourse with him. The ways in which this might work have been investigated in research in the last 10 years described next (see Baker and Bellis 1995; Baker 1996). Although much of the research on the sociobiological background of human sexual behaviour, including sperm warfare in humans, is quite new, and many of the hypotheses remain to be fully established and accepted, this research does have interesting potential implications for understanding the rewards which control human behaviour, and for this reason the research, and its potential implications, are considered here.

In the research by Baker and Bellis (1995) and others (see also Ridley 1993), it was found that if a woman has no orgasm, or if she has an orgasm more than a minute before the male ejaculates, relatively little sperm is retained in the woman. This is a low-retention orgasm. If she has an orgasm less that a minute before him or up to 45 min after him, then

---

[2] Something like this might actually occur in some promiscuous tribes, in which the men help to bring up their sisters' children, who will have some of their genes.

much more of the sperm stays in the woman, and some of it is essentially sucked up by the cervix during and just following the later stages of her perceived orgasm. This is a high-retention orgasm. (This effect, known as upsuck, does not literally mean that seminal fluid is sucked up physically into the womb, with a resulting low volume of fluid lost during the outflow from the woman 30–45 min later. Instead, the mechanism of sperm retention seems to be that in a high-retention orgasm, more sperm enter the channels in the cervical mucus, and either swim right through them into the womb, or stay in the cervical mucus. In both high- and low-retention orgasms, the volume of the outflow, which includes more than sperm, is similar, see Baker and Bellis 1995, p. 237.) After a high-retention orgasm, the woman is more likely to conceive (by that intercourse) even if she already has sperm in her reproductive tract left from intercourse in the previous 4 or so days. One way in which this occurs is that the upsuck may enable the newly ejaculated sperm to bypass the block of the cervical mucus channels which is produced by old 'blocker' sperm that remain blocking these channels for several days after a previous insemination (see Baker and Bellis 1995). This is one aspect of sperm competition. (Another is that the longer since she last had intercourse, the more sperm are retained by the woman (unless she has had a non-copulatory, i.e. probably masturbatory, orgasm).) Baker and Bellis then (using a questionnaire) found that in women who were faithful (having intercourse only with their husbands) about 55% of the orgasms were of the high-retention (i.e. most fertile) type. By contrast, in unfaithful women having intercourse with their husbands, only 45% of the copulations were high retention, but 70% of the copulations with the lover were of the high retention type. Moreover, the unfaithful women were having sex with their lovers at times of the month when they were most fertile, that is when they were just about to ovulate. The result in the research sample was that an unfaithful woman could have sex twice as often with her husband as with her lover, but was still slightly more likely to conceive a child by the lover than by the husband. Put another way, the women in this sample would be more than twice as likely to conceive during sex with their lover than with their partner[3]. Thus women appear to be able to influence to some extent who is the father of their children, not only by having intercourse with lovers, but also by influencing whether they will become pregnant by their lover. The ways in which reward mechanisms could help this process are described later in this chapter.

Another finding by Baker and Bellis indicates that men have evolved strategies to optimize the chances of their genes in this sperm selection process. One is that men ejaculate more sperm if they have not been for some time with the woman with whom they are having intercourse. The (evolutionary, adaptive) function of this may be for the man to increase the chances of his sperm in what could be a sperm war with the sperm of another man. The aim would be to outnumber the other sperm. Moreover, the man should do this as quickly as possible after returning from an absence, as time could be of the essence in

---

[3] Given that 14% of children are not the children of the male partner, this suggests (and not taking into account fertility factors such as the time of month, whether the woman is more likely to synchronize ovulation with a lover, and possible differences in contraceptives used) that the average across the whole population of the number of copulations women have with lovers rather than their partners could be in the order of 7.5%. When effects of fertility etc. are taken into account, it will be less than 7.5%.

determining which sperm get to the egg first if the woman has had intercourse with another man recently. The implication of this for reward mechanisms in men is that after an absence, having intercourse quite soon with the woman from whom the man has been absent should be very rewarding. Possible neural mechanisms for this are considered later. It even appears that there should be some reward value in having intercourse *very* soon with the woman after an absence, because the action of the glans penis, with its groove behind the head, may be to pull sperm already in the vagina out of it using repeated thrusting and pulling back (at least in some ancestors) (Baker and Bellis 1995). The potential advantage to this in the sperm warfare may be the biological function that during evolution results in thrusting and withdrawal of the penis during intercourse being rewarding (perhaps to both men and women). Such thrusting and withdrawal of the penis during intercourse should occur especially vigorously (and should therefore have evolved to become especially rewarding) after an absence by the man. The possible advantage in the sperm warfare that shaped our evolution could also result in its being rewarding for a man to have intercourse with a woman if he has just seen her having intercourse with another man. (This could be part of the biological background of why some men find videos showing sex rewarding.) However, large numbers of sperm from a previous man usually remain in the vagina for only up to 45 min after intercourse, after which a flowback of sperm and other fluids (the discharge of semen and other secretions) from the vagina usually occurs. Thus the evolutionary shaping of the glans penis, and the rewards produced by thrusting and withdrawing it and the shaft of the penis in the vagina, are likely to have adaptive value more in our ancestors than in us.

A second male strategy might be (see Baker and Bellis 1995 for their pioneering work which it would be helpful to see tested further) to ejaculate not only sperm that can potentially fertilize an egg, but also killer (or kamikaze) sperm that kill the sperm of another male, and blocker sperm that remain in the mucus at the entrance to the cervix blocking access through the channels in the mucus to other sperm. Given that (the majority of) sperm remain viable once out of the vagina (and acting as blockers in the cervical mucus channels or as killers or fertilizers in the uterus or Fallopian tubes) for up to about four days, it becomes important (read adaptive) for a man to have intercourse with his partner as least as often as say twice per week. So because of this function of sperm warfare, the brain should be built to make male intercourse with his partner rewarding approximately twice per week. For the sperm-blocking effect, and to help space children, it may not matter from this point of view if their intercourse does not lead to an orgasm by her. On the other hand, it is important (in the fitness sense) that a male should help his lover to have an orgasm, which should occur only just before or for 45 min after he has ejaculated for the upsuck effect to operate. (The orgasm causes the upsuck effect which causes the cervical mucus channel-blocking action of blocker sperm to be bypassed. This gives the woman some control over whether she will accept new sperm, even when she has had intercourse and has blocking sperm in her. The operation of this female 'strategy' is facilitated by the facts that sperm remain in the vagina only for a short time because of the flowback, and because the acidity of the vagina makes sperm viable in the vagina for less than 12 h. The result is that the upsuck effect with a lover can operate preferentially on his (recently ejaculated) sperm, because many of the sperm from previous intercourse will be ejected within 45 min in the flowback, and the majority in the vagina will be dead within 12 h.) For this reason, men should find intercourse with a lover very exciting and rewarding if this tends to increase the likelihood that their lover will have an orgasm. This biological function of an orgasm in women provides a general reason why men should find it rewarding when a woman has an orgasm (and should therefore try to produce orgasms in women, and be disappointed when they do not occur). This process might be helped if one factor that tended to produce ejaculation in men was knowledge that the woman was having an orgasm. Of course, the reverse may occur—a woman may be triggered to orgasm especially just after she receives an ejaculation especially if it is from a male with whom (presumably mainly subconsciously) she wishes to conceive. If she does not have an orgasm, she may fake an orgasm (as this is rewarding to the male), and this may be part of her deception mechanism.

Why do humans masturbate? Do they find it rewarding just because the rewards are somewhat similar to those involved in sexual behaviour? (Though presumably masturbation should not be as rewarding as intercourse between men and women, for that would be disastrous for fitness.) Or are there other factors that might influence the reward value of masturbation, and particularly might influence when it occurs? Similarly, are there adaptive reasons for ejaculation in men or orgasm in women during sleep. Interesting new light has been shed on these issues by the sperm competition hypothesis (Baker and Bellis 1995).

In women, masturbation or nocturnal orgasm can first increase the flow of mucus from the cervix to the vagina. This has an effect of removing old sperm which are no longer effective as blocker sperm from the cervical mucus, and at the same time has the effect of strengthening the cervical sperm filter (assuming that sperm are present in the cervical mucus), because the ejected viable sperm can re-enter the mucus and block any open channels in the mucus. The increased flow also disinfects by moving material out towards the outside, and also provides lubricant which sticks to the walls of the vagina, facilitating intercourse in future. (The masturbation would not lead to upsuck of sperm in the vagina unless occurring soon after insemination, because the sperm remain viable in the vagina for only approximately 12 h.) Second, the masturbation or nocturnal orgasm increases the acidity of the cervical mucus (using fluids from the acidic vagina). This tends to act as a barrier to sperm and infection (Baker and Bellis 1995). Both these effects would tend to reduce the likelihood that insemination in the next few days would result in fertilization (as the blocker sperm may be effective for up to about four days). Thus an effect of masturbation in women may be to help them control whether they will be fertilized at the next intercourse. It helps them control fertilization by reducing the probability that they will be fertilized, while leaving open to them the option of increasing the probability that they will be fertilized by a particular man in the future (the next 2–3 days) if they have an orgasm at the effective time during intercourse with him to lead to upsuck of his sperm, which effectively bypasses the effect of the cervical barrier. (The effective time for her orgasm to do this must, as described above, be either immediately before, or within 30–45 min of, ejaculation.) Thus masturbation (and nocturnal dreams) in women might have consequences for who fertilizes her, and it is possible that masturbation at particular times is especially rewarding and likely for this reason. If a woman masturbated this might make it less likely that she would be fertilized by her partner if she did not have an effective (or any) orgasm with him, and more likely that she would be fertilized by her lover if she has an effective orgasm with him. Having intercourse with her lover might, because of such a biological function, be more rewarding than having intercourse with her partner. Use of this strategy might potentially enable her to conceive by a particular man and thus obtain genes she has chosen.

Might masturbation in males also be rewarding not only because it has features in common with intercourse, but also because it is serving some biological function? This is a possibility suggested by Baker and Bellis (1995). Masturbation two days before sexual intercourse in a man can remove old sperm, so that at intercourse he will have many young sperm especially of the killer and fertilizing type, which will last for a long time after ejaculation. (His old sperm will not only not last for long, but are better suited for acting as blockers in the cervical mucus than for killing other sperm, or fertilizing an egg.) So masturbation perhaps two days before he ejaculates in a lover could serve a biological function, and for this reason might have evolved to be particularly rewarding as a preparation for such occasions. Of course, masturbation a shorter time before such an occasion might be less adaptive because it would deplete the number of sperm available, though it is interesting that the amount of sperm ejaculated by masturbation tends to be a constant amount, so does not deplete all resources, whereas the amount of ejaculate during intercourse does vary, being, for example, much larger with a lover whom the man presumably wants to impregnate than with a regular partner (Baker and Bellis 1995). (Another factor which might influence the outcome here is that recent masturbation might increase the time to ejaculation, which could itself have consequences for whether he is likely to fertilize the woman.) If masturbation in men had any effect on testosterone levels, perhaps increasing them, this might also have a biological consequence, by making him more aggressive and perhaps likely to find a lover. This could be another biological function that increases fitness thus leading during the course of evolution to masturbation being rewarding.

Having now outlined some of the functions at play in sexual behaviour we are in a better position later in this chapter to consider the brain processes that implement rewards to produce these different types of behaviour.

8.4 Individual differences in sexual rewards

Before considering how biological reward systems might have evolved in order to implement the types of behaviour just described, we first consider possible individual differences in these types of sexual behaviour, because these have implications for how the reward systems may differ in different individuals to produce these differences in sexual behaviour. We remind ourselves that genetic specification of different reward mechanisms could produce a polymorphic, fixed, evolutionarily stable strategy, as described in Footnote 1 of this chapter. An alternative mechanism is a conditional strategy (see Footnote 1), which can also be evolutionarily stable (Maynard-Smith 1982). In many of the examples discussed here, it is not clear which is the more likely. We should also note that many factors are likely to produce differences between the emotional behaviour of males and females. For example, in many species females are attracted to dominant males, thus further favouring male competitiveness. Further, females may be attracted to males favoured by other women. Both might be accounted for by their predictive relation to producing genetically successful male offspring.

8.4.1 Outline

Is the range of stimuli and situations related to sexual behaviour that different people find rewarding different, and can any differences be related to a biological function such as sperm warfare? It is plausible that there are such differences, and that they could be related to sperm warfare. Although experimental data on this issue in relation to an underlying function such as sperm competition are not yet available, the possibilities are sufficiently plausible that they are worth elaborating, in part as a guide to stimulating further concepts and experimental research in this area.

A hypothesis which seems plausible is that some individuals might be of the type that would specialize in sperm warfare. Such individuals might find especially rewarding the types of stimuli that would make them especially successful in sperm warfare, and their resulting behaviour might reflect the stimuli they find most rewarding. If men, they might be built to find variety in sexual partners especially rewarding, and to be ambitious and competitive. This could increase their fitness, by enabling them potentially to have many children with different women. A risk of this 'unfaithful' strategy, which would tend to keep it in check, is that the man might make insufficient investment in helping any of his lovers and her children by him to ensure that the children flourish and themselves reproduce successfully. Women might avoid such men if they were not already in receipt of sufficient resources to provide for their children, and the partners of such women might require that they be faithful, even to the extent of guarding them. Such 'unfaithful' individuals, who would be likely to specialize in sperm warfare, if women, might be unfaithful and as a result be fit if they had a tendency to choose genetically fit men to be the father of their children, while at the same time having as a partner to help bring up the children another man who was not necessarily as genetically fit as their lover, but would help to bring up the children. For this to be an evolutionarily stable strategy, it might be expected that at least some of the children would be children of the partner, otherwise the deception might be too obvious. Part of the risk of this strategy, which keeps it in balance with others in the population, is that if her deception is discovered, the woman risks losing the resources being provided for her and her children by her partner. Too great a tendency to unfaithfulness would also be unstable because of the associated risks of sexually transmitted disease.

Other individuals in the population might be genetically predisposed to use a different strategy, of being faithful to their partner. This could benefit a faithful woman's genes, because her children would have a partner who could be relied on to help bring up the children, and put all his resources into this (because he would be sure that his genes were in the children, and because he would not be tempted by other women). (In addition, he might not be very attractive or successful in life, and might not have the opportunity to be tempted away.) Her fitness would be increased by the fact that her children would be likely to survive, but reduced by the fact that the genes with which she has mated would not be optimal, and nor would she benefit from the effect of pure variety of genes with which to combine her own, which is part of the advantage of sexual reproduction. There could also be an advantage to a man's genes for him to be faithful, because in being faithful he would be less likely to catch a disease, and would be more likely to put sufficient resources into his children to ensure that they have a good start in life; and would be more likely to attract a faithful woman as his partner, so that the children in whom he invested would be more likely to be his. The cost of this strategy would be that he might have fewer children than if he were unfaithful, and his children might, if the behaviour is controlled genetically, be less likely themselves to have large numbers of children, because they would not be likely to be the unfaithful type.

It is suggested that these different strategies, because each has associated advantages and costs, could be retained in a stable balance in populations in which genetic factors at least partly predisposed the individual to be of the unfaithful or faithful type. Of course, in a real human population it might be expected that there would be continuous variation between individuals in the tendency to be faithful or unfaithful, and for the actual range of differences found in a population to be being constantly adjusted depending on the fitness of the different types of strategy, and on the environment too, such as the availability of resources (see Footnote 1 to this chapter). (The availability of resources could affect the balance. For example, if food and other resources were readily available, so that the advantage of care by both parents was less than in more harsh environments in which perhaps the man might be specialized for hunting, then the relative advantages of unfaithfulness in the population would be higher.)

Evidence that genetic factors do actually influence the likelihood of infidelity in different individuals comes from the recent finding of what might be called a 'promiscuity gene' (Hamer 1998). The research (conducted at the National Institutes of Cancer in Washington) has so far been conducted in men, but there could be a parallel in women. Very interestingly in relation to the points made about dopamine and reward in this book, the gene affects the D4 dopamine receptor, and in particular it comes in a long form or a short form. Approximately 30% of men in the study carried the long form of the gene, and they were likely to have 20% more sexual partners than those with the short form. Men with the long form were likely to have an average of 10 sexual partners in their lifetime, whereas those with the short form were less likely to have sought such variety. Hamer also described a gene that influences sex drive that is different to that for promiscuity. This is a serotonin (i.e. 5-hydroxytryptamine)-related gene which influences anxiety. Men with the high anxiety form of this gene had more frequent sex, and those with the calm, happy and optimistic form had less sex. These genetic findings, reported after the rest of this book was written, provide support for the suggestion made in this chapter that different strategies for sexual behaviour, and in particular a strategy to be faithful vs a strategy to be unfaithful, could be influenced at least in part by genes.

Next we will consider how natural selection might make different types of stimuli differently rewarding to different people in order to produce these different types of behaviour. This will just be a possible scenario, because I know of little actual evidence on this. Then we will consider what such evidence might look like when it does become available.

8.4.2 How might different types of behaviour be produced by natural selection altering the relative reward value of different stimuli in different individuals?

We will consider what could occur hypothetically in different types of women, predisposed to be unfaithful and faithful, and in different types of men, predisposed to be unfaithful and faithful, for clarity. We remember that in practice there would be likely to be a continuous distribution of these differences in a human population. (We note that in addition to the two types of evolutionarily stable strategy outlined in Footnote 1 of this chapter, the different behaviours do not have to be equally successful. One type of behaviour might just be 'making the best of a bad job'.)

First we consider women who are genetically predisposed to be unfaithful and promote sperm warfare. (Sometimes the shorthand used for this is 'unfaithful woman', but this should always be taken to mean 'genetically predisposed to be an unfaithful woman'.) We might suppose that they should be especially attractive to men, and may therefore tend to be youthful-looking and thin, to indicate that they are at a fertile period of their lives, and are not already pregnant. They should not be shy, might be extravert, and might be flirtatious in order to attract men. They should like (sexually) aggressive men (because this is an indicator that her sons with him would pass on her genes to women that they were able to take as lovers). They might even like a man aggressive to other men as in war, because in war his genes (potentially in his children with her) will tend to survive and to be passed on, and he will be a potential protection in war. Women with genes predisposing them to be unfaithful might be attracted to men with a 'reputation'—because this also indicates that they will produce sons who are good at passing on (her) genes; should be good at finding a partner for stability, to bring up her children, but also good at deceiving him; should like men with large testes (which could correlate with testosterone levels, and thus perhaps be indicated by secondary sexual characteristics such as body hair); should like men with a large penis (because this would be good at sperm warfare by sucking out other men's sperm, and thus is an indicator of genetic fitness in sperm warfare); should be able to assess men for sexual fitness, not necessarily fast but by evaluating his position in society, power, wealth, and bodily fitness (one index of which is the shape of the buttocks). She might herself be sexually aggressive, because it is important (in terms of fitness) that when she takes risks and is unfaithful, she chooses the right man, with genes that will make her children fit, and does not choose just any man. She might also be likely to control sexual behaviour, rather than be passive—she wants to control whether and when (in relation to whether she is fertile) a man impregnates her, and if and when in relation to his ejaculation she has an orgasm. (She might, for example, choose to have intercourse with a fit lover especially when she is most fertile, and to orgasm soon after him. She might choose to have intercourse with her partner at other times, and either not to have an orgasm, or to orgasm before he does, to prevent upsuck. For this reason, and partly to please her partner, she might fake her orgasms.) She might be especially attracted to novel men, and indeed might need some element of novelty to make her have an orgasm and thus be likely to conceive. In this respect, she should be built to be continually searching for something better. She might also for this reason, because it is advantageous to her to control when and with whom she has orgasms, appear to need more stimulation to have an orgasm, and be especially likely to have orgasms with novel men or in novel situations. She may also tend to reproduce young, because of the risk of disease. Such an unfaithful woman, because of the risk that her deception might be discovered, might use her attractiveness to make relationships with a number of men, and have backup policies with several men, as insurance and support for her young.

Second, we consider women whose genes might have built them to be faithful. She might be less attractive, and once with a partner might take fewer steps to be attractive (she might not be thin, and might be less worried about her weight; she might be less concerned with cosmetics and might dress sensibly rather than provocatively). She might be reliable, looking for domestic security (to provide reliable resources for her and her children, as she has chosen to put her resources into bringing up her children well, rather than taking risks and possibly having genetically more fit children with a lover but risking the support for all her children). She might be relatively passive during intercourse, and not try to control sex (because with only one male, she does not need to control whether/when a male ejaculates in her, and if/when she orgasms). Partly for this reason, she might find it relatively easy to have orgasms, because she does not need to control who fertilizes her, and because orgasms might promote attachment to the (same) partner. Multiple orgasms in this situation could help, though they might be especially useful if the woman was 'trying' to conceive. At the same time, having no orgasms for such a woman would not be disastrous, because this could help to space children. (This would be due to the sperm-blocking effect in the cervical mucus.) The main prediction here is that orgasms would be much more consistent (either present or not) than in women genetically predisposed to be unfaithful. The woman genetically predisposed to be faithful might tend to reproduce older, because she has less risk of disease. She might be shy, could be introvert, and might be expected not to be a flirtatious type. She should make very stable relationships with friends in a supporting society (to ensure care of her young, a high priority to her, and to listen to gossip, to learn of potentially threatening males or females). She should disapprove of women with a reputation, as they are a threat to her security, e.g. by attracting her partner and thus threatening her resources.

Men genetically predisposed to be unfaithful and to participate in sperm warfare might be built by their genes as follows. First, at the simple physical level, they might have large testes and a large penis, both good in sperm warfare (see above). Second, they should be successful with other women, as this indicates how well a woman's sons with them would pass her genes on to future generations. (This could be 'why' some women are interested in a man's reputation, and why this could help to make a man attractive.) These men could be competitive and aggressive (both sexually and in war, see above); have high testosterone (possibly indicated by bodily hair); be ambitious, wealthy, successful and powerful (because these indicate potential to provide resources); possibly creative, intellectual, musical, etc. because these may be ways to keep women interested, and may be used in courtship. (There is the suggestion that women are selecting men's brains to be good at courtship, so that a man's brain would parallel a peacock's 'tail', see Ridley 1993; and if so, this selection might be particularly evident in unfaithful men.) Such men might also be good at deceit, as this would be an advantage in deception of their partner and their lover's partner.

Men genetically predisposed to be faithful might have smaller testes and penes on average; and have lower concentrations of testosterone and be less aggressive, and even possibly less ambitious. They should be less interested in and attracted by women other than their partner, that is they should be built less to keep searching for novelty; they should be stable, reliable, good at providing a home, and truthful, all of which would appeal to a woman genetically predisposed to be faithful. He should denounce men (or women) with a reputation, because they, and that type of behaviour, are a threat to him, given that he is inclined to make his major investment in one woman, and it is to his genes' advantage that the children he helps to bring up are his.

8.4.3 How being tuned to different types of reward could help to produce individual differences in sexual behaviour

Given the hypotheses (and they are of course only hypotheses) discussed in Section 8.4.2, it is now possible to ask how differences in sexual behaviour *might* be produced by genes influencing the different types of stimulation and situation which different individuals find rewarding. (We remember that an alternative to a polymorphic fixed ESS is a conditional strategy, see Footnote 1 to this chapter. A conditional strategy might not alter what would be found inherently rewarding, but might alter how different types of reward were perceived.) As above, when the term 'unfaithful man or woman' is used, it is simply shorthand for the description 'man or woman predisposed to be unfaithful'.

1 Unfaithful women could be built to find external (relative to internal) stimulation of the genitals particularly necessary for reward, because this helps them to control impregnation.

2 Unfaithful women could be built to need much (external and sometimes adventurous and novel) stimulation to produce enough reward/pleasure for them to orgasm. (This would be part of the control of impregnation process, making it particularly likely that they would have an orgasm and facilitate fertilization with a lover, who would probably be more novel than a regular partner. It would also be part of the mechanism that would encourage them to keep searching for something better, because some novelty would tend to be arousing.)

3 It is possible that sensory-specific satiety, a reduction in sexual desire for a particular person with whom intercourse has just taken place, relative to other men, would be more pronounced in unfaithful women, as a mechanism to facilitate searching for new genes, and sperm competition.

4 Unfaithful women could be built to like control, both of whether and when sex occurs with a particular man, and during sex, partly by requiring particular types of stimulation (novel and external), and perhaps partly by making control per se rewarding and important to them.

5 Unfaithful women could be built to find social interactions, sometimes flirtatious and provocative, including clothes, cosmetics etc., with men (and with novel men perhaps especially), particularly rewarding, as a mechanism to attract and obtain potential lovers.

6 Unfaithful women could tend to be smaller, to keep their bodies in trim, and to age less than faithful women, in order to attract males with fit genes. In fact, sexual dimorphism should be especially pronounced in those predisposed to be unfaithful.

7 In a complementary way, women predisposed to be faithful could be tuned to internal vs external stimulation during intercourse, to need less stimulation and particularly less novel stimulation to have an orgasm, to show less sensory-specific satiety for the partner, to be more passive rather than controlling before and during sex, and to be less socially provocative.

8 In a corresponding way, men predisposed to be unfaithful might be tuned to find it rewarding to produce an orgasm in women (because this is a way to facilitate the chances of their sperm in a sperm war), and therefore be willing to work hard for this; to find vigorous thrusting during intercourse particularly rewarding (to serve the biological function of increasing their chances in sperm competition); to be especially attracted to attractive, novel, and interactive women (to serve the biological function of finding genes able to produce fit daughters who will themselves attract males); and to not be satisfied for long with the same situation, but continually be searching for new relationships and lovers.

9 Some genetically selected tendency to make homosexuality rewarding in some males might be that homosexual relations often tend to occur early in life, providing early experience in handling social relations that could provide advantageous skills when later setting up heterosexual relations (Baker and Bellis 1995).

10 Partial reinforcement (i.e. only sometimes giving a reinforcer or reward) by an unfaithful woman should be greatly reinforcing to an unfaithful man (beyond the normal partial reinforcement effect, which itself increases the amount a person will work for a reward), because this is a test of how motivated and successful the man is to pass on his genes, a quality which the unfaithful woman will value for her sons. The unfaithful woman may even titrate the partial reinforcement level to see just how persistent, and thus potentially fit, the man is.

It may be emphasized that the reward processes that have just been described might be those to which different people are predisposed, and probably operate primarily through an implicit or unconscious system for rewards. In addition to this implicit system with its predispositions, humans have an explicit processing system which can of course influence the actual choice that is made (see Chapter 9).

8.5 The neural reward mechanisms that might mediate some aspects of sexual behaviour

In Section 8.3 sociobiological research on sexual behaviour was described. In Section 8.4

we speculated about possible individual differences in such sexual behaviour. In both these sections we produced hypotheses about how genes might influence sexual behaviour by building particular reward systems and mechanisms into animals. We now consider how the brain might implement these different reward processes. Might there be a few principles of operation of the brain reward systems that could help to account for the quite complex sexual behaviour that is apparent in humans? How are these mechanisms implemented neurophysiologically in the brain? We consider what is known on these issues in this section. Although the actual brain mechanisms are not fully worked out, the intention of the approach being taken here is to suggest what could be implemented in the brain mechanisms that provide the rewards for sexual behaviour, to guide future research and thinking.

Examples of quite simple neurophysiological rules and processes that could govern the operation of reward mechanism for sexual behaviour and that could account for many of the effects discussed above are given next.

1   Repeated thrusting and withdrawal of the penis during intercourse should be reward-ing to the man (and possibly also to the woman), because it serves the biological function (in sperm warfare) of helping to remove from the vagina sperm which could remain from previous intercourse, possibly with another male, for up to 12 h. If the only aim was to deposit semen in the vagina, then there would be little point in this repeated thrusting and withdrawal, which typically occurs in males 100–500 times during intercourse in humans (see Baker and Bellis 1995). An implication for brain reward systems is that stimulation of the glans and of the shaft of the penis should be rewarding, but should only bring the man to ejaculate after a reasonable number of thrust and withdrawal cycles have been completed. Humans may emphasize this design feature, in that many more cycles are completed before ejaculation than in many other species such as macaques (and rats, an example of a species in which the male will ejaculate as soon as the hard cervical plug from previous copulation is removed).

2   Correspondingly, if the woman is to take advantage of the sperm retention effect she can use with a new lover, she should not be brought to orgasm by the first thrust or two, but only after the greater part of the thrusting has been completed should she be likely to be brought to orgasm. The woman may actually facilitate this process, by tightening her vagina during most of the thrusting (which would help the potential sperm-removal effect of the thrusting and withdrawal), and relaxing it later on during intercourse, soon before she has an orgasm. If she does have this relaxation later on, this would make it less likely that when the male ejaculates he would remove his own sperm if he keeps moving for a short time.

3   After ejaculation in a woman, a man's thrusting movements should no longer be rewarding (or he would tend to suck out his own sperm), and the penis should shrink quite soon and withdraw slowly so as not to suck out sperm. Moreover, he should not feel like intercourse with that woman for 30–45 min (as that is the time period within which significant amounts of his sperm remain in the vagina, before the flowback).

Thus when it occurs after ejaculation, satiety should be rapid, strong, and last for at least the next 30–45 min in men. The reward which rubbing the penis has before ejaculation is described as turning rapidly to being unpleasant or even painful after ejaculation, and this switch from pleasure to pain is what would be predicted by the biological function being performed. That this switch may not be a simple switch controlled only by whether the neural circuitry has recently produced ejaculation is that introduction of a new female (in many animals and in humans) may enable the whole circuitry to be reset, resulting in rapid re-erection, re-initiation of thrusting movements, and the reward or pleasure associated with rubbing the penis, and eventually in ejaculation again in the new female. The adaptive value of this novelty effect (sometimes known as the Coolidge effect after a remark made by President Coolidge of the United States[4]) in potentially enhancing fitness is clear. The sperm competition hypothesis would predict that intercourse with the man's partner would only need to become very rewarding again within about four days, as by this time the woman would need 'topping up' with his sperm, to act as blockers (Baker and Bellis 1995).

4　The rapid speed of a first ejaculation in a woman, and the slow last one (which could be useful in conditions such as group sex, see Baker 1996) could be due to the satiety mechanism having a longer time-course each time it is successively activated, perhaps as a result of some neural adaptation of the reward relative to the aversive aspects of the stimulation.

5　We would predict that it should be rewarding to a man to induce an orgasm in a woman, because of its (probably not consciously realized or intended) biological function of increasing the likelihood, at least under conditions of sperm warfare, that conception of his child would occur. (Such an unconscious function could be a factor that might contribute to the reward value in both men and women of sex without a condom.)

6　In women, orgasm should be particularly likely to occur under conditions when they 'want' (perhaps subconsciously) to conceive. For this biological function, particularly in women predisposed to be unfaithful and therefore possibly trying to manipulate using sperm warfare which person they are impregnated by, orgasm might generally be difficult; might not always be stimulated to occur with the regular partner; might be more likely to occur with the lover; and with the lover might be especially stimulated by his ejaculation so that the upsuck effect for his sperm occurs optimally. Neurophysiological predictions are that the reward systems in unfaithful women might (relative to those in faithful women) be less easily activated, but particularly

---

[4] The story is that Calvin Coolidge and his wife were touring a farm when Mrs Coolidge asked the farmer whether the continuous and vigorous sexual activity among the flock of hens was the work of only one rooster. The reply was yes. 'You might point that out to Mr Coolidge', she said. The President then asked the farmer whether a different hen was involved each time. The answer, again, was yes. 'You might point that out to Mrs Coolidge', he said.

stimulated by novelty, especially by a novel man with genes perceived to be fit. Indeed, women predisposed to be unfaithful may find variety in sex, and sexual adventurousness, especially rewarding. They may always need something new, because they are built to always be looking for better sexual and related stimulation—because this predicts how fit their sons will be. This may extend to the courtship battle, which some believe may have played a role in the rapid evolution of the human brain (see Ridley 1993). The argument is that the most creative brains intellectually, musically, and artistically will be successful in having many children with women, because they can provide the variety that unfaithful women are predisposed to want—the variety of all sorts of stimulation is needed to keep an unfaithful woman interested in continuing her relationship with him, and thus in passing his genes into the next generation. G. F. Miller's (1992, see Ridley 1993) suggestion that brain size has evolved for courtship, might be extended to be important also beyond initial courtship, to keeping a partner interested while children are raised.

7   In women, we might expect that refractoriness after orgasm might be stronger for unfaithful women, and to be at least partly sensory-specific (for the male with whom she has just had intercourse), because there may (at least in the past) have been an advantage to females to allow sperm competition to occur, implying intercourse with another male in the not too distant future. This would be less important for women predisposed to be faithful, in whom even multiple orgasms might occur, helping to reward her and her partner (see above) in the mutual relationship.

8   A neurophysiological mechanism operating in a man which made sex with a woman more rewarding if she was relatively novel could contribute to a number of phenomena. It could contribute to make the reward value of a particular woman for a man higher if he has not seen her for some time. The biological function of this is that then the chance is greater that she has had intercourse with another man, and a sperm competition situation, in which speed is of the essence, could be necessary. Evidence that men do have appropriate behaviour for this situation is that the volume a man ejaculates into a particular woman increases with the length of the time since he has last seen her (Baker and Bellis 1995). The same neurophysiological mechanism could contribute to a form of sensory-specific satiety in which even after intercourse and ejaculation with one woman, a man may be quickly aroused again by another woman. (Possibly it is partly because of this arousing effect of a novel potential lover that the sight of others having intercourse, e.g. in a video, might be arousing. Also possibly related is that the sperm warfare hypothesis might predict that if a man saw someone else having intercourse with his partner, a fit response might be to have intercourse with her too, to promote sperm warfare. However, this would not be an adaptive response if the woman had not yet had an orgasm, and did subsequently have one as a result of the second intercourse.) A similar neurophysiological mechanism could also contribute to making a man wish to have intercourse perhaps every four days, or sooner if he suspects infidelity.

9   There should be at least a small tendency to become attached to (find more

rewarding) a person with whom intercourse has occurred (especially if it leads to ejaculation in the woman). For the woman this is one way of seeking resources for her potential child, by becoming attached to a person who may now be disposed to provide resources to help his genes. For the man such an attachment mechanism is one way of increasing the probability that he will provide for his potential offspring with her, and thus for the success of his genes. (Evidence that this may actually occur comes from a rather surprising source. Baker and Bellis (1995) report that women who have actually been raped by a man are more likely to develop some form of social relationship with him afterwards than women with whom rape was attempted but not completed.)

10 The rewards produced by tactile stimulation are such that touch can be rewarding and feel pleasant, and this can occur in situations that are not explicitly sexual as well as in more sexual episodes. One example is grooming in monkeys, which may be rewarding because it serves a number of biological functions, including removing skin parasites, indicating commitment to another by the investment of time, or by trusting another to touch one, as a preliminary to more sexual touch, etc. Where in the brain is the pleasantness of touch made explicit? Is it in or before the somatosensory cortex of primates, or primarily after this in some of the connected areas such as the insula, orbitofrontal cortex, or amygdala (see Figs 4.1 and 4.2)? As shown in Section 4.2 and Figs 4.4 and 4.5, one area of the brain in which the pleasantness of touch is made explicit is in a part of the orbitofrontal cortex. The area of the orbitofrontal cortex in which pleasant touch is represented was different from the area in which taste and odour are represented (see Figs 2.21 and 2.22). This is an early indication that there may be brain mechanisms specialized for processing the affective or rewarding aspects of touch in humans. Doubtless there will be a number of brain regions in addition to the orbitofrontal cortex where such information is represented. Perhaps one function of the representation in the orbitofrontal cortex is to act as a representation of touch as a primary reinforcer or unconditioned stimulus in stimulus–reinforcement association learning (see Chapter 4). The orbitofrontal representation of pleasant touch may also be involved in the subjective affective feeling produced by the touch, for orbitofrontal cortex damage in humans does blunt the affective component of other affective stimuli such as pain (Melzack and Wall 1996). Aspects of touch that may make it particularly pleasant include slight unpredictability, and a psychological component which reflects what it is one believes is providing the touch, and who is performing the touching. It will be of interest to determine where in the somatosensory system such cognitive influences converge with inputs originating from touch receptors to alter the affective component of the touch.

With regard to tactile stimulation that women may find rewarding in the early stages of a relationship or sexual episode, gentle touch, hugging, and kissing on any part of the body may be rewarding, perhaps as an indicator of caring, protection, and investment of time offered by a man. Because of the importance to a woman of indicators of investment by a man, women also have fantasies and prefer literature which emphasizes romance, commitment, and attachment rather than explicit details of sexual encounters and the physical stimulation being exchanged (Ellis and Simons 1990). Stimulation of the nipples may be rewarding partly to promote the biological function of breast-feeding. Its sexually arousing effects might be related to the fact that such stimulation may cause the release of the hormone oxytocin, which stimulates movements or contractions of the uterus. The movements might have a biological function in relation to later orgasm and the upsuck effect.

With regard to more explicitly sexual genital stimulation in women, both external (clitoral and vulval) and internal (vaginal, including the G spot on the anterior wall of the vagina) stimulation can be rewarding and pleasant. The possibility that women predisposed to be unfaithful might require more such stimulation to produce an orgasm, might be especially stimulated by a novel lover with fit genes and by novelty in the situation, and might be biased towards finding external as compared with internal stimulation more rewarding has been introduced above, together with the biological functions that might be served by being made differentially sensitive to these different types of reward.

The active control of a sexual episode may be rewarding not only to men (because being in control of sex is likely to make his genes fit), but also particularly to women predisposed to be unfaithful, because they can then determine whether they proceed to intercourse with that particular man, and also whether they receive the right stimulation to have an orgasm with that particular man, with its biological function of controlling the likelihood of conception with that particular man. It is also possible that a lack of control could act as a reward sometimes in some women, because the feeling of being dominated by a particular man could indicate potential fitness in her sons with him (who might be likely to dominate other women).

The reward value which oral sex can have (in both males and females) could be related to the biological function of determining whether the other person is disease-free (using sight, smell, and taste), and, if performed randomly, of detecting infidelity in a partner (by smell, possibly reduced volume of ejaculate from a male, etc.) (see Ridley 1993).

11 The attractiveness, reward value, and beauty of women to men is determined by a number of factors to which the brain must be sensitive (see Buss 1989; Thornhill and Gangestad 1996; articles in Betzig 1997). One factor is a low waist-to-hip ratio. Waist-to-hip ratio in women correlates negatively with oestrogen, age, fertility, and health, and positively with age. Low waist-to-hip ratios (0.6–0.7) in women are maximally attractive to men. One of the obvious ways in which a low ratio indicates fertility is that it will reflect whether the woman is pregnant. It may be partly because of the biologically relevant signals given by a low waist-to-hip ratio that thinness and dieting are rewarding, and this may even be selecting for a small body build in women. Other indicators with similar biological signalling functions which are therefore rewarding to men and make women attractive include a youthful face (sometimes almost a baby face, with a small nose); slow ageing; symmetry (because symmetry is reduced by environmental insults, e.g. parasites and toxins, and genetic disruptions such as mutations and inbreeding, and so reflects fitness); smooth unblemished skin;

etc. All these signals of attractiveness and beauty might be selected for particularly in women predisposed to be unfaithful (because they must attract genetically fit men as lovers, even if they cannot have them as partners). Sexual restraint in women could make them attractive to men because this implies chastity and thus protection of the potential investment of a man in bringing up putatively his children with that woman. In addition, the relative reward value of different signals may vary as a function of the environment. Women who perceive that they are in an environment where men are not likely to invest, act and dress in a more sexually provocative manner, and use copulation to attract desirable men. That is, women may be designed to show sexual restraint (thus giving cues of paternity reliability) when investing males may be accessible, and less sexual restraint (to access material benefits) when each male can or will invest little.

An implication for brain mechanisms is that all these factors that reflect attractiveness, which include information from face analysis, must be used in the brain to determine reward value.

12 The attractiveness of men is influenced by their power, status in society, wealth, and ambition as a predictor of these. These factors are rewarding and attractive to women because they are an indication of the resources that can be provided by the man for the woman, to help bring up her children to maturity and reproduction. Aggressiveness and competitiveness with other men, and domination and success with other women, may be attractive because they indicate fitness (in terms of genetic potential) of the man's genes, and thus of hers in their children. (Aggression and competitiveness in men can thus be ascribed to women's choice.) Physical factors such as symmetry, firm buttocks and a muscular build also make men attractive to women because they serve as biological signals of health and fertility, and also possibly because they indicate that such men can cope well despite the 'handicap' of a high level of testosterone, which suppresses the immune system. These factors are reviewed by Buss (1989), Thornhill and Gangestad (1996), and in the articles in Betzig (1997). To a woman predisposed to be faithful, indicators of a man's potential parental investment in her children as indicated by caring, stability, and lack of reputation, should make a man attractive.

The operation of some of these factors can be understood in terms of a parental investment model. The parental investment model implies that the sex investing more (most commonly the female) will be most choosy; whereas the sex investing least (most commonly the male) should be most competitive (Kenrick *et al.* 1990). High male parental investment in humans contrasts with most other mammalian species. So the above may be less true of humans. The result is that when one measures patterns for what makes a stranger attractive, they are like those of other mammals; whereas when one measures what makes a long-term partner attractive, more similar selectivity should be found between males and females—that is, the requirements for marriage (high investment) are much more stringent than for dating (low investment), and the balance may shift under these conditions from males selecting females mainly on attractiveness to males selecting females as partners who will be faithful and protect their investment (Kenrick *et al.* 1990).

13 Olfactory rewards and pheromones. Pheromones, which are typically olfactory stimuli, can trigger a number of different types of sexual behaviour, and thus either affect what is rewarding or in some cases can act as rewards.

First, pheromones can affect reproductive cycles. They produce the Lee–Boot effect, in which the oestrous cycles of female mice housed together without a male slow down and eventually stop. They act in the Whitten effect, in which the mice start cycling again if they are exposed to the odour of a male or his urine. They act in the Vandenbergh effect, the acceleration in the onset of puberty in a female rodent caused by the odour of a male. They act in the Bruce effect, in which if a recently impregnated female mouse encounters a male mouse other than the one with which she mated, the pregnancy is very likely to fail. The new male can then mate with her. This form of genetic warfare happening after the sperm-warfare stage is clearly to the advantage of the new male's genes, and presumably to the advantage of the female's genes, because it means that her pregnancies will tend to be with males who are not only able to oust other males, but are with males who are with her, so that her offspring will not be harmed by the new male, and may even be protected. The pheromones which produce these effects are produced in males under the influence of testosterone (see Carlson 1994). These effects depend on an accessory olfactory system, the vomeronasal organ and its projections to the accessory olfactory bulb. The accessory olfactory bulb in turn projects to the medial nucleus of the amygdala, which in turn project to the preoptic area, anterior hypothalamus, and ventromedial hypothalamus. Pheromones can cause groups of women housed together to start cycling together.

Second, pheromones can act as attracting or rewarding signals. For example, pheromones present in the vaginal secretions of hamsters attract males. In some monkeys, bacteria in the vagina produce more of a pheromone under the influence of an androgen (male sex hormone) produced in small quantities in the adrenal glands, and this pheromone increases the attractiveness of the female to the male (Baum *et al.* 1977). (In this case, male sexual behaviour is induced by a male hormone produced in females!) Male rats also produce pheromones, which are attractive to females. In humans, body odours are not generally described as attractive, but there is a whole industry based on perfume, the odour of a mate may become attractive by conditioning, and there is some evidence that androstenol, a substance found in the underarm sweat of males especially, may increase the number of social interactions that women have with men (Cowley and Brooksbank 1991).

There is interesting recent research suggesting that pheromones may act in humans through the vomeronasal system. Monti-Bloch and colleagues (1994, 1998; see also Berliner *et al.* 1996) applied what they termed 'vomeropherins' to the vomeronasal system while they recorded negative potentials from the human vomeronasal organ. They found vomerpherins that activated the vomeronasal organ but not the olfactory epithelium. Conversely, conventional odourants activated the olfactory epithelium but not the vomeronasal organ. Interestingly, males and females were sensitive to different vomeropherins. In men, the vomeropherin pregna-4,20-diene-3,6-dione (PDD) in concentrations of 5×10^{-9} M activated the vomeronasal organ and reduced luteinizing-hormone pulsatility and levels, and follicle-stimulating hormone (FSH) pulsatility. The pheromone also reduced respiratory frequency, increased cardiac frequency, and produced changes in electrodermal activity and the EEG. No significant effects of this pheromone were produced in women. In women (but not in men) the vomeropherins PH56 and PH94B activated the vomeronasal organ, and increased electrodermal activity, skin temperature, and alpha-cortical (EEG) activity. These findings raise interesting possibilities requiring much further exploration about the function of the human vomeronasal organ and accessory olfactory system, including potential roles in acting as a reward, or in influencing reward systems.

In a different line of research, it has been suggested that the way in which animals including humans respond to pheromones as rewards or as aversive stimuli could be a molecular mechanism for producing genetic diversity by influencing those who are considered attractive as mates. In particular, major histocompatibility complex (MHC)-dependent abortion and mate choice, based on olfaction, can maintain MHC diversity and probably functions both to avoid genome-wide inbreeding and produce MHC-heterozygous offspring with increased immune responsiveness (Eggert *et al.* 1996; Apanius *et al.* 1997.

8.6 Conclusion

We can conclude this chapter by remembering that there is some evidence on how the brain produces sexual behaviour by being sensitive to certain rewards (Section 8.2), and that reward systems for rewards of the type described in Section 8.5 may have been built in the brain by genes as their way of increasing their fitness. It will be interesting to know how these different reward systems actually operate in the brain. In any case, the overall conclusion is that genes do appear to build reward systems that will lead to behaviour that will enhance their own survival in future generations. We return to this issue of the role of reward (and punishment) systems in brain design by genetic variation and natural selection in Chapter 10.

9 A theory of consciousness, and its application to understanding emotion and pleasure

9.1 Introduction

It might be possible to build a computer which would perform the functions of emotions described in Chapters 3 and 10, and yet we might not want to ascribe emotional *feelings* to the computer. We might even build the computer with some of the main processing stages present in the brain, and implemented using neural networks which simulate the operation of the real neural networks in the brain (see Chapter 4, the Appendix, and Rolls and Treves 1998), yet we might not still wish to ascribe emotional feelings to this computer. This point often arises in discussions with undergraduates, who may say that they follow the types of point made about emotion in Chapters 3 and 4, yet believe that almost the most important aspect of emotions, the feelings, have not been accounted for, nor their neural basis described. In a sense, the functions of reward and punishment in emotional behaviour are described in Chapters 3 and 10, but what about the subjective aspects of emotion, what about the pleasure?

A similar point arises in Chapters 2 and 7, where parts of the taste, olfactory, and visual systems in which the reward value of the taste, smell, and sight of food is represented are described. (One such brain region is the orbitofrontal cortex.) Although the neuronal representation in the orbitofrontal cortex is clearly related to the reward value of food, is this where the pleasantness (the subjective hedonic aspect) of the taste, smell, and sight of food is represented? Again, we could (in principle at least) build a computer with neural networks to simulate each of the processing stages for the taste, smell, and sight of food which are described in Chapter 2 (and more formally in terms of neural networks by Rolls and Treves 1998), and yet would probably not wish to ascribe feelings of pleasantness to the system we have simulated on the computer.

What is it about neural processing that makes it feel like something when some types of information processing are taking place? It is clearly not a general property of processing in neural networks, for there is much processing, for example that concerned with the control of our blood pressure and heart rate, of which we are not aware. Is it then that awareness arises when a certain type of information processing is being performed? If so, what type of information processing? And how do emotional feelings, and sensory events, come to feel like anything? These feels are called qualia. These are great mysteries that have puzzled philosophers for centuries. They are at the heart of the problem of consciousness, for why it should feel like something at all is the great mystery. Other aspects of consciousness, such as the fact that often when we 'pay attention' to events in the world, we can process those events in some better way, that is process or access as opposed to phenomenal aspects of consciousness, may be easier to analyse (Block 1995; Chalmers 1996; Allport 1988). The puzzle of qualia, that is of the phenomenal aspect of consciousness, seems to be rather different from normal investigations in science, in that there is no agreement on criteria by which to assess whether we have made progress. So, although the aim of this chapter is to address the issue of consciousness, especially of qualia, what is written cannot be regarded as being as firmly scientific as the previous chapters in this book. For most of the work in those, there is good evidence for most of the points made, and there would be no hesitation or difficulty in adjusting the view of how things work as new evidence is obtained. However, in the work on qualia, the criteria are much less clear. Nevertheless, the reader may well find these issues interesting, because although not easily solvable, they are very important issues to consider if we wish to really say that we understand some of the very complex and interesting issues about brain function, and ourselves.

With these caveats in mind, I consider in this chapter the general issue of consciousness and its functions, and how feelings, and pleasure, come to occur as a result of the operation of our brains. A view on consciousness, influenced by contemporary cognitive neuroscience, is outlined next. I outline a theory of what the processing is that is involved in consciousness, of its adaptive value in an evolutionary perspective, and of how processing in our visual and other sensory systems can result in subjective or phenomenal states, the 'raw feels' of conscious awareness. However, this view on consciousness that I describe is only preliminary, and theories of consciousness are likely to develop considerably. Partly for these reasons, this theory of consciousness, at least, should not be taken to have practical implications.

9.2 A theory of consciousness

A starting point is that many actions can be performed relatively automatically, without apparent conscious intervention. An example sometimes given is driving a car. Such actions could involve control of behaviour by brain systems which are old in evolutionary terms such as the basal ganglia. It is of interest that the basal ganglia (and cerebellum) do not have backprojection systems to most of the parts of the cerebral cortex from which they receive inputs (see, e.g., Rolls and Johnstone 1992; Rolls 1994a; Rolls and Treves 1998). In contrast, parts of the brain such as the hippocampus and amygdala, involved in functions such as episodic memory and emotion respectively, about which we can make (verbal) declarations (hence declarative memory, Squire 1992) do have major backprojection systems to the high parts of the cerebral cortex from which they receive forward projections (Rolls 1992b; Treves and Rolls 1994; Rolls and Treves 1998) (see Figs 9.1, 4.26 and 4.27). It may be that evolutionarily newer parts of the brain, such as the language areas and parts of the prefrontal cortex, are involved in an alternative type of control of behaviour, in which actions can be planned with the use of a (language) system which allows relatively arbitrary (syntactic) manipulation of semantic entities (symbols).

The general view that there are many routes to behavioural output is supported by the evidence that there are many input systems to the basal ganglia (from almost all areas of

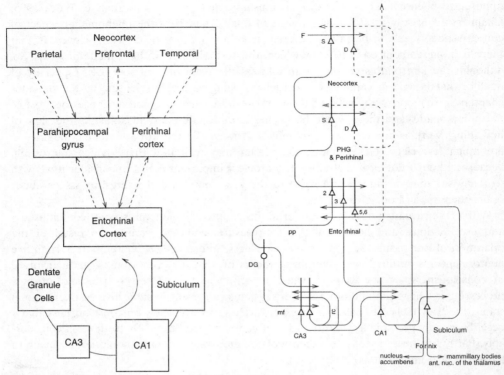

Fig. 9.1 Forward connections (solid lines) from areas of cerebral association neocortex via the parahip-pocampal gyrus and perirhinal cortex, and entorhinal cortex, to the hippocampus; and backprojections (dashed lines) via the hippocampal CA1 pyramidal cells, subiculum, and parahippocampal gyrus to the neocortex. There is great convergence in the forward connections down to the single network imple-mented in the CA3 pyramidal cells, and great divergence again in the backprojections. Left: block diagram. Right: more detailed representation of some of the principal excitatory neurons in the pathways. Abbrevia-tions: D: Deep pyramidal cells. DG: Dentate Granule cells. F: Forward inputs to areas of the association cortex from preceding cortical areas in the hierarchy. mf: mossy fibres. PHG: parahippocampal gyrus and perirhinal cortex. pp: perforant path. rc: recurrent collateral of the CA3 hippocampal pyramidal cells. S: Superficial pyramidal cells. 2: pyramidal cells in layer 2 of the entorhinal cortex. 3: pyramidal cells in layer 3 of the entorhinal cortex. The thick lines above the cell bodies represent the dendrites.

the cerebral cortex), and that neuronal activity in each part of the striatum reflects the activity in the overlying cortical area (Rolls and Johnstone 1992; Rolls 1994a; Rolls and Treves 1998). The evidence is consistent with the possibility that different cortical areas, each specialized for a different type of computation, have their outputs directed to the basal ganglia, which then select the strongest input, and map this into action (via outputs directed, for example, to the premotor cortex) (Rolls and Johnstone 1992; Rolls and Treves 1998). Within this scheme, the language areas would offer one of many routes to action, but a route particularly suited to planning actions, because of the syntactic manipulation of semantic entities which may make long-term planning possible. A schematic diagram of this suggestion is provided in Fig. 9.2. Consistent with the hypothesis of multiple routes to action, only some of which utilize language, is the evidence that split-brain patients may not be aware of actions being performed by the 'non-dominant' hemisphere (Gazzaniga and LeDoux 1978; Gazzaniga 1988, 1995). Also consistent with multiple, including non-verbal, routes to action, patients with focal brain damage, for example to the prefrontal cortex, may emit actions, yet comment verbally that they should not be performing those actions (Rolls, Hornak, Wade and McGrath 1994a). In both these types of patient, confabulation may occur, in that a verbal account of why the action was performed may be given, and this may not be related at all to the environmental event which actually triggered the action (Gazzaniga and LeDoux 1978; Gazzaniga 1988, 1995). It is possible that sometimes in normal humans when actions are initiated as a result of processing in a specialized brain region such as those involved in some types of rewarded behaviour, the language system may subsequently elaborate a coherent account of why that action was performed (i.e. confabulate). This would be consistent with a general view of brain evolution in which, as areas of the cortex evolve, they are laid on top of existing circuitry connecting inputs to outputs, and in which each level in this hierarchy of separate input–output pathways may control behaviour according to the specialized function it can perform (see schematic in Fig. 9.2). (It is of interest that mathematicians may get a hunch that something is correct, yet not be able to verbalize why. They may then resort to formal, more serial and language-like, theorems to prove the case, and these seem to require conscious processing. This is a further indication of a close association between linguistic processing, and consciousness. The linguistic processing need not, as in reading, involve an inner articulatory loop.)

We may next examine some of the advantages and behavioural functions that language, present as the most recently added layer to the above system, would confer. One major advantage would be the ability to plan actions through many potential stages and to evaluate the consequences of those actions without having to perform the actions. For this, the ability to form propositional statements, and to perform syntactic operations on the semantic representations of states in the world, would be important. Also important in this system would be the ability to have second-order thoughts about the type of thought that I have just described (e.g. I think that he thinks that ...), as this would allow much better modelling and prediction of others' behaviour, and therefore of planning, particularly planning when it involves others[1]. This capability for higher-order thoughts would also enable reflection on past events, which would also be useful in planning. In contrast, non-linguistic behaviour would be driven by learned reinforcement associations, learned rules etc., but not by flexible planning for many steps ahead involving a model of the world including others' behaviour. (For an earlier view which is close to this part of the argument see Humphrey 1980.) (The examples of behaviour from non-humans that may reflect planning may reflect much more limited and inflexible planning. For example, the dance of the honey-bee to signal to other bees the location of food may be said to reflect planning, but the symbol manipulation is not arbitrary. There are likely to be interesting examples of non-human primate behaviour, perhaps in the great apes, that reflect the

---

[1] Second-order thoughts are thoughts about thoughts. Higher-order thoughts refer to second-order, third-order, etc., thoughts about thoughts ...

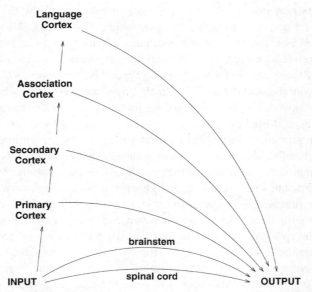

Fig. 9.2 Schematic illustration indicating many possible routes from input systems to action (output) systems. Cortical information-processing systems are organized hierarchically, and there are routes to output systems from most levels of the hierarchy.

evolution of an arbitrary symbol-manipulation system that could be useful for flexible planning, cf. Cheney and Seyfarth 1990.) It is important to state that the language ability referred to here is not necessarily human verbal language (though this would be an example). What it is suggested is important to planning is the syntactic manipulation of symbols, and it is this syntactic manipulation of symbols which is the sense in which language is defined and used here.

It is next suggested that this arbitrary symbol-manipulation using important aspects of language processing and used for planning but not in initiating all types of behaviour is close to what consciousness is about. In particular, consciousness may *be* the state which arises in a system that can think about (or reflect on) its own (or other peoples') thoughts, that is in a system capable of second- or higher-order thoughts (Rosenthal 1986, 1990, 1993; cf. Dennett 1991). On this account, a mental state is non-introspectively (i.e. non-reflectively) conscious if one has a roughly simultaneous thought that one is in that mental state. Following from this, introspective consciousness (or reflexive consciousness, or self consciousness) is the attentive, deliberately focused consciousness of one's mental states. It is noted that not all of the higher-order thoughts need themselves be conscious (many mental states are not). However, according to the analysis, having a higher-order thought about a lower-order thought is necessary for the lower-order thought to be conscious. A slightly weaker position than Rosenthal's on this is that a conscious state corresponds to a first-order thought that has the *capacity* to cause a second-order thought or judgement about it (Carruthers 1996). [Another position which is close in some respects to that of Carruthers and the present position is that of Chalmers (1996), that awareness is something that has *direct availability for behavioural control*, which amounts effectively for him in humans to saying that consciousness is what we can report (verbally) about[2].] This analysis is consistent with the points made above that the brain systems that are required for consciousness and language are similar. In particular, a system which can have second- or higher-order thoughts about its own operation, including its planning and linguistic operation, must itself be a language processor, in that it must be able to bind correctly to the symbols and syntax in the first-order system. According to this explanation, the feeling of anything is the state which is present when linguistic processing that involves second- or higher-order thoughts is being performed.

It might be objected that this captures some of the process aspects of consciousness, what it is good for in an information processing system, but does not capture the phenomenal aspect of consciousness. (Chalmers, following points made in his 1996 book, might make this point.) I agree that there is an element of 'mystery' that is invoked at this step of the argument, when I say that it feels like something for a machine with higher-order thoughts to be thinking about its own first- or lower-order thoughts. But the return point is the following: *if a human with second-order thoughts is thinking about its own first-order thoughts, surely it is very difficult for us to conceive that this would NOT feel like something?* (Perhaps the higher-order thoughts in thinking about the first-order thoughts would need to have in doing this some sense of continuity or self, so that the first-order thoughts would be related to the same system that had thought of something else a few minutes ago. But even this continuity aspect may not be a requirement for consciousness. Humans with anterograde amnesia cannot remember what they felt a few minutes ago, yet their current state does feel like something.)

It is suggested that part of the evolutionary adaptive significance of this type of higher-order thought is that is enables correction of errors made in first-order linguistic or in non-linguistic processing. Indeed, the ability to reflect on previous events is extremely important for learning from them, including setting up new long-term semantic structures. It was shown above that the hippocampus may be a system for such 'declarative' recall of recent memories. Its close relation to 'conscious' processing in humans (Squire has

---

[2] Chalmers (1996) is not entirely consistent about this. Later in the same book he advocates a view that *experiences are associated with information-processing systems*, e.g. experiences are associated with a thermostat (p. 297). He does not believe that the *brain* has experiences, but that he has experiences. This leads him to suggest that experiences are associated with information processing systems such as the thermostat in the same way as they are associated with him. "If there is experience associated with thermostats, there is probably experience *everywhere*: wherever there is a causal interaction, there is information, and wherever there is information, there is experience." (p. 297). He goes on to exclude rocks from having experiences, in that "a rock, unlike a thermostat, is not picked out as an information-processing system". My response to this is that of course there is mutual information between the physical world (e.g. the world of tastants, the chemical stimuli that can produce tastes) and the conscious world (e.g. of taste)—if there were not, the information represented in the conscious processing system would not be useful for any thoughts or operations on or about the world. And according to the view I present here, the conscious processing system is good at some specialized types of processing (e.g. planning ahead using syntactic processing with semantics grounded in the real world, and reflecting on and correcting such plans), for which it would need reliable information about the world. Clearly Chalmers' view on consciousness is very much weaker than mine, in that he allows thermostats to be associated with consciousness, and in contrast to the theory presented here, does not suggest any special criteria for the types of information processing to be performed in order for the system to be aware of its thoughts, and of what it is doing.

classified it as a declarative memory system) may be simply that it enables the recall of recent memories, which can then be reflected upon in conscious, higher-order, processing. Another part of the adaptive value of a higher-order thought system may be that by thinking about its own thoughts in a given situation, it may be able to understand better the thoughts of another individual in a similar situation, and therefore predict that individual's behaviour better (Humphrey 1980, 1986; cf. Barlow 1997).

As a point of clarification, I note that according to this theory, a language processing system is not *sufficient* for consciousness. What defines a conscious system according to this analysis is the ability to have higher-order thoughts, and a first-order language processor (that might be perfectly competent at language) would not be conscious, in that it could not think about its own or others' thoughts. One can perfectly well conceive of a system which obeyed the rules of language (which is the aim of much connectionist modelling), and implemented a first-order linguistic system, that would not be conscious. [Possible examples of language processing that might be performed non-consciously include computer programs implementing aspects of language, or ritualized human conversations, e.g. about the weather. These might require syntax and correctly grounded semantics (see Section 10.4), and yet be performed non-consciously. A more complex example, illustrating that syntax could be used, might be 'If A does X, then B will probably do Y, and then C would be able to do Z.' A first-order language system could process this statement. Moreover, the first-order language system could apply the rule usefully in the world, provided that the symbols in the language system (A, B, X, Y etc.) are grounded (have meaning) in the world.]

In line with the argument on the adaptive value of higher-order thoughts and thus consciousness given above, that they are useful for correcting lower-order thoughts, I now suggest that correction using higher-order thoughts of lower-order thoughts would have adaptive value primarily if the lower-order thoughts are sufficiently complex to benefit from correction in this way. The nature of the complexity is specific—that it should involve syntactic manipulation of symbols, probably with several steps in the chain, and that the chain of steps should be a one-off (or in American, "one-time", meaning used once) set of steps, as in a sentence or in a particular plan used just once, rather than a set of well learned rules. The first or lower-order thoughts might involve a linked chain of 'if' ... 'then' statements that would be involved in planning, an example of which has been given above. It is partly because complex lower-order thoughts such as these which involve syntax and language would benefit from correction by higher-order thoughts, that I suggest that there is a close link between this reflective consciousness and language. The hypothesis is that by thinking about lower-order thoughts, the higher-order thoughts can discover what may be weak links in the chain of reasoning at the lower-order level, and having detected the weak link, might alter the plan, to see if this gives better success. In our example above, if it transpired that C could not do Z, how might the plan have failed? Instead of having to go through endless random changes to the plan to see if by trial and error some combination does happen to produce results, what I am suggesting is that by thinking about the previous plan, one might, for example, using knowledge of the situation and the probabilities that operate in it, guess that the step where the plan failed was that B did not in fact do Y. So by thinking about the plan (the first- or lower-order thought), one might correct the original plan, in such a way that the weak link in that chain, that 'B will probably do Y', is circumvented. To draw a parallel with neural networks: there is a 'credit assignment' problem in such multistep syntactic plans, in that if the whole plan fails, how does the system assign credit or blame to particular steps of the plan? The suggestion is that this is the function of higher-order thoughts and is why systems with higher-order thoughts evolved. The suggestion I then make is that if a system were doing this type of processing (thinking about its own thoughts), it would then be very plausible that it should feel like something to be doing this. I even suggest to the reader that it is not plausible to suggest that it would not feel like anything to a system if it were doing this.

Two other points in the argument should be emphasized for clarity. One is that the system that is having syntactic thoughts about its own syntactic thoughts would have to have its symbols grounded in the real world for it to feel like something to be having higher-order thoughts. The intention of this clarification is to exclude systems such as a computer running a program when there is in addition some sort of control or even overseeing program checking the operation of the first program. We would want to say that in such a situation it would feel like something to be running the higher level control program only if the first-order program was symbolically performing operations on the world and receiving input about the results of those operations, and if the higher-order system understood what the first-order system was trying to do in the world. The issue of symbol grounding is considered further in Section 10.4. The second clarification is that the plan would have to be a unique string of steps, in much the same way as a sentence can be a unique and one-off string of words. The point here is that it is helpful to be able to think about particular one-off plans, and to correct them; and that this type of operation is very different from the slow learning of fixed rules by trial and error, or the application of fixed rules by a supervisory part of a computer program.

This analysis does not yet give an account for sensory qualia ('raw sensory feels', for example why 'red' feels red), for emotional qualia (e.g. why a rewarding touch produces an emotional feeling of pleasure), or for motivational qualia (e.g. why food deprivation makes us *feel* hungry). The view I suggest on such qualia is as follows. Information processing in and from our sensory systems (e.g. the sight of the colour red) may be relevant to planning actions using language and the conscious processing thereby implied. Given that these inputs must be represented in the system that plans, we may ask whether it is more likely that we would be conscious of them or that we would not. I suggest that it would be a very special-purpose system that would allow such sensory inputs, and emotional and motivational states, to be part of (linguistically based) planning, and yet remain unconscious. It seems to be much more parsimonious to hold that we would be conscious of such sensory, emotional, and motivational qualia because they would be being used (or are available to be used) in this type of (linguistically based) higher-order thought processing, and this is what I propose.

The explanation of emotional and motivational subjective feelings or qualia that this discussion has led towards is thus that they should be felt as conscious because they enter into a specialized linguistic symbol-manipulation system that is part of a higher-order thought system that is capable of reflecting on and correcting its lower-order thoughts involved for example in the flexible planning of actions. It would require a very special machine to enable this higher-order linguistically-based thought processing, which is conscious by its nature, to occur without the sensory, emotional and motivational states (which must be taken into account by the higher-order thought system) becoming felt qualia. The qualia are thus accounted for by the evolution of the linguistic system that can reflect on and correct its own lower-order processes, and thus has adaptive value.

This account implies that it may be especially animals with a higher-order belief and thought system and with linguistic symbol manipulation that have qualia. It may be that much non-human animal behaviour, provided that it does not require flexible linguistic planning and correction by reflection, could take place according to reinforcement-guidance (using, e.g., stimulus–reinforcement association learning in the amygdala and orbitofrontal cortex, Rolls 1990b, 1996d), and rule-following (implemented, e.g., using habit or stimulus–response learning in the basal ganglia—Rolls and Johnstone 1992; Rolls 1994a). Such behaviours might appear very similar to human behaviour performed in similar circumstances, but would not imply qualia. It would be primarily by virtue of a system for reflecting on flexible, linguistic, planning behaviour that humans (and animals close to humans, with demonstrable syntactic manipulation of symbols, and the ability to think about these linguistic processes) would be different from other animals, and would have evolved qualia.

In order for processing in a part of our brain to be able to reach consciousness, appropriate pathways must be present. Certain constraints arise here. For example, in the sensory pathways, the nature of the representation may change as it passes through a hierarchy of processing levels, and in order to be conscious of the information in the form in which it is represented in early processing stages, the early processing stages must have access to the part of the brain necessary for consciousness. An example is provided by processing in the taste system. In the primate primary taste cortex, neurons respond to taste independently of hunger, yet in the secondary taste cortex, food-related taste neurons (e.g. responding to sweet taste) only respond to food if hunger is present, and gradually stop responding to that taste during feeding to satiety (see Rolls 1989d, 1993, 1995a). Now the quality of the tastant (sweet, salt, etc.) and its intensity are not affected by hunger, but the pleasantness of its taste is reduced to zero (neutral) (or even becomes unpleasant) after we have eaten it to satiety. The implication of this is that for quality and intensity information about taste, we must be conscious of what is represented in the primary taste cortex (or perhaps in another area connected to it which bypasses the secondary taste cortex), and not of what is represented in the secondary taste cortex. In contrast, for the pleasantness of a taste, consciousness of this could not reflect what is represented in the primary taste cortex, but instead what is represented in the secondary taste cortex (or in an area beyond it). The same argument arises for reward in general, and therefore for emotion, which in primates is not represented early on in processing in the sensory pathways (nor in or before the inferior temporal cortex for vision), but in the areas to which these object analysis systems project, such as the orbitofrontal cortex, where the reward value of visual stimuli is reflected in the responses of neurons to visual stimuli (see Rolls 1990b, 1995a,c; Chapter 2). It is also of interest that reward signals (e.g. the taste of food when we are hungry) are associated with subjective feelings of pleasure (see Rolls

1990b, 1993, 1995a,c; Chapter 2). I suggest that this correspondence arises because pleasure is the subjective state that represents in the conscious system a signal that is positively reinforcing (rewarding), and that inconsistent behaviour would result if the representations did not correspond to a signal for positive reinforcement in both the conscious and the non-conscious processing systems.

Do these arguments mean that the conscious sensation of, e.g., taste quality (i.e. identity and intensity) is represented or occurs in the primary taste cortex, and of the pleasantness of taste in the secondary taste cortex, and that activity in these areas is sufficient for conscious sensations (qualia) to occur? I do not suggest this at all. Instead the arguments I have put forward above suggest that we are only conscious of representations when we have high-order thoughts about them. The implication then is that pathways must connect from each of the brain areas in which information is represented about which we can be conscious, to the system which has the higher-order thoughts, which as I have argued above, requires language. Thus, in the example given, there must be connections to the language areas from the primary taste cortex, which need not be direct, but which must bypass the secondary taste cortex, in which the information is represented differently (see Rolls 1989d, 1995a). There must also be pathways from the secondary taste cortex, not necessarily direct, to the language areas so that we can have higher-order thoughts about the pleasantness of the representation in the secondary taste cortex. There would also need to be pathways from the hippocampus, implicated in the recall of declarative memories, back to the language areas of the cerebral cortex (at least via the cortical areas which receive backprojections from the hippocampus, see Fig. 9.1, which would in turn need connections to the language areas). A schematic diagram incorporating this anatomical prediction about human cortical neural connectivity in relation to consciousness is shown in Fig. 9.3.

One question that has been discussed is whether there is a causal role for consciousness (e.g. Armstrong and Malcolm 1984). The position to which the above arguments lead is that indeed conscious processing does have a causal role in the elicitation of behaviour, but only under the set of circumstances when higher-order thoughts play a role in correcting or influencing lower-order thoughts. The sense in which the consciousness is causal is then, it is suggested, that the higher-order thought is causally involved in correcting the lower-order thought; and that it is a property of the higher-order thought system that it feels like something when it is operating. As we have seen, some behavioural responses can be elicited when there is not this type of reflective control of lower-order processing, nor indeed any contribution of language. There are many brain-processing routes to output regions, and only one of these involves conscious, verbally represented processing which can later be recalled (see Fig. 9.2 and Section 9.3).

It is of interest to comment on how the evolution of a system for flexible planning might affect emotions. Consider grief which may occur when a reward is terminated and no immediate action is possible (see Rolls 1990b, 1995c). It may be adaptive by leading to a cessation of the formerly rewarded behaviour and thus facilitating the possible identification of other positive reinforcers in the environment. In humans, grief may be particularly potent because it becomes represented in a system which can plan ahead, and understand the enduring implications of the loss. (Thinking about or verbally discussing emotional

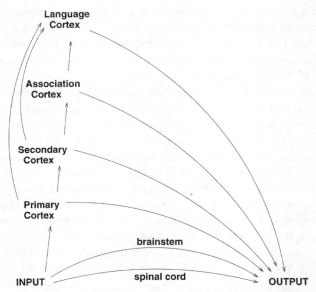

Fig. 9.3 Schematic illustration indicating that early cortical stages in information processing may need access to language areas which bypass subsequent levels in the hierarchy, so that consciousness of what is represented in early cortical stages, and which may not be represented in later cortical stages, can occur. Higher-order linguistic thoughts (HOLTs) could be implemented in the language cortex itself, and would not need a separate cortical area. Backprojections, a notable feature of cortical connectivity, with many probable functions including recall (Rolls 1989a,b, 1996a), probably reciprocate all the connections shown.

states may also in these circumstances help, because this can lead towards the identification of new or alternative reinforcers, and of the realization that, for example, negative consequences may not be as bad as feared.)

This account of consciousness also leads to a suggestion about the processing that underlies the feeling of free will. Free will would in this scheme involve the use of language to check many moves ahead on a number of possible series of actions and their outcomes, and then with this information to make a choice from the likely outcomes of different possible series of actions. (If in contrast choices were made only on the basis of the reinforcement value of immediately available stimuli, without the arbitrary syntactic symbol manipulation made possible by language, then the choice strategy would be much more limited, and we might not want to use the term free will, as all the consequences of those actions would not have been computed.) It is suggested that when this type of reflective, conscious, information processing is occurring and leading to action, the system performing this processing and producing the action would have to believe that it could cause the action, for otherwise inconsistencies would arise, and the system might no longer try to initiate action. This belief held by the system may partly underlie the feeling of free will. At other times, when other brain modules are initiating actions (in the implicit systems), the conscious processor (the explicit system) may confabulate and believe that it caused the action, or at least give an account (possibly wrong) of why the action was initiated. The fact that the conscious processor may have the belief even in these circumstances that it initiated the action may arise as a property of its being inconsistent for a system which can take overall control using conscious verbal processing to believe that it was over-ridden by another system. This may be the reason why confabulation occurs.

In the operation of such a free-will system, the uncertainties introduced by the limited information possible about the likely outcomes of series of actions, and the inability to use optimal algorithms when combining conditional probabilities, would be much more important factors than whether the brain operates deterministically or not. (The operation of brain machinery must be relatively deterministic, for it has evolved to provide reliable outputs for given inputs.)

Before leaving these thoughts, it may be worth commenting on the feeling of continuing self-identity that is characteristic of humans. Why might this arise? One suggestion is that if one is an organism that can think about its own long-term multistep plans, then for those plans to be consistently and thus adaptively executed, the goals of the plans would need to remain stable, as would memories of how far one had proceeded along the execution path of each plan. If one felt each time one came to execute, perhaps on another day, the next step of a plan, that the goals were different, or if one did not remember which steps had already been taken in a multistep plan, the plan would never be usefully executed. So, given that it does feel like something to be doing this type of planning using higher-order thoughts, it would have to feel as if one were the same agent, acting towards the same goals, from day to day. Thus it is suggested that the feeling of continuing self-identity falls out of a situation in which there is an actor with consistent long-term goals, and long-term recall. If it feels like anything to be the actor, according to the suggestions of the higher-order thought theory, then it should feel like the same thing from occasion to occasion to be the actor, and no special further construct is needed to account for self-identity. Humans without such a feeling of being the same person from day to day might be expected to have, for example, inconsistent goals from day to day, or a poor recall memory. It may be noted that the ability to recall previous steps in a plan, and bring them into the conscious, higher-order thought system, is an important prerequisite for long-term planning which involves checking each step in a multistep process.

These are my initial thoughts on why we have consciousness, and are conscious of sensory, emotional and motivational qualia, as well as qualia associated with first-order linguistic thoughts. However, as stated above, one does not feel that there are straightforward criteria in this philosophical field of enquiry for knowing whether the suggested theory is correct; so it is likely that theories of consciousness will continue to undergo rapid development; and current theories should not be taken to have practical implications (Rolls, 1997d).

9.3 Dual routes to action

According to the present formulation, there are two types of route to action performed in relation to reward or punishment in humans. Examples of such actions include emotional and motivational behaviour.

The first route is via the brain systems that have been present in non-human primates such as monkeys, and to some extent in other mammals, for millions of years. These systems include the amygdala and, particularly well-developed in primates, the orbitofrontal cortex. These systems control behaviour in relation to previous associations of stimuli with reinforcement. The computation which controls the action thus involves assessment of the reinforcement-related value of a stimulus. This assessment may be based on a number of different factors. One is the previous reinforcement history, which involves stimulus–reinforcement association learning using the amygdala, and its rapid updating especially in primates using the orbitofrontal cortex. This stimulus–reinforcement association learning may involve quite specific information about a stimulus, for example of the energy associated with each type of food, by the process of conditioned appetite and satiety (Booth 1985). A second is the current motivational state, for example whether hunger is present, whether other needs are satisfied, etc. A third factor which affects the computed reward value of the stimulus is whether that reward has been received recently. If it has been received recently but in small quantity, this may increase the reward value of the stimulus. This is known as incentive motivation or the 'salted peanut' phenomenon. The adaptive value of such a process is that this positive feedback of reward value in the early stages of working for a particular reward tends to lock the organism on to behaviour being performed for that reward. This means that animals that are for example almost equally hungry and thirsty will show hysteresis in their choice of action, rather than continually switching from eating to drinking and back with each mouthful of water or food. This introduction of hysteresis into the reward evaluation system makes action selection a much more efficient process in a natural environment, for constantly switching between different types of behaviour would be very costly if all the different rewards were not available in the same place at the same time. (For example, walking half a mile between a site where water was available and a site where food was available after every mouthful would be very inefficient.) The amygdala is one structure that may be involved in this increase in the reward value of stimuli early on in a series of presentations, in that lesions of the amygdala (in rats) abolish the expression of this reward-incrementing process which is normally evident in the increasing rate of working for a food reward early on in a meal (Rolls and Rolls 1973, 1982). A fourth factor is the computed absolute value of the reward or punishment expected or being obtained from a stimulus, e.g. the sweetness of the stimulus (set by evolution so that sweet stimuli will tend to be rewarding, because they are generally associated with energy sources), or the pleasantness of touch (set by evolution to be pleasant according to the extent to which it brings animals of the opposite sex together, and depending on the investment in time that the partner is willing to put into making the touch pleasurable, a sign which indicates the commitment and value for the partner of the relationship). After the reward value of the stimulus has been assessed in these ways, behaviour is then initiated based on approach towards or withdrawal from the stimulus. A critical aspect of the behaviour produced by this type of system is that it is aimed directly towards obtaining a sensed or expected reward, by virtue of connections to brain systems such as the basal ganglia which are concerned with the initiation of actions (see Fig. 9.4). The expectation may of course, involve behaviour to obtain stimuli associated with reward, which might even be present in a chain.

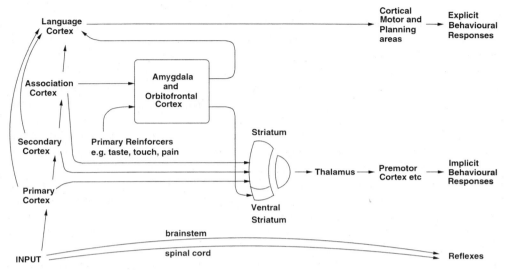

Fig. 9.4 Dual routes to the initiation of action in response to rewarding and punishing stimuli. The inputs from different sensory systems to brain structures such as the orbitofrontal cortex and amygdala allow these brain structures to evaluate the reward- or punishment-related value of incoming stimuli, or of remembered stimuli. The different sensory inputs enable evaluations within the orbitofrontal cortex and amygdala based mainly on the primary (unlearned) reinforcement value for taste, touch, and olfactory stimuli, and on the secondary (learned) reinforcement value for visual and auditory stimuli. In the case of vision, the 'association cortex' which outputs representations of objects to the amygdala and orbitofrontal cortex is the inferior temporal visual cortex. One route for the outputs from these evaluative brain structures is via projections directly to structures such as the basal ganglia (including the striatum and ventral striatum) to enable implicit, direct behavioural responses based on the reward- or punishment-related evaluation of the stimuli to be made. The second route is via the language systems of the brain, which allow explicit (verbalizable) decisions involving multistep syntactic planning to be implemented.

Now part of the way in which the behaviour is controlled with this first route is according to the reward value of the outcome. At the same time, the animal may only work for the reward if the cost is not too high. Indeed, in the field of behavioural ecology animals are often thought of as performing optimally on some cost–benefit curve (see, e.g., Krebs and Kacelnik 1991). This does not at all mean that the animal thinks about the rewards, and performs a cost–benefit analysis using a lot of thoughts about the costs, other rewards available and their costs, etc. Instead, it should be taken to mean that in evolution the system has evolved in such a way that the way in which the reward varies with the different energy densities or amounts of food and the delay before it is received, can be used as part of the input to a mechanism which has also been built to track the costs of obtaining the food (e.g. energy loss in obtaining it, risk of predation, etc.), and to then select given many such types of reward and the associated cost, the current behaviour that provides the most 'net reward'. Part of the value of having the computation expressed in this reward-minus-cost form is that there is then a suitable 'currency', or net reward value, to enable the animal to select the behaviour with currently the most net reward gain (or minimal aversive outcome).

The second route in humans involves a computation with many 'if ... then' statements, to implement a plan to obtain a reward. In this case, the reward may actually be *deferred* as part of the plan, which might involve working first to obtain one reward, and only then to work for a second more highly valued reward, if this was thought to be overall an optimal strategy in terms of resource usage (e.g., time). In this case, syntax is required, because the many symbols (e.g. names of people) that are part of the plan must be correctly linked or bound. Such linking might be of the form: 'if A does this, then B is likely to do this, and this will cause C to do this ...'. The requirement of syntax for this type of planning implies that an output to language systems in the brain is required for this type of planning (see Fig. 9.4). This the explicit language system in humans may allow working for deferred rewards by enabling use of a one-off, individual, plan appropriate for each situation. Another building block for such planning operations in the brain may be the type of short-term memory in which the prefrontal cortex is involved. This short-term memory may be, for example in non-human primates, of where in space a response has just been made. A development of this type of short-term response memory system in humans to enable multiple short-term memories to be held in place correctly, preferably with the temporal order of the different items in the short-term memory coded correctly, may be another building block for the multiple step 'if ... then' type of computation in order to form a multiple step plan. Such short-term memories are implemented in the (dorsolateral and inferior convexity) prefrontal cortex of non-human primates and humans (see Goldman-Rakic 1996; Petrides 1996), and may be part of the reason why prefrontal cortex damage impairs planning (see Shallice 1996).

Of these two routes (see Fig. 9.4), it is the second which I have suggested above is related to consciousness. The hypothesis is that consciousness is the state which arises by virtue of having the ability to think about one's own thoughts, which has the adaptive value of enabling one to correct long multistep syntactic plans. This latter system is thus the one in which explicit, declarative, processing occurs. Processing in this system is frequently associated with reason and rationality, in that many of the consequences of possible actions can be taken into account. The actual computation of how rewarding a particular stimulus or situation is or will be probably still depends on activity in the orbitofrontal cortex and amygdala, as the reward value of stimuli is computed and represented in these regions, and in that it is found that verbalized expressions of the reward (or punishment) value of stimuli are dampened by damage to these systems. (For example, damage to the orbitofrontal cortex renders painful input still identifiable as pain, but without the strong affective, 'unpleasant', reaction to it.) This language system which enables long-term planning may be contrasted with the first system in which behaviour is directed at obtaining the stimulus (including the remembered stimulus) which is currently most rewarding, as computed by brain structures that include the orbitofrontal cortex and amygdala. There are outputs from this system, perhaps those directed at the basal ganglia, which do not pass through the language system, and behaviour produced in this way is described as implicit, and verbal declarations cannot be made directly about the reasons for the choice made. When verbal declarations are made about decisions made in this first system, those verbal declarations may be confabulations, reasonable explanations or fabrications, of reasons why the choice was made. These reasonable explanations would be generated to be consistent with the sense of continuity and self that is a characteristic of reasoning in the language system.

The question then arises of how decisions are made in animals such as humans that have both the implicit, direct reward-based, and the explicit, rational, planning systems (see Fig. 9.4). One particular situation in which the first, implicit, system may be especially important is when rapid reactions to stimuli with reward or punishment value must be made, for then the direct connections from structures such as the orbitofrontal cortex to the basal ganglia may allow rapid actions. Another is when there may be too many factors to be taken into account easily by the explicit, rational, planning, system, when the implicit system may be used to guide action. In contrast, when the implicit system continually makes errors, it would then be beneficial for the organism to switch from automatic, direct, action based on obtaining what the orbitofrontal cortex system decodes as being the most positively reinforcing choice currently available, to the explicit conscious control system which can evaluate with its long-term planning algorithms what action should be performed next. Indeed, it would be adaptive for the explicit system to be regularly assessing performance by the more automatic system, and to switch itself in to control behaviour quite frequently, as otherwise the adaptive value of having the explicit system would be less than optimal. Another factor which may influence the balance between control by the implicit and explicit systems is the presence of pharmacological agents such as alcohol, which may alter the balance towards control by the implicit system, may allow the implicit system to influence more the explanations made by the explicit system, and may within the explicit system alter the relative value it places on caution and restraint vs commitment to a risky action or plan.

There may also be a flow of influence from the explicit, verbal system to the implicit system, in that the explicit system may decide on a plan of action or strategy, and exert an influence on the implicit system which will alter the reinforcement evaluations made by and the signals produced by the implicit system. An example of this might be that if a pregnant woman feels that she would like to escape a cruel mate, but is aware that she may not survive in the jungle, then it would be adaptive if the explicit system could suppress some aspects of her implicit behaviour towards her mate, so that she does not give signals that she is displeased with her situation. (In the literature on self-deception, it has been suggested that unconscious desires may not be made explicit in consciousness (or actually repressed), so as not to compromise the explicit system in what it produces; see, e.g., Alexander 1975, 1979; Trivers 1976, 1985; and the review by Nesse and Lloyd 1992). Another example might be that the explicit system might, because of its long-term plans, influence the implicit system to increase its response to for example a positive reinforcer. One way in which the explicit system might influence the implicit system is by setting up the conditions in which, for example, when a given stimulus (e.g. person) is present, positive reinforcers are given, to facilitate stimulus–reinforcement association learning by the implicit system of the person receiving the positive reinforcers. Conversely, the implicit system may influence the explicit system, for example by highlighting certain stimuli in the environment that are currently associated with reward, to guide the attention of the explicit system to such stimuli.

However, it may be expected that there is often a conflict between these systems, in that the first, implicit, system is able to guide behaviour particularly to obtain the greatest immediate reinforcement, whereas the explicit system can potentially enable immediate rewards to be deferred, and longer-term, multistep, plans to be formed. This type of conflict will occur in animals with a syntactic planning ability, that is in humans and any other animals that have the ability to process a series of 'if ... then' stages of planning. This is a property of the human language system, and the extent to which it is a property of non-human primates is not yet fully clear. In any case, such conflict may be an important aspect of the operation of at least the human mind, because it is so essential for humans to decide correctly, at every moment, whether to invest in a relationship or a group that may offer long-term benefits, or whether to pursue immediate benefits directly (Nesse and Lloyd 1992). As Nesse and Lloyd (1992) describe, analysts have come to a somewhat similar position, for they hold that intrapsychic conflicts usually seem to have two sides, with impulses on one side and inhibitions on the other. Analysts describe the source of the impulses as the *id*, and the modules that inhibit the expression of impulses, because of external and internal constraints, the *ego* and *superego* respectively (Leak and Christopher 1982; Trivers 1985; see Nesse and Lloyd 1992, p. 613). The superego can be thought of as the conscience, while the ego is the locus of executive functions that balance satisfaction of impulses with anticipated internal and external costs. A difference of the present position is that it is based on identification of dual routes to action implemented by different systems in the brain, each with its own selective advantage.

Some investigations on deception in non-human primates have been interpreted as showing that animals can plan to deceive others (see, e.g., Griffin 1992), that is to utilize 'Machiavellian intelligence'. For example, a baboon might 'deliberately' mislead another animal in order to obtain a resource such as food (e.g. by screaming to summon assistance in order to have a competing animal chased from a food patch) or sex (e.g. a female baboon who very gradually moved into a position from which the dominant male could not see her grooming a subadult baboon) (see M. Dawkins 1993). The attraction of the Machiavellian argument is that the behaviour for which it accounts seems to imply that there is a concept of another animal's mind, and that one animal is trying occasionally to mislead another, which implies some planning. However, such observations tend by their nature to be field-based, and may have an anecdotal character, in that the previous experience of the animals in this type of behaviour, and the reinforcements obtained, are not known (M. Dawkins 1993). It is possible, for example, that some behavioural responses that appear to be Machiavellian may have been the result of previous instrumental learning in which reinforcement was obtained for particular types of response, or of observational learning, with again learning from the outcome observed. However, in any case, most examples of Machiavellian intelligence in non-human primates do not involve multiple stages of 'if ... then' planning requiring syntax to keep the symbols apart (but may involve learning of the type 'if the dominant male sees me grooming a subadult male, I will be punished') (see M. Dawkins 1993). Nevertheless, the possible advantage of such Machiavellian *planning* could be one of the adaptive guiding factors in evolution which provided advantage to a multistep, syntactic system which enables long-term planning, the best example of such a system being human language. However, another, not necessarily exclusive, advantage of the evolution of a linguistic multistep planning system could well be not Machiavellian planning, but planning for social co-operation and advantage. Perhaps in general an 'if ... then' multistep syntactic planning ability is useful primarily in evolution in social situations of the type: 'if X does this, then Y does that; then I would/should do that, and the outcome would be ... '. It is not yet at all clear whether such planning is required in order to explain the social behaviour of social animals such as hunting dogs, or socializing monkeys (M. Dawkins 1993). However, in humans there is evidence that members of 'primitive' hunting tribes spend hours recounting tales of recent events (perhaps who did what, when; who then did what, etc.), perhaps to help learn from experience about good strategies, necessary for example when physically weak men take on large animals (see Pinker and Bloom 1992). Thus, social co-operation may be as powerful a driving force in the evolution of syntactical planning systems as Machiavellian intelligence. What is common to both is that they involve social situations. However, such a syntactic planning system would have advantages not only in social systems, for such planning may be useful in obtaining resources purely in a physical (non-social) world. An example might be planning how to cross terrain given current environmental constraints in order to reach a particular place[3].

The thrust of this argument thus is that much complex animal, including human, behaviour can take place using the implicit, non-conscious, route to action. We should be very careful not to postulate intentional states (i.e. states with intentions, beliefs, and desires) unless the evidence for them is strong, and it seems to me that a flexible, one-off, linguistic processing system that can handle propositions is needed for intentional states. What the explicit, linguistic, system does allow is exactly this flexible, one-off, multistep planning-ahead type of computation, which allows us to defer immediate rewards based on such a plan.

This discussion of dual routes to action has been with respect to the behaviour produced. There is of course in addition a third output of brain regions such as the orbitofrontal cortex and amygdala involved in emotion, that is directed to producing autonomic and endocrine responses. Although it has been argued in Chapter 3 that the autonomic system is not normally in a circuit through which behavioural responses are produced (i.e. against the James–Lange and related theories), there may be some influence from effects produced through the endocrine system (and possibly the autonomic system, through which some endocrine responses are controlled) on behaviour, or on the dual systems just discussed which control behaviour. For example, during female orgasm the hormone oxytocin may be released, and this may influence the implicit system to help develop positive reinforcement associations and thus attachment to her lover.

---

[3] Tests of whether such multistep planning might be possible in even non-human primates are quite difficult to devise. One example might be to design a multistep maze. On a first part of the trial, the animal might be allowed to choose for itself, given constraints set on that trial to ensure trial unique performance, a set of choices through a maze. On the second part of that trial, the animal would be required to run through the maze again, remembering and repeating every choice just made in the first part of that trial. This part of the design is intended to allow recall of a multistep plan. To test on probe occasions whether the plan is being recalled, and whether the plan can be corrected by a higher-order thought process, the animal might be shown after the first part of its trial that one of its previous free choices was not now available. The test would be to determine whether the animal can make a set of choices that indicate corrections to the multistep plan, in which the trajectory has to be altered before the now unavailable choice point is reached.

9.4 Discussion

Some ways in which the current theory may be different from other related theories follow. The current theory holds that it is higher-order *linguistic* thoughts (HOLTs) that are closely associated with consciousness, and this might differ from Rosenthal's higher-order thoughts (HOTs) theory (Rosenthal 1986, 1990, 1993) in the emphasis in the current theory on language. Language in the current theory is defined by syntactic manipulation of symbols, and does not necessarily imply verbal language. The reason that strong emphasis is placed on language is that it is as a result of having a multistep flexible 'on the fly' reasoning procedure that errors which cannot be easily corrected by reward or punishment received at the end of the reasoning, need 'thoughts about thoughts', that is some type of supervisory and monitoring process, to detect where errors in the reasoning have occurred. This suggestion on the adaptive value in evolution of such a higher-order linguistic thought process for multistep planning ahead, and correcting such plans, may also be different from earlier work. Put another way, this point is that credit assignment when reward or punishment are received is straightforward in a one-layer network (in which the reinforcement can be used directly to correct nodes in error, or responses), but is very difficult in a multistep linguistic process executed once 'on the fly'. Very complex mappings in a multilayer network can be learned if hundreds of learning trials are provided. But once these complex mappings are learned, their success or failure in a new situation on a given trial cannot be evaluated and corrected by the network. Indeed, the complex mappings achieved by such networks (e.g. backpropagation nets) mean that after training they operate according to fixed rules, and are often quite impenetrable and inflexible. In contrast, to correct a multistep, single occasion, linguistically based plan or procedure, recall of the steps just made in the reasoning or planning, and perhaps related episodic material, needs to occur, so that the link in the chain which is most likely to be in error can be identified. This may be part of the reason why there is a close relationship between declarative memory systems, which can explicitly recall memories, and consciousness.

Some computer programs may have supervisory processes. Should these count as higher-order linguistic thought processes? My current response to this is that they should not, to the extent that they operate with fixed rules to correct the operation of a system which does not itself involve linguistic thoughts about symbols grounded semantically in the external world. If on the other hand it were possible to implement on a computer such a high-order linguistic thought-supervisory correction process to correct first-order one-off linguistic thoughts with symbols grounded in the real world, then this process would *prima facie* be conscious. If it were possible in a thought experiment to reproduce the neural connectivity and operation of a human brain on a computer, then *prima facie* it would also have the attributes of consciousness. It might continue to have those attributes for as long as power was applied to the system.

Another possible difference from earlier theories is that raw sensory feels are suggested to arise as a consequence of having a system that can think about its own thoughts. Raw sensory feels, and subjective states associated with emotional and motivational states, may not necessarily arise first in evolution.

A property often attributed to consciousness is that it is *unitary*. The current theory would account for this by the limited syntactic capability of neuronal networks in the brain, which renders it difficult to implement more than a few syntactic bindings of symbols simultaneously (see Rolls and Treves 1998; McLeod, Plunkett and Rolls 1998). This limitation makes it difficult to run several 'streams of consciousness' simultaneously. In addition, given that a linguistic system can control behavioural output, several parallel streams might produce maladaptive behaviour (apparent as, e.g., indecision), and might be selected against. The close relationship between, and the limited capacity of, both the stream of consciousness, and auditory–verbal short-term memory, may be that both implement the capacity for syntax in neural networks. Whether syntax in real neuronal networks is implemented by temporal binding (see von der Malsburg 1990) is still very much an unresolved issue (Rolls and Treves 1998). [For example, the code about which visual stimulus has been shown can be read off from the end of the visual system without taking the temporal aspects of the neuronal firing into account; much of the information about which stimulus is shown is available in short times of 30–50 ms, and cortical neurons need fire for only this long during the identification of objects (Tovee, Rolls, Treves and Bellis 1993; Rolls and Tovee 1994; Tovee and Rolls 1995; Rolls and Treves 1998) (these are rather short time-windows for the expression of multiple separate populations of synchronized neurons); and oscillations, at least, are not an obvious property of neuronal firing in the primate temporal cortical visual areas involved in the representation of faces and objects (Tovee and Rolls 1992; see further Rolls and Treves 1998).] However, the hypothesis that syntactic binding is necessary for consciousness is one of the postulates of the theory I am describing (for the system I describe must be capable of correcting its own syntactic thoughts), and the fact that the binding must be implemented in neuronal networks may well place limitations on consciousness which lead to some of its properties, such as its unitary nature. The postulate of Crick and Koch (1990) that oscillations and synchronization are necessary bases of consciousness could thus be related to the present theory if it turns out that oscillations or neuronal synchronization are the way the brain implements syntactic binding. However, the fact that oscillations and neuronal synchronization are especially evident in anaesthetized cats does not impress as strong evidence that oscillations and synchronization are critical features of consciousness, for most people would hold that anaesthetized cats are *not* conscious. The fact that oscillations and synchronization are much more difficult to demonstrate in the temporal cortical visual areas of awake behaving monkeys might just mean that during evolution to primates the cortex has become better able to avoid parasitic oscillations, as a result of developing better feedforward and feedback inhibitory circuits (see Rolls and Treves 1998).

The current theory holds that consciousness arises by virtue of a system that can think linguistically about its own linguistic thoughts. The advantages for a system of being able to do this have been described, and this has been suggested as the reason why consciousness evolved. The evidence that consciousness arises by virtue of having a system that can perform higher-order linguistic processing is however, and I think might remain, circumstantial. (Why must it feel like something when we are performing a certain type of information processing? The evidence described here suggests that it does feel like something when we are performing a certain type of information processing, but does not produce a strong reason for why it has to feel like something. It just does, when we are using this linguistic processing system capable of higher-order thoughts.) The evidence, summarized above, includes the points that we think of ourselves as conscious when, for example, we recall earlier events, compare them with current events, and plan many steps ahead. Evidence also comes from neurological cases, from, for example, split-brain patients (who may confabulate conscious stories about what is happening in their other, non-language, hemisphere; and from cases such as frontal lobe patients who can tell one consciously what they should be doing, but nevertheless may be doing the opposite. (The force of this type of case is that much of our behaviour may normally be produced by routes about which we cannot verbalize, and are not conscious about.) This raises the issue of the causal role of consciousness. Does consciousness cause our behaviour?[4] The view that I currently hold is that the information processing which is related to consciousness (activity in a linguistic system capable of higher-order thoughts, and used for planning and correcting the operation of lower-order linguistic systems) can play a causal role in producing our behaviour (see Fig. 9.2). It is, I postulate, a *property* of processing in this system (capable of higher-order thoughts) that it feels like something to be performing that type of processing. It is in this sense that I suggest that consciousness can act causally to influence our behaviour—consciousness is the property that occurs when a linguistic system is thinking about its lower-order thoughts. The hypothesis that it does feel like something when this processing is taking place is at least to some extent testable: humans performing this type of higher-order linguistic processing, for example recalling episodic memories and comparing them with current circumstances, who denied being conscious, would *prima facie* constitute evidence against the theory. Most humans would find it very implausible though to posit that they could be thinking about their own thoughts, and reflecting on their own thoughts, without being conscious. This type of processing does appear, for most humans, to be necessarily conscious.

Finally, I provide a short specification of what might have to be implemented in a neural network to implement conscious processing. First, a linguistic system, not necessarily verbal, but implementing syntax between symbols implemented in the environment would be needed. Then a higher-order thought system also implementing syntax and able to think about the representations in the first-order language system, and able to correct the reasoning in the first-order linguistic system in a flexible manner, would be needed. So my view is that consciousness can be implemented in neural networks, (and that this is a topic worth discussing), but that the neural networks would have to implement the type of higher-order linguistic processing described in this chapter.

---

[4] This raises the issue of the causal relation between mental events and neurophysiological events, part of the mind–body problem. My view is that the relationship between mental events and neurophysiological events is similar (apart from the problem of consciousness) to the relationship between the program running in a computer and the hardware of the computer. In a sense, the program causes the logic gates to move to the next state. This move causes the program to move to its next state. Effectively, we are looking at different levels of what is overall the operation of a *system*, and causality can usefully be understood as operating both within levels (causing one step of the program to move to the next), as well as between levels (e.g. software to hardware and vice versa). This is the solution I propose to this aspect of the mind–body (or mind–brain) problem.

9.5   Conclusion

It is suggested that it feels like something to be an organism or machine that can think about its own (linguistic and semantically based) thoughts. It is suggested that qualia, raw sensory, and emotional feels, arise secondarily to having evolved such a higher-order thought system, and that sensory and emotional processing feels like something because it would be unparsimonious for it to enter the planning, higher-order thought, system and *not* feel like something. The adaptive value of having sensory and emotional feelings, or qualia, is thus suggested to be that such inputs are important to the long-term planning, explicit, processing system. Raw sensory feels, and subjective states associated with emotional and motivational states, may not necessarily arise first in evolution.

10   Reward, punishment, and emotion in brain design

10.1   Introduction

We now confront the fundamental issue of why we, and other animals, are built to use rewards and punishments to guide or determine our behaviour. Why are we built to have emotions, as well as motivational states? Is there any reasonable alternative around which evolution could have built complex animals? In Section 10.2 I outline several types of brain design, with differing degrees of complexity, and suggest that evolution can operate with only some of these types of design.

10.2   Brain design

10.2.1   Taxes, rewards, and punishments
10.2.1.1   Taxes

A simple design principle is to incorporate mechanisms for taxes into the design of organisms. Taxes consist at their simplest of orientation towards stimuli in the environment, for example the bending of a plant towards light which results in maximum light collection by its photosynthetic surfaces. (When just turning rather than locomotion is possible, such responses are called tropisms.) With locomotion possible, as in animals, taxes include movements towards sources of nutrient, and movements away from hazards such as very high temperatures. The design principle here is that animals have, through a process of natural selection, built receptors for certain dimensions of the wide range of stimuli in the environment, and have linked these receptors to response mechanisms in such a way that the stimuli are approached or avoided.

10.2.1.2   Reward and punishment

As soon as we have approach to stimuli at one end of a dimension (e.g. a source of nutrient) and away from stimuli at the other end of the dimension (in this case lack of nutrient), we can start to wonder when it is appropriate to introduce the terms rewards and punishers for the stimuli at the different ends of the dimension. By convention, if the response consists of a fixed response to obtain the stimulus (e.g. locomotion up a chemical gradient), we shall call this a taxis not a reward. On the other hand, if an arbitrary operant response can be performed by the animal in order to approach the stimulus, then we will call this rewarded behaviour, and the stimulus which the animal works to obtain a reward.

(The arbitrary operant response can be thought of as any arbitrary response the animal will perform to obtain the stimulus. It can be thought of as an action.) This criterion, of an arbitrary operant response, is often tested by bidirectionality. For example, if a rat can be trained to either raise its tail, or lower its tail, in order to obtain a piece of food, then we can be sure that there is no fixed relationship between the stimulus (e.g. the sight of food) and the response, as there is in a taxis. Some authors reserve the term *motivated behaviour* for that in which an arbitrary operant response will be performed to obtain a reward or to escape from or avoid a punishment. If this criterion is not met, and only a fixed response can be performed, then the term *drive* can be used to describe the state of the animal when it will work to obtain or escape from the stimulus.

We can thus distinguish a first level of approach/avoidance mechanism complexity in a taxis, with a fixed response available for the stimulus, from a second level of complexity in which any arbitrary response can be performed, in which case we use the term reward when a stimulus is being approached, and punishment when the response is to escape from or avoid the stimulus.

The role of natural selection in this process is to guide animals to build sensory systems that will respond to dimensions of stimuli in the natural environment along which responses of the animals can lead to better survival to enable genes to be passed on to the next generation, that is, can increase fitness. The animals must be built by such natural selection to make responses that will enable them to obtain more rewards, that is to work to obtain stimuli that will increase their fitness. Correspondingly, animals must be built to make responses that will enable them to escape from, or avoid when learning mechanisms are introduced, stimuli that will reduce their fitness. There are likely to be many dimensions of environmental stimuli along which responses of the animal can alter fitness. Each of these dimensions may be a separate reward–punishment dimension. An example of one of these dimensions might be food reward. It increases fitness to be able to sense nutrient need, to have sensors that respond to the taste of food, and to perform behavioural responses to obtain such reward stimuli when in that need or motivational state. Similarly, another dimension is water reward, in which the taste of water becomes rewarding when there is body-fluid depletion (see B. Rolls and Rolls 1982).

One aspect of the operation of these reward/punishment systems that these examples illustrate is that with very many reward/punishment dimensions for which actions may be performed, there is a need for a selection mechanism for actions performed to these different dimensions. In this sense, rewards and punishers provide a *common currency* which provides one set of inputs to response selection mechanisms. Evolution must set the magnitudes of each of the different reward systems so that each will be chosen for action in such a way as to maximize overall fitness. Food reward must be chosen as the aim for action if some nutrient depletion is present, but water reward as a target for action must be selected if current water depletion poses a greater threat to fitness than does the current degree of food depletion. This indicates that for a competitive selection process for rewards, each reward must be carefully calibrated in evolution to have the right common currency in the selection process. Other types of behaviour, such as sexual behaviour, must be selected sometimes, but probably less frequently, in order to maximize fitness (as measured by gene transmission into the next generation). There are many processes which contribute to increasing the chances that a wide set of different environmental rewards will be chosen over a period of time, including not only need-related satiety mechanisms which reduce the rewards within a dimension, but also sensory-specific satiety mechanisms, which facilitate switching to another reward stimulus (sometimes within and sometimes outside the same main dimension), and attraction to novel stimuli. (As noted in Section 4.4.4, attraction to novel stimuli, i.e. finding them rewarding, is one way that organisms are encouraged to explore the multidimensional space within which their genes are operating. The suggestion is that animals should be built to find somewhat novel stimuli rewarding, for this encourages then to explore new parts of the environment in which their genes might do better than others' genes. Unless animals are built to find novelty somewhat rewarding, the multidimensional genetic space being explored by genes in the course of evolution might not find the appropriate environment in which they might do better than others' genes.)

10.2.1.3 Stimulus–response learning reinforced by rewards and punishers

In this second level of complexity, involving reward or punishment, learning may occur. If an organism performs trial-and-error responses, and as the result of performing one particular response is more likely to obtain a reward, then the response may become linked by a learning process to that stimulus as a result of the reward received. The reward is said to reinforce the response to that stimulus, and we have what is described as stimulus–response or habit learning. The reward acts as a positive reinforcer in that it increases the probability of a response on which it is made contingent. A punisher acts as a negative reinforcer in that it reduces the probability of a response on which it is made contingent. (It should be noted that this is an operational definition, and that there is no implication that the punishment feels like anything—it just has in the learning mechanism to reduce the probability of responses followed by the punisher.) This type of stimulus–response, S–R, or habit learning was extensively studied in the 1930s and 1940s by such scientists as Hull and Spence, and later by Skinner—see Mackintosh 1974; Dickinson 1980; Pearce 1996).

10.2.2 Stimulus–reinforcement association learning, and two–factor learning theory

Two-process learning, introduced in Section 3.1.5 (see also J. Gray 1975), introduces a third level of complexity and capability into the ways in which behaviour can be guided. Rewards and punishers still provide the basis for guiding behaviour within a dimension, and for selecting the dimension towards which action should be directed. The first stage of the learning is stimulus–reinforcement association learning, in which the reinforcement value of a previously neutral, e.g. visual or auditory, stimulus is learned because of its association with a primary reinforcer, such as a sweet taste or a painful touch. This learning is similar to classical conditioning. This stimulus–reinforcer learning can be very fast, in as little as one trial. For example, if a new visual stimulus is placed in the mouth and a sweet taste is obtained, a simple approach response such as reaching for the object will be made on the next trial. Moreover, this stimulus–reinforcement association learning can be reversed very rapidly. For example, if subsequently the object is made to taste of salt, then approach no longer occurs to the stimulus, and the stimulus is even likely to be actively pushed away. The second process or stage in this type of learning is instrumental learning of an operant response made in order to obtain the stimulus now associated with reward (or avoid a stimulus associated by learning with punishment). This stage may be much slower, for it may involve trial-and-error learning of which response is successful in enabling the animal to obtain the stimulus now associated with reward or avoid the stimulus now associated with punishment. However, this second stage may be greatly speeded if an operant response or strategy that has been learned previously to obtain a different type of reward (or avoid a different punishment) can be used to obtain (or avoid) the new stimulus now known to be associated with reinforcement. It is in this flexibility of the response that two-factor learning has a great advantage over stimulus–response learning. The advantage is that any response (even, at its simplest, approach or with-drawal) can be performed once an association has been learned between a stimulus and a primary reinforcer. This flexibility in the response is much more adaptive (and could provide the difference between survival or not) than no learning, as in taxes, or stimulus–response learning.

Another key advantage of this type of two-stage learning is that after the first stage the different rewards and punishers available in an environment can be compared in a selection mechanism, using the common currency of rewards and punishers for the comparison and selection process. In this type of system, the many dimensions of reward and punishment are again the basis on which the selection of a behaviour to perform is made.

Part of the process of evolution can be seen as identifying the factors or dimensions which affect the fitness of an animal, and providing the animal with sensors which lead to rewards and punishers that are tuned to the environmental dimensions that influence fitness. The example of sweet taste receptors being set up by evolution to provide reward when physiological nutrient need is present has been given above.

We can ask whether there would need to be a separate sensing mechanism tuned to provide primary (unlearned) reinforcement for every dimension of the environment to which it may be important to direct behaviour. (The behaviour has to be directed to climb up the reward gradient to obtain the best reward, or to climb a gradient up and away from punishment.) It appears that there may not be. For example, in the case of the so-called specific appetites, for perhaps a particular vitamin lacking in the diet, it appears that a type of stimulus–reinforcement association learning may actually be involved, rather than having every possible flavour set up to be a primary reward or punisher. The way this happens is by a form of association learning. If an animal deficient in one nutrient is fed a food with that nutrient, it turns out that the animal 'feels better' some time after ingesting the new food, and associates this 'feeling better' with the taste of that particular food. Later, that food will be chosen. The point here is that the first time the animal is in the deficient state and tastes the new food, that food may not be chosen instead of other foods. It is only after the post-ingestive conditioning that, later, that particular food will be selected (Rozin and Kalat 1971). Thus in addition to a number of specific primary (unlearned) reward systems (e.g. sweet taste for nutrient need, salt taste for salt deficiency, pain for potentially damaging somatosensory stimulation), there may be great opportunity for other arbitrary sensory stimuli to become rewarding or punishing by association with some quite general change in physiological state. Another example to clarify this might be the way in which a build-up of carbon dioxide is aversive. If we are swimming deep, we may need to come to the surface in order to expel carbon dioxide (and obtain oxygen), and we may indeed find it very rewarding to obtain the fresh air. Does this mean that we have a specific reward/punishment system for carbon dioxide? It may be that too much carbon dioxide has been conditioned to be a negative reinforcer or punisher, because we feel so much better after we have breathed out the carbon dioxide. Another example might be social reinforcers. It would be difficult to build in a primary reinforcement system for every possible type of social reinforcer. Instead, there may be a number of rather general primary social reinforcers, such as acceptance within a group, approbation, greeting, face expression, and pleasant touch which are among the primary rewards by association with which other stimuli become secondary social reinforcers.

To help specify the way in which stimulus-reinforcement association learning operates, a list of what may be in at least some species primary reinforcers follows (in Table 10.1). The reader will doubtless be able to add to this list, and it may be that some of the reinforcers in the following list are actually secondary reinforcers. The reinforcers are categorized where possible by modality, to help the list to be systematic. Possible dimensions to which each reinforcer is tuned are suggested.

10.2.3 Explicit systems, language, and reinforcement

A fourth level of complexity to the way in which behaviour is guided is by processing that includes syntactic operations on semantically grounded symbols (see Section 9.2). This allows multistep one-off plans to be formulated. Such a plan might be: if I do this, then B is likely to do this, C will probably do this, and then X will be the outcome. Such a process cannot be performed by an animal that works just to obtain a reward, or secondary reinforcers. *The process may enable an available reward to be deferred for another reward that a particular multistep strategy could lead to.* What is the role of reward and punishment in such a system?

The language system can still be considered to operate to obtain rewards and avoid punishers. This is not merely a matter of definition, for many of the rewards and punishments will be the same as those described above, those which have been tuned by evolution to the dimensions of the environment that can enable an animal to increase fitness. The processing afforded by language can be seen as providing a new type of strategy to obtain such rewards or avoid such punishers. If this were not the case, then the use of the language system would not be adaptive: it would not increase fitness.

However, once a language system has evolved, a consequence may be that certain new types of reward become possible. These may be related to primary reinforcers already present, but may develop beyond them. For example, music may have evolved from the system of non-verbal communication that enables emotional states to be communicated to others. An example might be that lullabies could be related to emotional messages that can be sent from parents to offspring to soothe them. Music with a more military character might be related to the sounds given as social signals to each other in situations in which fighting (or co-operation in fighting) might occur. Then on top of this, the intellectualization afforded by linguistic (syntactic) processing would contribute further aspects to music. A point here is that solving problems by intellectual means should itself be a primary reinforcer as a result of evolution, for this would encourage the use of intellectual abilities which have potential advantage if used.

10.2.4 Special purpose design by an external agent vs evolution by natural selection

The above mechanisms, which operate in an evolutionary context to enable animals' behaviour to be tuned to increase fitness by evolving reward/punishment systems tuned to dimensions in the environment which increase fitness, may be contrasted with typical engineering design. In the latter, we may want to design a robot to work on an assembly line. Here there is an external designer, the engineer, who defines the function to be performed by the robot (e.g. picking a nut from a box, and attaching it to a particular bolt in the object being assembled). The engineer then produces special-purpose design features which enable the robot to perform this task, by for example providing it with sensors and an arm to enable it to select a nut, and to place the nut in the correct position in the 3D space of the object to enable the nut to be placed on the bolt and tightened. This contrast with a real animal allows us to see important differences between these types of control for the behaviour of the system. In the case of the animal, there is a multidimensional space within which many optimizations to increase fitness must be performed. The solution to this is to evolve reward/punishment systems to be tuned to each dimension in the environment which can lead to an increased fitness if the animal performs the appropriate actions. Natural selection guides evolution to find these dimensions. In contrast, in the robot arm, there is an externally defined behaviour to be performed, of placing the nut on the bolt, and the robot does not need to tune itself to find the goal to be performed. The contrast is between design by evolution which is 'blind' to the purpose of the animal, and design by a designer who specifies the job to be performed (cf. R. Dawkins 1986). Another contrast is that for the animal the space will be high-dimensional, so that selection of the most appropriate reward for current behaviour (taking into account the costs of obtaining each reward) is needed, whereas for the robot arm, the function to perform at any one time is specified by the designer. Another contrast is that the behaviour, that is the operant response, that is most appropriate to obtain the reward must be selected by the animal, whereas the movement to be made by the robot arm is specified by the design engineer.

The implication of this comparison is that operation by animals using reward and punishment systems tuned to dimensions of the environment that increase fitness provides a mode of operation which can work in organisms that evolve by natural selection. It is clearly a natural outcome of Darwinian evolution to operate using reward and punishment systems tuned to fitness-related dimensions of the environment, if arbitrary responses are to be made by the animals, rather than just preprogrammed movements such as are

Table 10.1
Some primary reinforcers, and the dimensions of the environment to which they are tuned

Taste	
Salt taste	+ reinforcer in salt deficiency
Sweet	+ reinforcer in energy deficiency
Bitter	− reinforcer, indicator of possible poison
Sour	− reinforcer
Umami	+ reinforcer, indicator of protein; produced by monosodium glutamate and inosine monophosphate; see Rolls et al. 1996b
Tannic acid	− reinforcer, it prevents absorption of protein; found in old leaves; probably somatosensory rather than strictly gustatory; see Critchley and Rolls 1996c

Odour	
Putrefying odour	− reinforcer; hazard to health
Pheromones	+ reinforcer (depending on hormonal state)

Somatosensory	
Pain	− reinforcer
Touch	+ reinforcer
Grooming	+ reinforcer; to give grooming may also be a primary reinforcer
Washing	+ reinforcer
Temperature	+ reinforcer if tends to help maintain normal body temperature; otherwise −

Visual	
Snakes, etc.	− reinforcer for, e.g., primates
Youthfulness	+ reinforcer, associated with mate choice
Beauty	+ reinforcer
Secondary sexual characteristics	+ reinforcers
Face expression	+ (e.g. smile) and −(e.g. threat) reinforcer
Blue sky, cover, open space	+ reinforcer, indicator of safety
Flowers	+ reinforcer (indicator of fruit later in the season?)

Auditory	
Warning call	− reinforcer
Aggressive vocalization	− reinforcer
Soothing vocalization	+ reinforcer (part of the evolutionary history of music, which at least in its origins taps into the channels used for the communication of emotions)

Table 10.1—*continued*

Reproduction

courtship	+ reinforcer
sexual behaviour	+ reinforcer (a number of different reinforcers, including a low waist-to-hip ratio, and attractiveness influenced by symmetry and being found attractive by members of the other sex, are discussed in Chapter 8)
mate guarding	+ reinforcer for a male to protect his parental investment; jealousy results if his mate is courted by another male, because this may ruin his parental investment
nest building	+ reinforcer (when expecting young)
parental attachment	+ reinforcer
infant attachment to parents	+ reinforcer
crying of infant	− reinforcer to parents; produced to promote successful development

Other

Novel stimuli	+ reinforcers (encourage animals to investigate the full possibilities of the multidimensional space in which their genes are operating)
Sleep	+ reinforcer; minimizes nutritional requirements and protects from danger
Altruism to genetically related individuals (kin altruism)	+ reinforcer
Altruism to other individuals (reciprocal altruism)	+ reinforcer while the altruism is reciprocated in a 'tit-for-tat' reciprocation; − reinforcer when the altruism is not reciprocated
Group acceptance	+ reinforcer (social greeting might indicate this)
Control over actions	+ reinforcer
Play	+ reinforcer
Danger, stimulation, excitement	+ reinforcer if not too extreme (adaptive because practice?)
Exercise	+ reinforcer (keeps the body fit for action)
Mind reading	+ reinforcer; practice in reading others' minds, which might be adaptive
Solving an intellectual problem	+ reinforcer (practice in which might be adaptive)
Storing, collecting	+ reinforcer (e.g. food)
Habitat preference, home, territory	+ reinforcer
Some responses	+ reinforcer (e.g. pecking in chickens, pigeons; adaptive because it is a simple way in which eating grain can be programmed for a relatively fixed type of environmental stimulus)
Breathing	+ reinforcer

involved in tropisms and taxes. Is there any alternative to such a reward/punishment-based system in this evolution by natural selection situation? I am not clear that there is. This may be the reason why we are built to work for rewards, avoid punishers, have emotions, and feel needs (motivational states). These concepts start to bear on developments in the field of artificial life (see, e.g., Balkenius 1995; Boden 1996).

The sort of question that some philosophers might ponder is whether if life evolved on Mars it would have emotions. My answer to this is 'Yes', if the organisms have evolved genetically by natural selection, and the genes have elaborated behavioural mechanisms to maximize their fitness in a flexible way, which as I have just argued would imply that they have evolved reward and punishment systems which guide behaviour. They would have emotions in the sense introduced in Chapter 3, in that they would have states that would be produced by rewards or punishers, or by stimuli associated with rewards and punishers. It is of course a rather larger question to ask whether our extraterrestrial organisms would have emotional feelings. My answer to this arises out of the theory of consciousness introduced in Chapter 9, and would be 'Only if the organisms have a linguistic system that can think about and correct their first order linguistic thoughts'. However, even if such higher-order thought processes are present, it is worth considering whether emotional feelings might not be present. After all, we know that much behaviour can be guided unconsciously, implicitly, by rewards and punishments. My answer to this issue is that the organisms would have emotional feelings; for as suggested above, the explicit system has to work in general for rewards of the type that are rewarding to the implicit system, and for the explicit system to be guided towards solutions that increase fitness, it should feel good when the explicit system works to a correct solution. Otherwise, it is difficult to explain how the explicit system is guided towards solutions that are not only solutions to problems, but that are also solutions that tend to have adaptive value. If the system has evolved so that it feels like something when it is performing higher-order thought processing, then it seems likely that it would feel like something when it obtained a reward or punishment, for this is the way that the explicit, conscious, thoughts would be guided.

10.3   Selection of behaviour: cost–benefit 'analysis'

One advantage of a design based on reward and punishment is that the decoding of stimuli to a reward or punishment value provides a common currency for the mechanism that selects which behavioural action should be performed. Thus, for example, a moderately sweet taste when little hunger is present would have a smaller reward value than the taste of water when thirst is present. An action-selection mechanism could thus include in its specification competition between the different rewards, all represented in a common currency, with the most rewarding stimulus being that most likely to be selected for action. As described above, to make sure that different types of reward are selected when appropriate, natural selection would need to ensure that different types of reward would operate on similar scales (from minimum to maximum), so that each type of reward would be selected if it reaches a high value on its scale. Mechanisms such as sensory-specific satiety can be seen as contributing usefully to this mechanism which ensures that different types of reward will be selected for action.

However, the action selection mechanisms must take into account not only the relative value of each type of reward, but also the cost of obtaining each type of reward. If there is a very high cost of obtaining a particular reward, it may be better, at least temporarily, until the situation changes, to select an action which leads to a smaller reward, but is less costly. It appears that animals do operate according to such a cost–benefit analysis, in that if there is a high cost for an action, that action is less likely to be performed. One example of this comes from the fighting of deer. A male deer is less likely to fight another if he is clearly inferior in size or signalled prowess (M. Dawkins 1995). There may also be a cost to switching behaviour. If the sources of food and water are very distant, it would be costly to switch behaviour (and perhaps walk a mile) every time a mouthful of food or a mouthful of water was swallowed. This may be part of the adaptive value of incentive motivation or the 'salted peanut' phenomenon—that after one reward is given early on in working for that reward the incentive value of that reward may increase. This may be expressed in the gradually increasing rate of working for food early on in a meal. By increasing the reward value of a stimulus for the first minute or two of working for it, hysteresis may be built into the behaviour selection mechanism, to make behaviour 'stick' to one reward for at least a short time once it is started.

When one refers to a 'cost–benefit analysis', one does not necessarily mean at all that the animal thinks about it and plans with 'if ... then' multistep linguistic processing the benefits and costs of each possible course of action. Instead, in many cases 'cost–benefit analysis' is likely to be built into animals to be performed with simple implicit processing or rules. One example would be the incentive motivation just described, which provides a mechanism for an animal to persist for at least a short time in one behaviour without having to explicitly plan to do this by performing as an individual a cost–benefit analysis of the relative advantage and cost of continuing or switching. Another example might be the way in which the decision to fight is made by male deer: the decision may be based on simple processes such as reducing the probability of fighting if the other individual is larger, rather than thinking through the consequences of fighting or not on this occasion. Thus, many of the costs and benefits or rewards that are taken into account in the action selection process may in many animals operate according to simply evaluated rewards and costs built in by natural selection during evolution (Krebs and Kacelnik 1991; M. Dawkins 1995). Animals may take into account, for example, quite complex information, such as the mean and variance of the rewards available from different sources, in making their selection of behaviour, yet the actual selection may then be based on quite simple rules of thumb, such as, 'if resources are very low, choose a reliable source of reward'. It may only be in some animals, for example humans, that explicit, linguistically based multistep cost–benefit analysis can be performed. It is important when interpreting animal behaviour to bear these arguments in mind, and to be aware that quite complex behaviour can result from very simple mechanisms. It is important not to over-interpret the factors that underlie any particular example of behaviour.

Reward and punishment signals provide a common currency for different sensory inputs, and can be seen as important in the selection of which actions are performed. Evolution ensures that the different reward and punishment signals are made potent to the extent that each will be chosen when appropriate. For example, food will be rewarding when hungry, but as hunger falls, the current level of thirst may soon become sufficient to make the reward produced by the taste of water greater than that produced by food, so that water is ingested. If however a painful input occurs or is signalled at any time during the feeding or drinking, this may be a stronger signal in the common currency, so that behaviour switches to that appropriate to reduce or avoid the pain. After the painful stimulus or threat is removed, the next most rewarding stimulus in the common currency might be the taste of water, and drinking would therefore be selected. The way in which a part of the brain such as the striatum and rest of the basal ganglia may contribute to the selection of behaviour by implementing competition between the different rewards and punishers available, all expressed in a common currency, is described by Rolls and Treves (1998, Chapter 9).

Many of the rewards for behaviour consist of stimuli, or remembered stimuli. Examples of some primary reinforcers are included in Table 10.1. However, for some animals, evolution has built-in a reward value for certain types of response. For example, it may be reinforcing to a pigeon or chicken to peck. The adaptive value of this is that for these animals, simply pecking at their environment may lead to the discovery of rewards. Another example might be exercise, which may have been selected to be rewarding in evolution because it keeps the body physically fit, which could be adaptive. While for some animals making certain responses may thus act as primary reinforcers (see Glickman and Shiff 1967), this is likely to be adaptive only if animals operate in limited environmental niches. If one is built to find pecking very rewarding, this may imply that other types of response are less able to be made, and this tends to restrict the animal to an environmental niche. In general, animals with a wide range of behavioural responses and strategies available, such as primates, are able to operate in a wider range of environments, are in this sense more general-purpose, are less likely to find that particular responses are rewarding per se, and are more likely to be able to select behaviour based on which of a wide range of stimuli is most rewarding, rather than based on which response-type they are pre-adapted to select.

The overall aim of the cost–benefit analysis in animals is to maximize fitness. By fitness we mean the probability that an animal's genes will be passed on into the next generation. To maximize this, there may be many ways in which different stimuli have been selected during evolution to be rewards and punishments (and among punishments we could include costs). All these rewards and punishers should operate together to ensure that over the lifetime of the animal there is a high probability of passing on genes to the next generation; but in doing this, and maximizing fitness in a complex and changing environment, all these rewards and punishments may be expected to lead to a wide variety of behaviour.

Once language enables rewards and punishments to be intellectualized, so that, for example, solving complex problems in language, mathematics, or music becomes rewarding, behaviour might be less obviously seen as adapted for fitness. However, it was suggested above that the ability to solve complex problems may be one way in which fitness, especially in a changing environment, can be maximized. Thus we should not be surprised that working at the level of ideas, to increase understanding, should in itself be rewarding. These circumstances, that humans have developed language and other complex intellectual abilities, and that natural selection in evolution has led problem-solving to be rewarding, may lead to the very rapid evolution of ideas.

10.4   Content and meaning in representations: How are representations grounded in the world?

It is possible to show that the firing of populations of neurons encodes information about stimuli in the world (see Rolls and Treves 1998). For example, from the firing rates of small numbers of neurons in the primate inferior temporal visual cortex, it is possible to know which of 20 faces has been shown to the monkey (Abbott, Rolls and Tovee 1996; Rolls, Treves and Tovee 1997c). Similarly, a population of neurons in the anterior part of the macaque temporal lobe visual cortex has been discovered that has a view-invariant representation of objects (Booth and Rolls 1998). From the firing of a small ensemble of neurons in the olfactory part of the orbitofrontal cortex, it is possible to know which of eight odours was presented (Rolls, Critchley and Treves 1996c). From the firing of small ensembles of neurons in the hippocampus, it is possible to know where in allocentric space a monkey is looking (Rolls, Treves, Robertson, Georges-François and Panzeri 1998b). In each of these cases, the number of stimuli that is encoded increases exponentially with the number of neurons in the ensemble, so this is a very powerful representation (Rolls and Treves 1998). What is being measured in each example is the mutual information between the firing of an ensemble of neurons and which stimuli are present in the world. In this sense, one can read off the code that is being used at the end of each of these sensory systems. However, what sense does the representation make to the animal? What does the firing of each ensemble of neurons 'mean'? What is the content of the representation? In the visual system, for example, it is suggested that the representation is built by a series of appropriately connected competitive networks, operating with a modified Hebb-learning rule (Rolls 1992a, 1994d; Wallis and Rolls 1997; Rolls and Treves 1998). Now competitive networks categorize their inputs without the use of a teacher. So which neurons fire to represent a particular object or stimulus is arbitrary. What meaning, therefore, does the particular ensemble that fires to an object have? How is the representation grounded in the real world? The fact that there is mutual information (see Rolls and Treves 1998, Appendix 2) between the firing of the ensemble of cells in the brain and a stimulus or event in the world does not answer this question.

One answer to this question is that there may be meaning in the case of objects and faces that it is an object or face, and not just a particular view. This is the case in that the representation may be activated by any view of the object or face. This is a step, suggested to be made possible by a short-term memory in the learning rule which enables different views of objects to be associated together (see Rolls and Treves 1998). But it still does not provide the representation with any meaning in terms of the real world. What actions might one make, or what emotions might one feel, if that arbitrary set of temporal cortex visual cells was activated?

This leads to one of the answers I propose. I suggest that one type of meaning of representations in the brain is provided by their reward (or punishment) value—activation of these representations is the goal of actions. In the case of primary reinforcers such as the taste of food or pain, the activation of these representations would have meaning in the sense that the animal would work to obtain the activation of the taste of food cells when hungry, and to escape from stimuli that cause the cells representing pain to be activated. Evolution has built the brain in such a way that the animal will work to produce activation of the taste of food reward cells when hungry, and to escape from situations which cause the activation of the cells that respond to pain. In the case of other ensembles of cells in, for example, the visual cortex which respond to objects with the colour and shape of a banana, and which 'represent' the sight of a banana in that their activation is always and uniquely produced by the sight of a banana, such representations come to have meaning only by association with a primary reinforcer, involving the process of stimulus–reinforcement association learning.

The second sense in which a representation may be said to have meaning is by virtue of sensory-motor correspondences in the world. For example, the touch of a solid object such as a table might become associated with evidence from the motor system that attempts to walk through the table result in cessation of movement. The representation of the table in the inferior temporal visual cortex might have 'meaning' only in the sense that there is mutual information between the representation and the sight of the table until the table is seen just before and while it is touched, when sensory–sensory association between inputs from different sensory modalities will be set up that will enable the visual representation to become associated with its correspondences in the touch and movement worlds. In this second sense, meaning will be conferred on the visual sensory representation because of its associations in the sensory–motor world. Thus it is suggested that there are two ways by which sensory representations can be said to be grounded, that is to have meaning, in the real world.

It is suggested that the symbols used in language become grounded in the real world by the same two processes. In the first, a symbol such as the word 'banana' has meaning because it is associated with primary reinforcers such as the flavour of the banana and with secondary reinforcers such as the sight of the banana. In the second process, the word 'table' may have meaning because it is associated with sensory stimuli produced by tables such as their touch, shape, and sight, as well as other functional properties, such as, for example, being load-bearing (see p. 250).

10.5 An afterthought: what is the sociobiological background to moral issues?

There are many reasons why people have particular moral beliefs, and believe that it is good to act in particular ways. It is possible that biology can help to explain why certain types of behaviour are adopted perhaps implicitly by humans, and become incorporated for consistency into explicit rules for conduct. This approach does not, of course, replace other approaches to what is moral, but it may help in implementing moral beliefs held for other reasons to have some insight into some of the directions that the biological underpinnings of human behaviour might lead. Humans may be better able to decide explicitly what to do when they have knowledge and insight into the biological underpinnings. It is in this framework that the following points are made, with no attempt made to lead towards any suggestions about what is 'right' or 'wrong'. The arguments that follow are based on the hypothesis that there are biological underpinnings based on the types of reward and punishment systems that have been built into our genes during evolution for at least some of the types of behaviour held to be moral.

One type of such biological underpinning is kin selection. This would tend to produce supportive behaviour towards individuals likely to be related, especially towards children, grandchildren, siblings etc., depending on how closely they are genetically related. This does tend to occur in human societies, and is part of what is regarded as 'right', and indeed it is a valued 'right' to be able to pass on goods, possessions, wealth, etc., to children. The underlying basis here would be genes for kin altruism[1]. Another such underpinning might be the fact that many animals, and especially primates, co-operate with others in order to achieve ends which turn out to be on average to their advantage, including genetic advantage. One example includes the coalitions formed by groups of males in order to obtain a female for one of the groups, followed by reciprocation of the good turn later (see Ridley 1996). This is an example of reciprocal altruism, in this case by groups of primates, which is to the advantage of both groups or individuals provided that neither individual or group cheats, in which case the rules for social interaction must change to keep the strategy stable. Another such underpinning, in this case for property 'rights', might be the territory guarding behaviour which is so common from fish to primates. Another such underpinning might be the jealousy and guarding of a partner shown by males who invest parental care in their partner's offspring. This occurs in many species of birds, and also in humans, with both exemplars showing male paternal invest-ment because of the immaturity of the children (due to their brain size). This might be a biological underpinning to the 'right' to fidelity in a female partner. The suggestion I make is that in all these cases, and in many others, there are biological underpinnings that determine what we find rewarding or punishing, designed into genes by evolution to lead to appropriate behaviour which helps to increase the fitness of the genes. When these implicit systems for rewards and punishers start to be expressed explicitly (in language) in humans, the explicit rules, rights, and laws which are formalized are those which set out in language what the biological underpinnings 'want' to occur. Clearly in formulating the explicit rights and laws, some compromise is necessary in order to keep the society stable. When the rights and laws are formulated in small societies, it is likely that individuals in that society will have many of the same genes, and rules such as help your neighbour (but make war with 'foreigners') will probably be to the advantage of one's genes. However, when the society increases in size beyond a small village (in the order of 1000), then the explicitly formalized rules, rights, and laws may no longer produce behaviour that turns out to be to the advantage of an individual's genes. In addition, it may no longer be possible to keep track of individuals in order to maintain the stability of 'tit-for-tat' co-operative social strategies (Dunbar 1996; Ridley 1996)[2]. In such cases, other factors doubtless come into play to additionally influence what groups hold to be right. For

---

[1] Kin selection genes spread because of kin altruism. Such genes direct their bodies to aid relatives because those relatives have a high chance of having the same relative-helping gene. This is a specific mechanism, and it happens to be incorrect to think that genes direct their bodies to aid relatives because those bodies 'share genes' in general (see Hamilton 1964; M. Dawkins 1995, chapter on inclusive fitness).

[2] A limit on the size of the group for reciprocal altruism might be set by the ability both to have direct evidence for and remember person–reinforcer associations for large numbers of different individual people. In this situation, reputation passed on verbally from others who have the direct experience of whether an individual can be trusted to reciprocate might be a factor in the adaptive value of language and gossip (Dunbar 1996).

example, a group of subjects in a society might demand the 'right' to free speech because it is to their economic advantage.

Thus overall it is suggested that many aspects of what a society holds as right and moral, and of what becomes enshrined in explicit 'rights' and laws, are related to biological underpinnings, which have usually evolved because of the advantage to the individual's genes, but that as societies develop other factors also start to influence what is believed to be 'right' by groups of individuals, related to socioeconomic factors. In both cases, the laws and rules of the society develop so that these 'rights' are protected, but often involving compromise in such a way that a large proportion of the society will agree to, or can be made subject to, what is held as right. To conclude this discussion, we note that what is natural does not necessarily imply what is 'right' (the naturalistic fallacy, pointed out by G. E. Moore) (see, e.g., Singer 1981). However, our notions of what we think of as right may be related to biological underpinnings, and the point of this discussion is that it can only give helpful insight into human behaviour to realize this.

Other ways in which a biological approach, based on what our brains have evolved to treat as rewarding or punishing, can illuminate moral issues, and rights, follow.

'Pain is a worse state than no pain.' This is a statement held as true by some moral philosophers, and is said to hold with no reference to biological underpinnings. It is a self-evident truth, and certain implications for behaviour may follow from the proposition. A biological approach to pain is that the elicitation of pain has to be punishing (in the sense that animals will work to escape or avoid it), as pain is the state elicited by stimuli signalling a dimension of environmental conditions which reduces survival and fitness.

'Incest is morally wrong. One should not marry a brother or sister. One should not have intercourse with any close relation.' The biological underpinning is that children of close relations have an increased chance of having double-recessive genes, which are sometimes harmful to the individual and reduce fitness. In addition, breeding out may produce hybrid vigour. It is presumably for this reason that many animals as well as humans have behavioural strategies (produced by the properties of reward systems) that reduce inbreeding. At the same time, it may be adaptive (for genes) to pair with another animal that has many of the same genes, for this may help complex gene sequences to be passed intact into the next generation. This may underlie the fact that quails have mechanisms which enable them to recognize their cousins, and make them appear attractive, an example of kin selection. In humans, if one were part of a strong society (in which one's genes would have a good chance not to be eliminated by other societies), then it could be advantageous (whether male or female) to invest resources with someone else who would provide maximum genetic and resource potential for one's children, which on average across a society of relatively small size and not too mobile would be a person with relatively similar genes and resources (wealth, status etc.) to oneself. In an exception to this, in certain societies there has been a tradition of marrying close relations (e.g. the Pharaohs of Egypt), and part of the reason for this could be maintaining financial and other resources within the (genetic) family.

There may be several reasons why particular behavioural conduct may be selected. A first is that the conduct may be good for the individual and for the genes of the individual, at least on average. An example might be a prohibition on killing others in the same society (while at the same time defending that kin group in times of war). The advantage here could be one's own genes, which would be less at risk in a society without large numbers of killings. A second reason is that particular codes of conduct might effectively help one's genes by making society stable. An example here might be a prohibition on theft, which would serve to protect property. A third reason is that the code of conduct might actually be to other, powerful, individuals' advantage, and might have been made for that reason into a rule that others in society are persuaded to follow. A general rule in society might be that honesty is a virtue, but the rule might be given a special interpretation or ignored by members of society too powerful to challenge.

As discussed in Chapter 8, different aspects of behaviour could have different importance for males and females. This could lead men and women to put different stress on different rules of society, because they have different importance for men and women. One example might be being unfaithful. Because this could be advantageous to men's genes, this may be treated by men as a less serious error of conduct than by women. However, within men there could be differential condemnation, with men predisposed to being faithful being more concerned about infidelity in other men, because it is a potential threat to them. In the same way, powerful men who can afford to have liaisons with many women may be less concerned about infidelity than less powerful men, whose main genetic investment may be with one woman.

Society may set down certain propositions of what is 'right'. One reason for this is that it may be too difficult on every occasion, and for everyone, to work out explicitly what all the payoffs of each rule of conduct are. A second reason is that what is promulgated as 'right' could actually be to someone else's advantage, and it would not be wise to expose this fully. One way to convince members of society not to do what is apparently in their immediate interest is to promise a reward later. Such deferred rewards are often offered by religions. The ability to work for a deferred reward using a one-off plan in this way becomes possible, it was suggested in Chapter 9, with the evolution of the explicit, propositional, system.

The overall view that one is led to is that some of our moral beliefs may be an explicit, verbal formulation of what may reflect factors built genetically by kin selection into behaviour, namely a tendency to favour kin, because they are likely to share some of an individual's genes. In a small society this explicit formulation may be 'appropriate' (from the point of view of the genes), in that many members of that society will be related to that individual. When the society becomes larger, the relatedness may decrease, yet the explicit formulation of the rules or laws of society may not change. In such a situation, it is presumably appropriate for society to make it clear to its members that its rules for what is acceptable and 'right' behaviour are set in place so that individuals can live in safety, and with some expectation of help from society in general. Other factors that can influence what is held to be right might reflect socioeconomic advantage to groups or alliances of individuals. It would be then in a sense up to individuals to decide whether they wished to accept the rules, with the costs and benefits provided by the rules of that society, in a form of social contract. Individuals who did not agree to the social contract might wish to transfer to another society with a different place on the continuum of costs and potential benefits to the individuals, or to influence the laws and policies of their own society. Individuals who attempt to cheat the system would be expected to pay a cost in terms of punishment meted out by the society in accordance with its rules.

10.6 Emotion and literature

Those interested in literature are sometimes puzzled by the following situation, which can perhaps be clarified by the theory of emotion developed here. The puzzle is that emotions often seem very intense in humans, indeed sometimes so intense that they produce behaviour which does not seem to be adaptive, such as fainting instead of producing an active escape response, or freezing instead of avoiding, or vacillating endlessly about emotional situations and decisions, or falling hopelessly in love even when it can be predicted to be without hope or to bring ruin. The puzzle is not only that the emotion is so intense, but also that even with our rational, reasoning, capacities, humans still find themselves in these situations, and may find it difficult to produce reasonable and effective behaviour for resolving the situation.

The reasons for this include, I suggest, the following. In humans, the reward and punishment systems may operate implicitly in comparable ways to those in other animals. But in addition to this, humans have the explicit system, which enables us consciously to look and predict many steps ahead (using language and syntax) the consequences of environmental events, and also to reflect on previous events (see Chapter 9). The consequence of this explicit processing is that we can see the full impact of rewarding and punishing events, both looking ahead to see how this will impact us, and reflecting back to previous situations which we can see may never be repeated. For example, in humans grief occurs with the loss of a loved one, and this may be much more intense than might occur simply because of failure to receive a positively reinforcing stimulus, because we can look ahead to see that the person will never be present again, can process all the possible consequences of that, and can remember all the previous occasions with that person. In another example, someone may faint at the sight of blood, and this is more likely to occur in humans because we appreciate the full consequences of major loss of blood, which we all know is life-threatening. Thus what happens is that reinforcing events can have a very much greater reinforcing value in humans than in other animals, because we have so much cognitive, especially linguistic, processing which leads us to evaluate and appreciate many reinforcing events far more fully than can other animals. Thus humans may decode reinforcers to have supernormal intensity relative to what is usual in other animals, and the supernormal appreciated intensity of the decoded reinforcers leads to super-strong emotions. The emotional states can then be so strong that they are not necessarily adaptive, and indeed language has brought humans out of the environmental conditions under which our emotional systems evolved. For example, the autonomic responses to the sight of blood may be so strong, given that we know the consequences of loss of blood, that we faint rather than helping. Another example is that panic and anxiety states can be exacerbated by feeling the heart pounding, because we are able to use our explicit processing system to think and worry about all the possible causes. One can think of countless other examples from life, and indeed make up other examples, which of course is part of what novelists do.

A second reason for such strong emotions in humans is that the stimuli that produce emotions may be much stronger than those in which our emotional systems evolved. For example, with man-made artefacts such as cars and guns the sights which can be produced in terms of damage to humans are much more intense that those present when our emotional systems evolved. In this way, the things we see can produce super-strong emotions. Indeed, the strength and sometimes maladaptive consequences of human emotions have preoccupied literature and literary theorists for the last 2,400 years, since Aristotle.

A third reason for the intensely mobilizing, and sometimes immobilizing, effects of emotions in humans is that we can evaluate linguistically, with reasoning, the possible courses of action open to us in emotional situations. Because we can evaluate the possible effects of reinforcers many steps ahead in our plans, and because language enables us to produce flexible one-off plans for actions, and enables us to work for deferred rewards based on one-off plans (see Chapter 9), the ways in which reinforcers are used in decision-making becomes much more complex than in animals that cannot produce similar one-off plans using language. The consequence of this is that decision-making can become very difficult, with so many potential but uncertain reinforcement outcomes, that humans may vacillate. They are trying to compute by this explicit method the most favourable outcome of each plan in terms of the net reinforcements received, rather than using reinforcement implicitly to select the highest currently available reinforcer.

A fourth reason for complexity in the human emotional system is that there are, it is suggested, two routes to action for emotions in humans, an implicit (unconscious) and an explicit route (see Chapter 9). These systems may not always agree. The implicit system may tend to produce one type of behaviour, typically for immediately available rewards. The explicit system may tend to produce another planned course of action to produce better deferred rewards. Conflict between these systems can lead to many difficult situations, will involve conscience (what is right as conceived by the explicit system) and the requirement to abide by laws (which assume a rational explicit system responsible for our actions). It appears that the implicit system does often control our behaviour, as shown by the effects of frontal lobe damage in humans, which may produce deficits in reward-reversal tasks, even when the human can explicitly state the correct behaviour in the situation (see Chapters 4 and 9). The conflicts which arise between these implicit and explicit systems are again some of the very stuff on which literature often capitalizes.

A fifth reason for complexity in the human emotional system is that we, as social animals, with major investments in our children which benefit from long-term parental co-operation, and with advantages to be gained from social alliances if the partners can be trusted, may be built to try to estimate the goals and reliability of those we know. For example, it may matter to a woman with children whether her partner has been attracted by/is in love with/a different woman, as this could indicate a reduction of help and provision. Humans may thus be very interested in the emotional lives of each other, as this may impact on their own lives. Indeed, humans will, for this sort of reason, be very interested in who is co-operating with whom, and gossip about this may even have acted as a selective pressure for the evolution of language (Dunbar 1996). In these circumstances, fascination with unravelling the thoughts and emotions of others would have adaptive value, though it is difficult computationally to model the minds and interactions of groups of other people, and to keep track of who knows what about whom, as this requires many levels of nested syntactical reference. Our resulting fascination with this, and perhaps the value of experience of as wide a range of situations as possible, may then be another reason why human emotions, and guessing others' emotions in complex social situations, may also be part of the stuff of novelists, playwrights, and poets.

10.7 Coda and apostasis

Let us evaluate where we have reached in this book.

1   We have a scientific approach to emotion, its nature, and its functions (Chapter 3). It has been shown that this approach can help with classifying different emotions (Chapter 3), and in understanding *what* information processing systems in the brain are involved in emotion, and *how* they are involved (Chapter 4).

2   We have reached a quite specific view about how brains are designed around reward and punishment evaluation systems, because this is the way that genes can build a complex system that will produce appropriate but flexible behaviour to increase their fitness, as described earlier in this chapter. The way natural selection does this is to build us with reward and punishment systems that will direct our behaviour towards goals in such a way that survival and in particular fitness are achieved. By specifying goals, rather than particular behavioural patterns of responses, genes leave much more open the possible behavioural strategies that might be required to increase their fitness. Specifying particular behavioural responses would be inefficient in terms of behavioural flexibility as environments change during evolution, and also would be more genetically costly to specify (in terms of the information to be encoded and the possibility of error). This view of the evolutionarily adaptive value for genes to build organisms using reward- and punishment-decoding and action systems in the brain places one squarely in line as a scientist from Darwin. It helps us to understand much of sensory information processing in the brain, followed by reward- and punishment-evaluation, followed by behaviour-selection and -execution to obtain the goals identified by the sensory systems.

3   The importance of reward and punishment systems in brain design helps us to understand not only the significance and importance of emotion, but also of motivational behaviour, which frequently involves working to obtain goals which are specified by the current state of internal signals to achieve homeostasis (see Chapter 2 on hunger and Chapter 7 on thirst) or are influenced by internal hormonal signals (Chapter 8 on sexual behaviour).

4   We have outlined in Chapters 2 (on hunger) and 4 (on emotion) what may be the fundamental architectural and design principles of the brain for sensory, reward, and punishment information processing in primates. These architectural principles include the following:

   (a)   For potential secondary reinforcers, analysis is to the stage of invariant object identification before reward and punishment associations are learned. The reason for this is to enable correct generalization to other instances of the same or similar objects, even when a reward or punishment has been associated with one instance previously.

(b)   The representation of the object is (appropriately) in a form which is ideal as an input to pattern associators which allow the reinforcement associations to be learned. The representations are appropriately encoded in that they can be decoded by dot product decoding of the type that is very neuronally plausible, are distributed so allowing excellent generalization and graceful degradation, and have relatively independent information conveyed by different neurons in the ensemble thus allowing very high capacity, and allowing the information to be read off very quickly, in periods of 20–50 ms (see Chapter 4, the Appendix, and Rolls and Treves 1998).

(c)   An aim of processing in the ventral visual system (that projects to the inferior temporal visual cortex) is to help select the goals, or objects with reward or punishment associations, for actions. Action is concerned with the identification and selection of goals, for action, in the environment. The ventral visual system is crucially involved in this. I thus disagree with Milner and Goodale (1995) that the dorsal visual system is for the control of action, and the ventral for 'perception', e.g. perceptual and cognitive representations. The ventral visual system is concerned with selecting the goals for action. It does this by providing invariant representations of objects, with a representation which is appropriate for interfacing to systems (such as the amygdala and orbitofrontal cortex, see Chapters 4 and 6, and Figs. 4.2, 4.3 and 9.4 in which association cortex would correspond in vision to the inferior temporal visual cortex) which determine using pattern association the reward or punishment value of the object, as part of the process of selecting which goal is appropriate for action. Some of the evidence for this described in Chapter 4 is that large lesions of the temporal lobes (which damage the ventral visual system and some of its outputs such as the amygdala) produce the Kluver-Bucy syndrome, in which monkeys select objects indiscriminately, independently of their reward value, and place them in their mouths. The dorsal visual system helps with executing those actions, for example with shaping the hand appropriately to pick up a selected object. (Often this type of sensori-motor operation is performed implicitly, i.e. without conscious awareness.) In so far as explicit planning about future goals and actions requires knowledge of objects and their reward or punishment associations, it is the ventral visual system that provides the appropriate input for planning future actions. Further, for the same reason, I propose that when explicit, or conscious planning is required, activity in the ventral visual system will be closely related to consciousness, because it is about objects, represented in the ventral visual system, about which we normally plan.

(d)   For primary reinforcers, the reward decoding may occur after several stages of processing, as in the primate taste system in which reward is decoded only after the primary taste cortex. The architectural principle here is that in primates there is one main taste information-processing stream in the brain, via the thalamus to the primary taste cortex, and the information about the identity of the taste is not contaminated with modulation by how good the taste is before this so that the taste representation in the primary cortex can be used for purposes which are not reward-dependent. One example might be learning where a particular taste can be found in the environment, even when the primate is not hungry so that the taste is not pleasant. In the case of other sensory systems, the reinforcement value may be made explicit early on in sensory processing. This occurs, for example, in the pain system. The architectural basis of this is that there are different channels (nerve fibres) for pain and touch, so that the affective value and the identity of a tactile stimulus can be carried by separate parallel information channels, allowing separate representation and processing of each.

(e) In non-primates including, for example, rodents the design principles may involve less sophisticated design features, because the stimuli being processed are simpler. For example, view-invariant object recognition is probably much less developed in non-primates, with the recognition that is possible being based more on physical similarity in terms of texture, colour, simple features, etc. (see Rolls and Treves 1998, Section 8.8). It may be because there is less sophisticated cortical processing of visual stimuli in this way that other sensory systems are also organized more simply, with, for example, some (but not total, only perhaps 30%) modulation of taste processing by hunger early in sensory processing in rodents (see T. Scott and Giza 1992; T. Scott, Yan and Rolls 1995). Further, while it is appropriate usually to have emotional responses to well-processed objects (e.g. the sight of a particular person), there are instances, such as a loud noise or a pure tone associated with punishment, where it may be possible to tap off a sensory representation early in sensory information processing that can be used to produce emotional responses, and this may occur, for example, in rodents, where the subcortical auditory system provides afferents to the amygdala (see Chapter 4 on emotion).

(f) Another design principle is that the outputs of the reward and punishment systems must be treated by the action system as being the goals for action. The action systems must be built to try to maximize the activation of the representations produced by rewarding events, and to minimize the activation of the representations produced by punishers or stimuli associated with punishers. Drug addiction produced by the psychomotor stimulants such as amphetamine and cocaine can be seen as activating the brain at the stage where the outputs of the amygdala and orbitofrontal cortex, which provide representations of whether stimuli are associated with rewards or punishers, are fed in the ventral striatum as goals for the action system. The fact that addiction is persistent may be related to the fact that because the outputs of the amygdala and orbitofrontal cortex are after the stage of stimulus-reinforcer learning, the action system has to be built to interpret the representations they provide as meaning that reward actually is available.

5 Especially in primates, the visual processing in emotional and social behaviour requires sophisticated representation of individuals, and for this there are many neurons devoted to face processing. In addition, there is a separate system that encodes face gesture, movement, and view, as all are important in social behaviour, for interpreting whether a particular individual, with his or her own reinforcement associations, is producing threats or appeasements.

6 After mainly unimodal processing to the object level, sensory systems then project into convergence zones. Those especially important for reward and punishment, emotion and motivation, are the orbitofrontal cortex and amygdala, where primary reinforcers are represented. These parts of the brain appear to be especially important in emotion and motivation not only because they are the parts of the brain where

in primates the primary (unlearned) reinforcing value of stimuli is represented, but also because they are the parts of the brain that perform pattern-association learning between potential secondary reinforcers and primary reinforcers. They are thus the parts of the brain involved in learning the emotional and motivational value of stimuli.

7   The reward evaluation systems have tendencies to self-regulate, so that on average they can operate in a common currency which leads on different occasions, often depending on modulation by internal signals, for different rewards to be selected.

8   A principle that assists the selection of different behaviours is sensory-specific satiety, which builds up when a reward is repeated for a number of minutes. A principle that helps behaviour to lock on to one goal for at least a useful period is incentive motivation, the process by which early on in the presentation of a reward there is potentiation. There are probably simple neurophysiological bases for these time-dependent processes in the reward (as opposed to the early sensory) systems which involve neuronal habituation and facilitation respectively.

9   With the advances made in the last 30 years in understanding the brain mechanisms involved in reward and punishment, and emotion and motivation, the basis for addiction to drugs is becoming clearer, and it is hoped that there is a foundation for improving understanding of depression and anxiety and their pharmacological and non-pharmacological treatment, in terms of the particular brain systems that are involved in these emotional states (Chapter 6).

10 Although the architectural design principles of the brain to the stage of the representation of rewards and punishments seems apparent, it is much less clear how selection between the reward and punishment signals is made, how the costs of actions are taken into account, and how actions are selected. Some of the processes that may be involved are sketched in Chapters 4 and 6, but much remains to be understood.

11 In addition to the implicit system for action selection, in humans there is also an explicit system that can use language to compute actions to obtain deferred rewards using a one-off plan. The language system enables one-off multistep plans which require the syntactic organization of symbols to be formulated in order to obtain rewards and avoid punishments. There are thus two separate systems for producing actions to rewarding and punishing stimuli in humans. These systems may weight different courses of action differently, in that each can produce behaviour for different goals (immediate vs deferred).

12 It is possible that emotional feelings, part of the much larger problem of consciousness, arise as part of a process that involves thoughts about thoughts, which have the adaptive value of helping to correct multistep plans. This is the approach described in Chapter 9, but there seems to be no clear way to choose which theory of consciousness is moving in the right direction, and caution must be exercised here.

A la recherche à faire[3]

---

[3] To the research remaining to do (towards which I hope that this book will lead). (This contrasts with the search for time past that was the aim of Marcel Proust in his book 'A la recherche du temps perdu'.)

Appendix
Neural networks and emotion-related learning

A.1 Neurons in the brain, the representation of information, and neuronal learning mechanisms

A.1.1 Introduction

In Chapters 3 and 4, the type of learning that is very important in learned emotional responses was characterized as stimulus–reinforcement association learning. This is a particular case of pattern-association learning, in which the to-be-associated or conditioned stimulus is the potential secondary reinforcer, and the unconditioned stimulus is the primary reinforcer (see Fig. 4.6). In Chapter 4, it was indicated that many of the properties required of emotional learning (e.g. generalization and graceful degradation) arise in pattern associators if the correct type of distributed representation is present (Sections 4.3.1, 4.4). In this appendix the relevant properties of biologically plausible pattern-association memories (such as may be present in the orbitofrontal cortex and amygdala) are presented more formally, to provide a foundation for future research into the neural basis of emotional learning. A fuller analysis of these neural networks and their properties, and of other neural networks which, for example, build representations of sensory stimuli, is provided by Rolls and Treves (1998).

Before starting the description of pattern-association neuronal networks, a brief review of the evidence on synaptic plasticity, and the rules by which synaptic strength is modified, much based on studies with long-term potentiation, is provided.

After describing pattern-association neural networks, an overview of another learning algorithm, called reinforcement learning, which might be relevant to learning in systems that receive rewards and punishments and which has been supposed to be implemented using the dopamine pathways (Barto 1995; Schultz *et al.* 1995b; Houk *et al.* 1995), is provided.

A.1.2 Neurons in the brain, and their representation in neuronal networks

Neurons in the vertebrate brain typically have large dendrites, extending from the cell body, which receive inputs from other neurons through connections called synapses. The synapses operate by chemical transmission. When a synaptic terminal receives an all-or-nothing action potential from the neuron of which it is a terminal, it releases a transmitter which crosses the synaptic cleft and produces either depolarization or hyperpolarization in the postsynaptic neuron, by opening particular ion channels. (A textbook such as Kandel *et al.* 1998 gives further information on this process.) Summation of a number of such depolarization or excitatory inputs within the time constant of the receiving neuron, which is typically 20–30 ms, produces sufficient depolarization that the neuron fires an action potential. There are often 5000–20 000 inputs per neuron. An example of a neuron found in the brain is shown in Fig. A.1.1, and there are further examples in Rolls and Treves (1998), Chapter 10. Once firing is initiated in the cell body (or axon initial segment of the cell body), the action potential is conducted in an all-or-nothing way to reach the synaptic terminals of the neuron, whence it may affect other neurons. Any inputs the neuron receives which cause it to become hyperpolarized make it less likely to fire (because the membrane potential is moved away from the critical threshold at which an action potential is initiated); these are described as inhibitory. The neuron can thus be thought of in a simple way as a computational element which sums its inputs within its time-constant and, whenever this sum, minus any inhibitory effects, exceeds a threshold, produces an action potential which propagates to all of its outputs. This simple idea is incorporated in many neuronal-network models using a formalism of a type described in the next section.

A.1.3   A formalism for approaching the operation of single neurons in a network

Let us consider a neuron i as shown in Fig. A.1.2 which receives inputs from axons which we label j through synapses of strength w_{ij}. The first subscript (i) refers to the receiving neuron, and the second subscript (j) to the particular input[1]. j counts from 1 to C, where C is the number of synapses or connections received. The firing rate of the ith neuron is denoted r_i, and of the jth input to the neuron r'_j. (The prime is used to denote the input or presynaptic term. The letter r is used to indicate that the inputs and outputs of real neurons are firing rates.) To express the idea that the neuron makes a simple linear summation of the inputs it receives, we can write the activation of neuron i, denoted h_i, as

$$h_i = \sum_j r'_j w_{ij} \qquad\qquad (A.1.1)$$

where $\sum_j$ indicates that the sum is over the C input axons indexed by j. The multiplicative form here indicates that activation should be produced by an axon only if it is firing, and depending on the strength of the synapse w_{ij} from input axon j on to the dendrite of the receiving neuron i. Eqn (A.1.1) indicates that the strength of the activation reflects how fast the axon j is firing (that is r'_j), and how strong the synapse w_{ij} is. The sum of all such activations expresses the idea that summation (of synaptic currents in real neurons) occurs along the length of the dendrite, to produce activation at the cell body, where the activation h_i is converted into firing r_i. This conversion can be expressed as

$$r_i = f(h_i) \qquad\qquad (A.1.2)$$

---

[1] This convention, that i refers to the receiving neuron, and j refers to a particular input to that neuron via a synapse of weight w_{ij}, is used here except where otherwise stated.

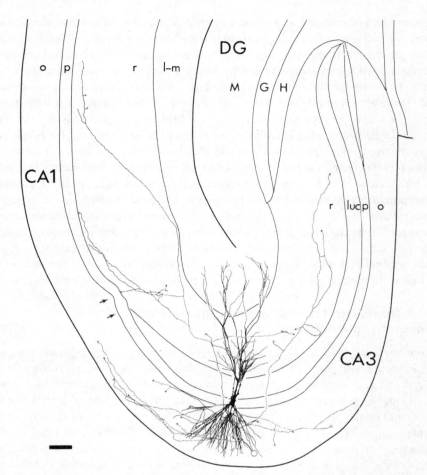

Fig. A.1.1 An example of a real neuron found in the brain. The neuron is a CA3 neuron from the hippocampus. The thick extensions from the cell body or soma are the dendrites, which form an extensive dendritic tree receiving in this case approximately 12 000 synapses. The axon is the thin connection leaving the cell. It divides into a number of collateral branches. Two axonal branches can be seen in the plane of the section to travel to each end of the population of CA3 cells. One branch (on the left) continues to connect to the next group of cells, the CA1 cells. The junction between the CA3 and CA1 cells is shown by the two arrows. The diagram shows a camera lucida drawing of a single CA3 pyramidal cell intracellularly labelled with horseradish peroxidase. DG, dentate gyrus. The small letters refer to the different strata of the hippocampus. (Reprinted with permission from Ishizuka, Weber and Amaral 1990.)

which indicates that the firing rate is a function of the postsynaptic activation. The function is called the activation function in this case. The function at its simplest could be linear, so that the firing rate would be proportional to the activation (see Fig. A.1.3a). Real neurons have thresholds, with firing occurring only if the activation is above the threshold. A threshold linear activation function is shown in Fig. A.1.3b. This has been useful in formal analysis of the properties of neural networks. Neurons also have firing rates which become saturated at a maximum rate, and we could express this as the sigmoid activation function shown in Fig. A.1.3c. Another simple activation function, used in some models of neural networks, is the binary threshold function (Fig. A.1.3d), which indicates that if the activation is below threshold, there is no firing, and that if the activation is above threshold, the neuron fires maximally. Some non-linearity in the activation function is an advantage, for it enables many useful computations to be performed in neuronal networks, including removing interfering effects of similar memories, and enabling neurons to perform logical operations, such as firing only if several inputs are present simultaneously.

A.1.4 Synaptic modification

For a neuronal network to perform useful computation, that is to produce a given output when it receives a particular input, the synaptic weights must be set up appropriately. This is often performed by synaptic modification occurring during learning.

A simple learning rule that was originally presaged by Donald Hebb (1949) proposes that synapses increase in strength when there is conjunctive presynaptic and postsynaptic activity. The Hebb rule can be expressed more formally as follows:

$$\delta w_{ij} = k r_i r_j' \qquad\qquad (A.1.3)$$

where δw_{ij} is the change of the synaptic weight w_{ij} which results from the simultaneous (or conjunctive) presence of presynaptic firing r_j' and postsynaptic firing r_i (or strong depolarization), and k is a learning rate-constant which specifies how much the synapses alter on any one pairing. The presynaptic and postsynaptic activity must be present approximately simultaneously (to within perhaps 100–500 ms in the real brain).

The Hebb rule is expressed in this multiplicative form to reflect the idea that *both* presynaptic and postsynaptic activity must be present for the synapses to increase in strength. The multiplicative form also reflects the idea that strong pre- and postsynaptic firing will produce a larger change of synaptic weight than smaller firing rates. The Hebb rule thus captures what is typically found in studies of associative long-term potentiation (LTP) in the brain, described in Section A.1.5.

One useful property of large neurons in the brain, such as cortical pyramidal cells, is that with their short electrical length, the postsynaptic term, r_i, is available on much of the dendrite of a cell. The implication of this is that once sufficient postsynaptic activation has been produced, any active presynaptic terminal on the neuron will show synaptic strengthening. This enables associations between coactive inputs, or correlated activity in input axons, to be learned by neurons using this simple associative learning rule.

A.1.5 Long-term potentiation and long-term depression as biological models of synaptic modifications that occur in the brain

Long-term potentiation (LTP) and long-term depression (LTD) provide useful models of some of the synaptic modifications that occur in the brain. The synaptic changes found appear to be synapse-specific, and to depend on information available locally at the synapse. LTP and LTD may thus provide a good model of biological synaptic modification involved in real neuronal network operations in the brain. We next, therefore, describe

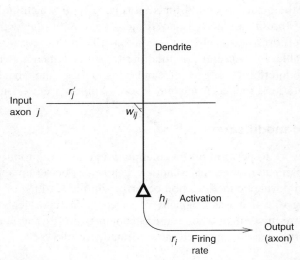

Fig. A.1.2 Notation used to describe an individual neuron in a network model. By convention, we generally represent the dendrite as thick, and vertically oriented (as this is the normal way that neuroscientists view cortical pyramidal cells under the microscope); and the axon as thin. The cell body or soma is indicated between them. The firing rate we also call the (firing rate) activity of the neuron.

some of the properties of LTP and LTD, and evidence which implicates them in learning in at least some brain systems. Even if they turn out not to be the basis for the synaptic modifications that occur during learning, they have many of the properties that would be needed by some of the synaptic-modification systems used by the brain.

Long-term potentiation (LTP) is a use-dependent and sustained increase in synaptic strength that can be induced by brief periods of synaptic stimulation. It is usually measured as a sustained increase in the amplitude of electrically evoked responses in specific neural pathways following brief trains of high-frequency stimulation (see Fig. A.1.4b). For example, high-frequency stimulation of the Schaffer collateral inputs to the hippocampal CA1 cells results in a larger response recorded from the CA1 cells to single test pulse stimulation of the pathway. LTP is *long-lasting*, in that its effect can be measured for hours in hippocampal slices, and in chronic in vivo experiments in some cases may last for months. LTP becomes evident rapidly, typically in less than 1 min. LTP is in some brain systems *associative*. This is illustrated in Fig. A.1.4c, in which a weak input to a group of cells (e.g. the commissural input to CA1) does not show LTP unless it is given at the same time as (i.e. associatively with) another input (which could be weak or strong) to the cells. The associativity arises because it is only when sufficient activation of the postsynaptic neuron to exceed the threshold of NMDA (N-methyl-D-aspartate) receptors (see below) is produced that any learning can occur. The two weak inputs summate to produce sufficient depolarization to exceed the threshold. This associative property is shown very clearly in experiments in which LTP of an input to a single cell only occurs if the cell membrane is depolarized by passing current through it at the same time as the input arrives at the cell. The depolarization alone or the input alone is not sufficient to produce the LTP, and the LTP is thus associative. Moreover, in that the presynaptic input and the postsynaptic depolarization must occur at about the same time (within approximately 500 ms), the LTP requires *temporal contiguity*. LTP is also *synapse-specific*, in that, for example, an inactive input to a cell does not show LTP even if the cell is strongly activated by other inputs (Fig. A.1.4b, input B).

These spatiotemporal properties of LTP can be understood in terms of actions of the inputs on the postsynaptic cell, which in the hippocampus has two classes of receptor, NMDA and K–Q (kainate–quisqualate), activated by the glutamate released by the presynaptic terminals. Now the NMDA-receptor channels are normally blocked by Mg^{2+}, but when the cell is strongly depolarized by strong tetanic stimulation of the type necessary to induce LTP, the Mg^{2+} block is removed, and Ca^{2+} entering via the NMDA-receptor channels triggers events that lead to the potentiated synaptic transmission (see Fig. A.1.5). Part of the evidence for this is that NMDA antagonists such as AP5 (D-2-amino-5-phosphonopentanoate) block LTP. Further, if the postsynaptic membrane is voltage-clamped to prevent depolarization by a strong input, then LTP does not occur. The voltage-dependence of the NMDA-receptor channels introduces a threshold and thus a non-linearity which contributes to a number of the phenomena of some types of LTP, such as co-operativity (many small inputs together produce sufficient depolarization to allow the NMDA receptors to operate), associativity (a weak input alone will not produce sufficient depolarization of the postsynaptic cell to enable the NMDA receptors to be activated, but the depolarization will be sufficient if there is also a strong input), and temporal contiguity between the different inputs that show LTP (in that if inputs occur non-conjunctively, the depolarization shows insufficient summation to reach the required level, or some of the inputs may arrive when the depolarization has decayed). Once the LTP has become established (which can be within 1 min of the strong input to the cell), the LTP is expressed through the K–Q receptors, in that AP5 blocks only the establishment of LTP, and not its subsequent expression (see further Bliss and Collingridge 1993; Nicoll and Malenka 1995; Fazeli and Collingridge 1996).

There are several possibilities about what change is triggered by the entry of Ca^{2+} to the postsynaptic cell to mediate LTP. One possibility is that somehow a messenger reaches the presynaptic terminals from the postsynaptic membrane and, if the terminals are active, causes them to release more transmitter in future whenever they are activated by an action potential. Consistent with this possibility is the observation that after LTP has been induced more transmitter appears to be released from the presynaptic endings. Another possibility is that the postsynaptic membrane changes just where Ca^{2+} has entered, so that K–Q receptors become more responsive to glutamate released in future. Consistent with this possibility is the observation that after LTP, the postsynaptic cell may respond more to locally applied glutamate (using a microiontophoretic technique).

The rule which underlies associative LTP is thus that synapses connecting two neurons become stronger if there is conjunctive presynaptic and (strong) postsynaptic activity. This learning rule for synaptic modification is sometimes called the Hebb rule, after Donald Hebb of McGill University who drew attention to this possibility, and its potential importance in learning, in 1949.

In that LTP is long-lasting, develops rapidly, is synapse-specific, and is in some cases associative, it is of interest as a potential synaptic mechanism underlying some forms of

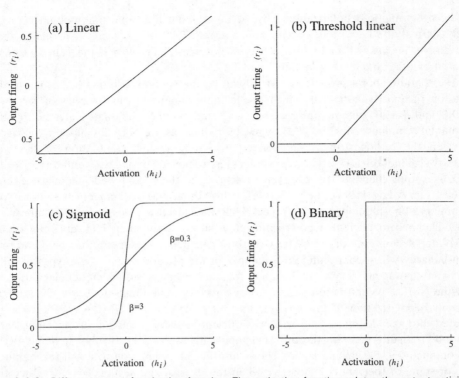

Fig. A.1.3 Different types of activation function. The activation function relates the output activity (or firing rate), r_i, of the neuron (i) to its activation, h_i. (a) Linear. (b) Threshold linear. (c) Sigmoid. (One mathematical exemplar of this class of activation function is $r_i = 1/(1 + \exp(-2\beta h_i))$. The output of this function, also sometimes known as the logistic function, is 0 for an input of $-\infty$, 0.5 for 0, and 1 for $+\infty$. The function incorporates a threshold at the lower end, followed by a linear portion, and then an asymptotic approach to the maximum value at the top end of the function. The parameter β controls the steepness of the almost linear part of the function round $h_i = 0$. If β is small, the output goes smoothly and slowly from 0 to 1 as h_i goes from $-\infty$ to $+\infty$. If β is large, the curve is very steep, and approximates a binary threshold activation function.) (d) Binary threshold.

memory. Evidence linking it directly to some forms of learning comes from experiments in which it has been shown that the drug AP5 infused so that it reaches the hippocampus to block NMDA receptors blocks spatial learning mediated by the hippocampus (see Morris 1989). The task learned by the rats was to find the location relative to cues in a room of a platform submerged in an opaque liquid (milk). Interestingly, if the rats had already learned where the platform was, then the NMDA infusion did not block performance of the task. This is a close parallel to LTP, in that the learning, but not the subsequent expression of what had been learned, was blocked by the NMDA antagonist AP5. Although there is still some uncertainty about the experimental evidence that links LTP to learning (see, e.g., Morris 1996), there is a need for a synapse-specific modifiability of synaptic strengths on neurons if neuronal networks are to learn (see Rolls 1996a and examples throughout Rolls and Treves 1998), and if LTP is not always an exact model of the synaptic modification that occurs during learning, then something with many of the properties of LTP is nevertheless needed, and is likely to be present in the brain given the functions known to be implemented in many brain regions (see Rolls and Treves 1998, Chapters 6–10).

In another model of the role of LTP in memory, Davis (1992) has studied the role of the amygdala in learning associations to fear-inducing stimuli. He has shown that blockade of NMDA synapses in the amygdala interferes with this type of learning, consistent with the idea that LTP provides a useful model of this type of stimulus-reinforcement association learning too (see further Chapter 4).

Long-term depression (LTD) can also occur. It can in principle be associative or non-associative. In associative LTD, the alteration of synaptic strength depends on the pre- and postsynaptic activities. There are two types. Heterosynaptic LTD occurs when the postsynaptic neuron is strongly activated, and there is low presynaptic activity (see Fig. A.1.4b input B, and Table A.2.1). Heterosynaptic LTD is so-called because the synapse that weakens is other than (hetero-) the one through which the postsynaptic neuron is activated. Heterosynaptic LTD is important in associative neuronal networks (see Rolls and Treves 1998, Chapters 2 and 3), and in competitive neuronal networks (see Rolls and Treves 1998, Chapter 4). In competitive neural networks it would be helpful if the degree of heterosynaptic LTD depended on the existing strength of the synapse, and there is some evidence that this may be the case (see Rolls and Treves 1998, Chapter 4). Homosynaptic LTD occurs when the presynaptic neuron is strongly active, and the postsynaptic neuron has some, but low, activity (see Fig. A.1.4d and Table A.1). Homosynaptic LTD is so-called because the synapse that weakens is the same as (homo-) the one that is active. Heterosynaptic and homosynaptic LTD are found in the neocortex (Artola and Singer 1993; Singer 1995) and hippocampus (Christie 1996 and other papers in *Hippocampus*, (1996), **6**, (1)), and in many cases are dependent on activation of NMDA receptors (see also Fazeli and Collingridge 1996). LTD in the cerebellum is evident as weakening of active parallel fibre to Purkinje cell synapses when the climbing fibre connecting to a Purkinje cell is active (see Ito 1984, 1989, 1993a,b).

The learning rules implicit in long-term potentiation and long-term depression (see eqns (A.1.3) and (A.2.7)) are local learning rules, in that the change in synaptic weight depends on factors local to the synapse, the presynaptic activity and the postsynaptic activation (see Section A.2.4.6). This is an important aspect of this type of learning rule, for it does not require errors to be computed from many places in the network and brought back as an individual error of teaching signal appropriate for each neuron in the network, which would require enormous numbers of special-purpose connections and computations (see Rolls and Treves 1998). Instead, a local learning rule is used in pattern associators as described in Section A.2, and is biologically very plausible given the findings on long-term potentiation and long-term depression just described.

A.1.6 Distributed representations

When considering the operation of many neuronal networks in the brain, it is found that many useful properties arise if each input to the network (arriving on the axons, r') is encoded in the activity of an ensemble or population of the axons or input lines (distributed encoding), and is not signalled by the activity of a single input, which is called

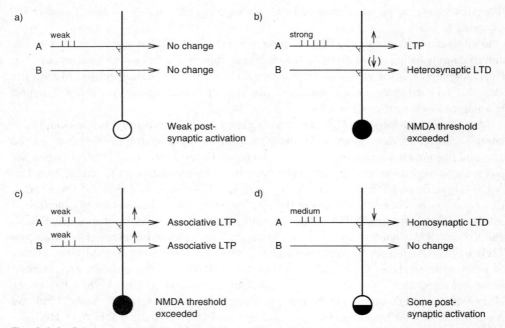

Fig. A.1.4 Schematic illustration of synaptic modification rules as revealed by long-term potentiation (LTP) and long-term depression (LTD). The activation of the postsynaptic neuron is indicated by the extent to which its soma is black. There are two sets of inputs to the neuron: A and B. (a) A weak input (indicated by three spikes) on the set A of input axons produces little postsynaptic activation, and there is no change in synaptic strength. (b) A strong input (indicated by five spikes) on the set A of input axons produces strong postsynaptic activation, and the active synapses increase in strength. This is LTP. It is homosynaptic in that the synapses that increase in strength are the same as those through which the neuron is activated. LTP is synapse-specific, in that the inactive axons, B, do not show LTP. They either do not change in strength, or they may weaken. The weakening is called heterosynaptic LTD, because the synapses that weaken are other than those through which the neuron is activated (*hetero-* is Greek for other). (c) Two weak inputs present simultaneously on A and B summate to produce strong postsynaptic activation, and both sets of active synapses show LTP. (d) Intermediate strength firing on A produces some activation, but not strong activation, of the postsynaptic neuron. The active synapses become weaker. This is homosynaptic LTD, in that the synapses that weaken are the same as those through which the neuron is activated (*homo-* is Greek for same).

local encoding. We start off with some definitions, and then highlight some of the differences, and summarize some evidence which shows the type of encoding used in some brain regions. Then we show below how many of the useful properties of the neuronal networks described depend on distributed encoding. Rolls and Treves (1998, Chapter 10), review evidence on the encoding actually found in different regions of the cerebral cortex.

A.1.6.1 Definitions

A *local* representation is one in which all the information that a particular stimulus or event occurred is provided by the activity of one of the neurons. In a famous example, a single neuron might be active only if one's grandmother was being seen. This would imply that most neurons in the brain regions where objects or events are represented would fire only very rarely. A problem with this type of encoding is that a new neuron would be needed for every object or event that has to be represented. There are many other disadvantages of this type of encoding, many of which are discussed by Rolls and Treves (1998). Moreover, there is evidence that objects are represented in the brain by a different type of encoding (see Section 4.3.4.6 and Rolls and Treves 1998).

A *fully distributed* representation is one in which all the information that a particular stimulus or event occurred is provided by the activity of the full set of neurons. If the neurons are binary (e.g. either active or not), the most distributed encoding is when half the neurons are active for any one stimulus or event.

A *sparse distributed* representation is a distributed representation in which a small proportion of the neurons is active at any one time. In a sparse representation with binary neurons, less than half of the neurons are active for any one stimulus or event. For binary neurons, we can use as a measure of the sparseness the proportion of neurons in the active state. For neurons with real, continuously variable, values of firing rates, the sparseness of the representation a can be measured, by extending the binary notion of the proportion of neurons that are firing, as

$$a = \left(\sum_{i=1,N} r_i/N \right)^2 \bigg/ \sum_{i=1,N} (r_i^2/N) \qquad (A.1.4)$$

where r_i is the firing rate of the ith neuron in the set of N neurons (Treves and Rolls 1991; Rolls and Treves 1998).

Coarse coding utilizes overlaps of receptive fields, and can compute positions in the input space using differences between the firing levels of coactive cells (e.g. colour-tuned cones in the retina). The representation implied is distributed. *Fine coding* (in which, for example, a neuron may be 'tuned' to the exact orientation and position of a stimulus) implies more local coding.

A.1.6.2 Advantages of different types of coding

One advantage of distributed encoding is that the similarity between two representations can be reflected by the correlation between the two patterns of activity which represent the different stimuli. We have already introduced the idea that the input to a neuron is represented by the activity of its set of input axons r_j', where j indexes the axons, numbered from $j = 1, C$ (see Fig. A.1.2 and eqn (A.1.1)). Now the set of activities of the input axons is a vector (a vector is an ordered set of numbers; Appendix 1 of Rolls and Treves 1998, provides a summary of some of the concepts involved). We can denote as $\mathbf{r}_1'$ the vector of axonal activity that represents stimulus 1, and $\mathbf{r}_2'$ the vector that represents stimulus 2. Then the similarity between the two vectors, and thus the two stimuli, is reflected by the correlation between the two vectors. The correlation will be high if the activity of each axon in the two representations is similar, and will become more and more different as the activity of more and more of the axons differs in the two representations. Thus the similarity of two inputs can be represented in a graded or continuous way if (this type of) distributed encoding is used. This enables generalization to similar stimuli, or to

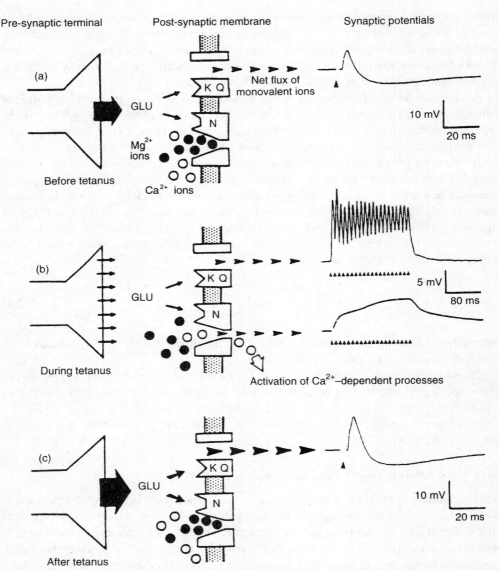

Fig. A.1.5 The mechanism of induction of LTP in the CA1 region of the hippocampus. (a) Neurotransmitter (e.g. L-glutamate) is released and acts upon both K–Q (kainate–quisqualate) and NMDA (N) receptors. The NMDA receptors are blocked by magnesium and the excitatory synaptic response (EPSP) is therefore mediated primarily by ion-flow through the channels associated with K–Q receptors. (b) During high-frequency activation, the magnesium block of the ion channels associated with NMDA receptors is released by depolarization. Activation of the NMDA receptor by transmitter now results in ions moving through the channel. In this way, calcium enters the postsynaptic region to trigger various intracellular mechanisms which eventually result in an alteration of synaptic efficacy. (c) Subsequent low-frequency stimulation results in a greater EPSP. See text for further details. (Reprinted with permission from Collingridge and Bliss 1987.)

incomplete versions of a stimulus (if it is, for example, partly seen or partly remembered), to occur. With a local representation, either one stimulus or another is represented, and similarities between different stimuli are not encoded.

Another advantage of distributed encoding is that the number of different stimuli that can be represented by a set of C components (e.g. the activity of C axons) can be very large. A simple example is provided by the binary encoding of an 8-element vector. One component can code for which of two stimuli has been seen, two components (or bits in a computer byte) for four stimuli, three components for eight stimuli, eight components for 256 stimuli, etc. That is, the number of stimuli increases exponentially with the number of components (or in this case, axons) in the representation. (In this simple binary illustrative case, the number of stimuli that can be encoded is 2^C.) Put the other way round, even if a neuron has only a limited number of inputs (e.g. a few thousand), it can nevertheless receive a great deal of information about which stimulus was present. This ability of a neuron with a limited number of inputs to receive information about which of potentially very many input events is present is probably one factor that makes computation by the brain possible. With local encoding, the number of stimuli that can be encoded increases only linearly with the number C of axons or components (because a different component is needed to represent each new stimulus). (In our example, only eight stimuli could be represented by eight axons.)

In the real brain, there is now good evidence that in a number of brain systems, including the high-order visual and olfactory cortices, and the hippocampus, distributed encoding with the above two properties, of representing similarity and of exponentially increasing encoding capacity as the number of neurons in the representation increases, is found (Rolls and Tovee 1995a; Abbott, Rolls and Tovee 1996; Rolls, Treves and Tovee 1997c; Rolls, Treves, Robertson, Georges-Franois and Panzeri 1998b; Booth and Rolls 1998). For example, in the high-order visual cortex in the temporal lobe of the primate brain, the number of faces that can be represented increases approximately exponentially with the number of neurons in the population (see Fig. 4.9c). If we plot instead the information about which stimulus is seen, we see that this rises approximately linearly with the number of neurons in the representation (Fig. 4.9a). This corresponds to an exponential rise in the number of stimuli encoded, because information is a log measure (see Rolls and Treves 1998, Appendix A2). A similar result has been found for the encoding of position in space by the primate hippocampus (Rolls, Treves, Robertson, Georges-Franois and Panzeri 1998b). It is particularly important that the information can be read from the ensemble of neurons using a simple measure of the similarity of vectors, the correlation (or dot product, see Rolls and Treves 1998, Appendix 1) between two vectors. The importance of this is that it is essentially vector similarity operations that characterize the operation of many neuronal networks (see, e.g., Rolls and Treves 1998, Chapters 2–4 and Appendix 1). The neurophysiological results show that both the ability to reflect similarity by vector correlation, and the utilization of exponential coding capacity, are a property of real neuronal networks found in the brain.

To emphasize one of the points being made here, although the binary encoding used in the 8-bit vector described above has optimal capacity for binary encoding, it is not optimal for vector similarity operations. For example, the two very similar numbers 127 and 128 are represented by 01111111 and 10000000 with binary encoding, yet the correlation or bit overlap of these vectors is 0. The brain in contrast uses a code which has the attractive property of exponentially increasing capacity with the number of neurons in the representation, though it is different from the simple binary encoding of numbers used in computers, and at the same time codes stimuli in such a way that the code can be read off with simple dot product or correlation-related decoding, which is what is specified for the elementary neuronal network operation shown in eqn (A.2.1) (Rolls and Tovee 1995a; Abbott, Rolls and Tovee 1996; Rolls, Treves and Tovee 1997c; Rolls, Treves, Robertson *et al.* 1998b; Booth and Rolls 1998; Rolls and Treves 1998).

A.2   Pattern-association memory

A fundamental operation of most nervous systems is to learn to associate a first stimulus with a second which occurs at about the same time, and to retrieve the second stimulus when the first is presented. The first stimulus might be the sight of food whereby it becomes a conditioned stimulus or secondary reinforcer, and the second stimulus the taste of food, an example of a primary reinforcer. After the association has been learned, the sight of food would enable its taste to be retrieved. In classical conditioning, the taste of food might elicit an unconditioned response of salivation, and if the sight of the food is paired with its taste, then the sight of that food would by learning come to produce salivation. More abstractly, if one idea is associated by learning with a second, then when the first idea occurs again, the second idea will tend to be associatively retrieved.

A.2.1   Architecture and operation

The essential elements necessary for pattern association, forming what could be called a prototypical pattern associator network, are shown in Fig. A.2.1. What we have called the second or unconditioned stimulus pattern is applied through unmodifiable synapses generating an input to each unit which, being external with respect to the synaptic matrix we focus on, we can call the external input e_i for the ith neuron. (We can also treat this as a vector, **e**, as indicated in the legend to Fig. A.2.1. Vectors and simple operations performed with them are summarized in Rolls and Treves 1998, Appendix A1). This unconditioned stimulus is dominant in producing or forcing the firing of the output neurons (r_i for the ith neuron, or the vector **r**). At the same time, the first or conditioned stimulus pattern r'_j for the jth axon (or equivalently the vector **r**′) present on the horizontally running axons in Fig. A.2.1 is applied through *modifiable* synapses w_{ij} to the dendrites of the output neurons. The synapses are modifiable in such a way that if there is presynaptic firing on an input axon r'_j paired during learning with postsynaptic activity on neuron i, then the strength or weight w_{ij} between that axon and the dendrite increases. This simple learning rule is often called the Hebb rule, after Donald Hebb who in 1949 formulated the hypothesis that if the firing of one neuron was regularly associated with another, then the strength of the synapse or synapses between the neurons should

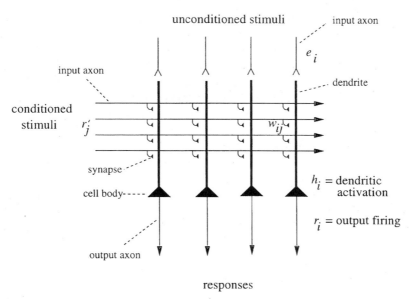

Fig. A.2.1 A pattern-association memory. An unconditioned stimulus has activity or firing rate e_i for the ith neuron, and produces firing r_i of the ith neuron. An unconditioned stimulus may be treated as a vector, across the set of neurons indexed by i, of activity **e**. The firing rate response can also be thought of as a vector of firing **r**. The conditioned stimuli have activity or firing rate r'_j for the jth axon, which can also be treated as a vector **r**'.

increase. (In fact, the terms in which Hebb put the hypothesis were a little different from an association memory, in that he stated that if one neuron regularly comes to elicit firing in another, then the strength of the synapses should increase. He had in mind the building of what he called cell assemblies. In a pattern associator, the conditioned stimulus need not produce before learning any significant activation of the output neurons. The connections must simply increase if there is associated pre- and post-synaptic firing when, in pattern association, most of the postsynaptic firing is being produced by a different input.) After learning, presenting the pattern **r**' on the input axons will activate the dendrite through the strengthened synapses. If the cue or conditioned stimulus pattern is the same as that learned, the postsynaptic neurons will be activated, even in the absence of the external or unconditioned input, as each of the firing axons produces through a strengthened synapse some activation of the postsynaptic element, the dendrite. The total activation h_i of each postsynaptic neuron i is then the sum of such individual activations. In this way, the 'correct' output neurons, that is those activated during learning, can end up being the ones most strongly activated, and the second or unconditioned stimulus can be effectively recalled. The recall is best when only strong activation of the postsynaptic neuron produces firing, that is if there is a threshold for firing, just like real neurons. The reasons for this arise when many associations are stored in the memory, as will soon be shown.

Next we introduce a more precise description of the above by writing down explicit mathematical rules for the operation of the simple network model of Fig. A.2.1, which will help us to understand how pattern association memories in general operate. (In this description we introduce simple vector operations, and, for those who are not familiar with these, the reader is referred to Rolls and Treves 1998, in which Appendix A1 provides a concise summary of the operations most relevant to simple neural networks.) We have denoted above a conditioned stimulus input pattern as $\mathbf{r}'$. Each of the axons has a firing rate, and if we count or index through the axons using the subscript j, the firing rate of the first axon is r'_1, of the second r'_2, of the jth r'_j, etc. The whole set of axons forms a vector, which is just an ordered (1, 2, 3, etc.) set of elements. The firing rate of each axon r'_j is one element of the firing rate vector $\mathbf{r}'$. Similarly, using i as the index, we can denote the firing rate of any output neuron as r_i, and the firing rate output vector as $\mathbf{r}$. With this terminology, we can then identify any synapse on to neuron i from neuron j as w_{ij} (see Fig. A.2.1). In this notation, the first index, i, always refers to the receiving neuron (and thus signifies a dendrite), while the second index, j, refers to the sending neuron (and thus signifies a conditioned stimulus input axon in Fig. A.2.1). We can now specify the learning and retrieval operations as follows:

A.2.1.1 Learning

The firing rate of every output neuron is forced to a value determined by the unconditioned (or external or forcing stimulus) input. In our simple model this means that for any one neuron i,

$$r_i = f(e_i) \tag{A.2.1}$$

which indicates that the firing rate is a function of the dendritic activation, taken in this case to reduce essentially to that resulting from the external forcing input (see Fig. A.2.1). The function f is called the activation function (see Fig. A.1.3), and its precise form is irrelevant, at least during this learning phase. For example, the function at its simplest could be taken to be linear, so that the firing rate would be just proportional to the activation.

The Hebb rule can then be written as follows:

$$\delta w_{ij} = k r_i r'_j \tag{A.2.2}$$

where δw_{ij} is the change of the synaptic weight w_{ij} which results from the simultaneous (or conjunctive) presence of presynaptic firing r'_j and postsynaptic firing or activation r_i, and k is a learning rate-constant which specifies how much the synapses alter on any one pairing.

The Hebb rule is expressed in this multiplicative form to reflect the idea that *both* presynaptic and postsynaptic activity must be present for the synapses to increase in strength. The multiplicative form also reflects the idea that strong pre-and post-synaptic firing will produce a larger change of synaptic weight than smaller firing rates. It is also assumed for now that before any learning takes place, the synaptic strengths are small in relation to the changes that can be produced during Hebbian learning. We will see that this assumption can be relaxed later when a modified Hebb rule is introduced that can lead to a reduction in synaptic strength under some conditions.

A.2.1.2 Recall

When the conditioned stimulus is present on the input axons, the total activation h_i of a neuron i is the sum of all the activations produced through each strengthened synapse w_{ij} by each active neuron r'_j. We can express this as

$$h_i = \sum_j r'_j w_{ij} \qquad (A.2.3)$$

where $\sum_j$ indicates that the sum is over the C input axons (or connections) indexed by j. The multiplicative form here indicates that activation should be produced by an axon only if it is firing, and only if it is connected to the dendrite by a strengthened synapse. It also indicates that the strength of the activation reflects how fast the axon r'_j is firing, and how strong the synapse w_{ij} is. The sum of all such activations expresses the idea that summation (of synaptic currents in real neurons) occurs along the length of the dendrite, to produce activation at the cell body, where the activation h_i is converted into firing r_i. This conversion can be expressed as

$$r_i = f(h_i) \qquad (A.2.4)$$

where the function f is again the activation function. The form of the function now becomes more important. Real neurons have thresholds, with firing occurring only if the activation is above the threshold. A threshold linear activation function is shown in Fig. A.1.3b. This has been useful in formal analysis of the properties of neural networks. Neurons also have firing rates which become saturated at a maximum rate, and we could express this as the sigmoid activation function shown in Fig. A.1.3c. Yet another simple activation function, used in some models of neural networks, is the binary threshold function (Fig. A.1.3d), which indicates that if the activation is below threshold, there is no firing, and that if the activation is above threshold, the neuron fires maximally. Whatever the exact shape of the activation function, some non-linearity is an advantage, for it enables small activations produced by interfering memories to be minimized, and it can enable neurons to perform logical operations, such as to fire or respond only if two or more sets of inputs are present simultaneously.

A.2.2 A simple model

An example of these learning and recall operations is provided in a very simple form as follows. The neurons will have simple firing rates, which can be 0 to represent no activity, and 1 to indicate high firing. They are thus binary neurons, which can assume one of two firing rates. If we have a pattern associator with six input axons and four output neurons, we could represent the network before learning, with the same layout as in Fig. A.2.1, as:

```
                    UCS
                 1  1  0  0
                 ↓  ↓  ↓  ↓
       CS
       1 →       0  0  0  0
       0 →       0  0  0  0
       1 →       0  0  0  0
       0 →       0  0  0  0  .
       1 →       0  0  0  0
       0 →       0  0  0  0
```

Fig. A.2.2

where r' or the conditioned stimulus (CS) is 101010, and r or the firing produced by the unconditioned stimulus (UCS) is 1100. (The arrows indicate the flow of signals.) The synaptic weights are initially all 0. After pairing the CS with the UCS during one learning trial, some of the synaptic weights will be incremented according to eqn (A.2.2), so that after learning this pair the synaptic weights will become:

```
                    UCS
                 1  1  0  0
                 ↓  ↓  ↓  ↓
       CS
       1 →       1  1  0  0
       0 →       0  0  0  0
       1 →       1  1  0  0
       0 →       0  0  0  0
       1 →       1  1  0  0
       0 →       0  0  0  0
```

Fig. A2.3

We can represent what happens during recall, when, for example, we present the CS that has been learned, as follows:

```
       CS
       1 →       1  1  0  0
       0 →       0  0  0  0
       1 →       1  1  0  0
       0 →       0  0  0  0
       1 →       1  1  0  0
       0 →       0  0  0  0
                 ↓  ↓  ↓  ↓

                 3  3  0  0     Activation $h_i$
                 1  1  0  0     Firing $r_i$
```

Fig. A.2.4

The activation of the four output neurons is 3300, and if we set the threshold of each output neuron to 2, then the output firing is 1100 (where the binary firing rate is 0 if below threshold, and 1 if above). The pattern associator has thus achieved recall of the pattern 1100, which is correct.

We can now illustrate how a number of different associations can be stored in such a pattern associator, and retrieved correctly. Let us associate a new CS pattern 110001 with the UCS 0101 in the same pattern associator. The weights will become as shown next in Fig. A.2.5 after learning:

$$
\begin{array}{cccc}
 & & \text{UCS} & \\
 & 0 & 1 & 0 & 1 \\
 & \downarrow & \downarrow & \downarrow & \downarrow \\
\text{CS} & & & \\
1 \rightarrow & 1 & 2 & 0 & 1 \\
1 \rightarrow & 0 & 1 & 0 & 1 \\
0 \rightarrow & 1 & 1 & 0 & 0 \\
0 \rightarrow & 0 & 0 & 0 & 0 \\
0 \rightarrow & 1 & 1 & 0 & 0 \\
1 \rightarrow & 0 & 1 & 0 & 1 \\
\end{array}
$$

Fig. A.2.5

If we now present the second CS, the retrieval is as follows:

$$
\begin{array}{cccc}
\text{CS} & & & \\
1 \rightarrow & 1 & 2 & 0 & 1 \\
1 \rightarrow & 0 & 1 & 0 & 1 \\
0 \rightarrow & 1 & 1 & 0 & 0 \\
0 \rightarrow & 0 & 0 & 0 & 0 \\
0 \rightarrow & 1 & 1 & 0 & 0 \\
1 \rightarrow & 0 & 1 & 0 & 1 \\
 & \downarrow & \downarrow & \downarrow & \downarrow \\
 & 1 & 4 & 0 & 3 & \quad \text{Activation } h_i \\
 & 0 & 1 & 0 & 1 & \quad \text{Firing } r_i \\
\end{array}
$$

Fig. A.2.6

The binary output firings were again produced with the threshold set to 2. Recall is perfect. This illustration shows the value of some threshold non-linearity in the activation function of the neurons. In this case, the activations did reflect some small cross-talk or interference from the previous pattern association of CS1 with UCS1, but this was removed by the threshold operation, to clean up the recall firing. The example also shows that when further associations are learned by a pattern associator trained with the Hebb rule, eqn (A.2.2), some synapses will reflect increments above a synaptic strength of 1. It is left as an exercise to the reader to verify that recall is still perfect to CS1, the vector 101010. (The output activation vector $\mathbf{h}$ is 3401, and the output firing vector r with the same threshold of 2 is 1100, which is perfect recall.)

A.2.3 The vector interpretation

The way in which recall is produced, eqn (A.2.3), consists for each output neuron i in multiplying each input firing rate r'_j by the corresponding synaptic weight w_{ij} and summing the products to obtain the activation h_i. Now we can consider the firing rates r'_j where j varies from 1 to N', the number of axons, to be a vector. (A vector is simply an ordered set of numbers; more detail on vector operations in neural networks is provided by Rolls and Treves 1998, Appendix A1.) Let us call this vector $\mathbf{r'}$. Similarly, on a neuron i, the synaptic weights can be treated as a vector, $\mathbf{w}_i$. (The subscript i here indicates that this is the weight vector on the ith neuron.) The operation we have just described to obtain the output activation can now be seen to be a simple multiplication operation of two vectors to produce a single output value (called a scalar output). This is the inner product or dot product of two vectors, and can be written

$$h_i = \mathbf{r'} \cdot \mathbf{w}_i \qquad \text{(A.2.5)}$$

The inner product of two vectors indicates how similar they are. If two vectors have corresponding elements the same, then the dot product will be maximal. If the two vectors are similar but not identical, then the dot product will be high. If the two vectors are completely different, the dot products will be 0, and the vectors are described as orthogonal. (The term orthogonal means at right angles, and arises from the geometric interpretation of vectors, which is summarized in Rolls and Treves 1998, Appendix A1.) Thus the dot product provides a direct measure of how similar two vectors are. It can now be seen that a fundamental operation many neurons perform is effectively to compute how similar an input pattern vector $\mathbf{r'}$ is to a stored weight vector. The similarity measure they compute, the dot product, is a very good measure of similarity, and indeed, the standard (Pearson product-moment) correlation coefficient used in statistics is the same as a normalized dot product with the mean subtracted from each vector, as shown in Appendix 1 of Rolls and Treves (1998). (The normalization used in the correlation coefficient results in the coefficient varying always between $+1$ and -1, whereas the actual scalar value of a dot product depends on the length of the vectors from which it is calculated.)

With these concepts, we can now see that during learning, a pattern associator adds to its weight vector a vector $\delta \mathbf{w}_i$ that has the same pattern as the input pattern $\mathbf{r'}$, if the postsynaptic neuron i is strongly activated. Indeed, we can express eqn (A.2.2) in vector form as

$$\delta \mathbf{w}_i = k \cdot r_i \cdot \mathbf{r'} \qquad \text{(A.2.6)}$$

We can now see that what is recalled by the neuron depends on the similarity of the recall cue vector $\mathbf{r'}_r$ to the originally learned vector $\mathbf{r'}$. The fact that during recall the output of each neuron reflects the similarity (as measured by the dot product) of the input pattern $\mathbf{r'}_r$ to each of the patterns used originally as $\mathbf{r'}$ inputs (conditioned stimuli in Fig. A.2.1) provides a simple way to appreciate many of the interesting and biologically useful properties of pattern associators, as described next.

A.2.4 Properties
A.2.4.1 Generalization

During recall, pattern associators generalize, and produce appropriate outputs if a recall cue vector $\mathbf{r}'_r$ is similar to a vector that has been learned already. This occurs because the recall operation involves computing the dot (inner) product of the input pattern vector $\mathbf{r}'_r$ with the synaptic weight vector $\mathbf{w}_i$, so that the firing produced, r_i, reflects the similarity of the current input to the previously learned input pattern $\mathbf{r}'$. (Generalization will occur to input cue or conditioned stimulus patterns $\mathbf{r}'_r$ which are incomplete versions of an original conditioned stimulus $\mathbf{r}'$, although the term completion is usually applied to the autoassociation networks described in Chapter 3 of Rolls and Treves 1998.)

This is an extremely important property of pattern associators, for input stimuli during recall will rarely be absolutely identical to what has been learned previously, and automatic generalization to similar stimuli is extremely useful, and has great adaptive value in biological systems.

Generalization can be illustrated with the simple binary pattern associator considered above. (Those who have appreciated the vector description just given might wish to skip this illustration.) Instead of the second CS, pattern vector 110001, we will use the similar recall cue 110100.

CS

$1 \rightarrow$		1	2	0	1
$1 \rightarrow$		0	1	0	1
$0 \rightarrow$		1	1	0	0
$1 \rightarrow$		0	0	0	0
$0 \rightarrow$		1	1	0	0
$0 \rightarrow$		0	1	0	1
		$\downarrow$	$\downarrow$	$\downarrow$	$\downarrow$

		1	3	0	2	Activation h_i
		0	1	0	1	Firing r_i

Fig. A.2.7

It is seen that the output firing rate vector, 0101, is exactly what should be recalled to CS2 (and not to CS1), so correct generalization has occurred. Although this is a small network trained with few examples, the same properties hold for large networks with large numbers of stored patterns, as described more quantitatively in the section on capacity below and in Appendix A3 of Rolls and Treves (1998).

A.2.4.2 Graceful degradation or fault tolerance

If the synaptic weight vector $\mathbf{w}_i$ has synapses missing (e.g. during development), or loses synapses, then the output activation h_i or $\mathbf{h}$ is still reasonable, because h_i is the dot product (correlation) of $\mathbf{r}'$ with $\mathbf{w}_i$. The result, especially after passing through the output activation function, can frequently be perfect recall. The same property arises if, for example, one or some of the CS input axons are lost or damaged. This is a very important property of associative memories, and is not a property of conventional computer memories, which produce incorrect data if even only one storage location (for one bit or binary digit of data) of their memory is damaged or cannot be accessed. This property of graceful degradation is of great adaptive value for biological systems.

We can illustrate this with a simple example. If we damage two of the synapses in Fig. A.2.2 to produce the synaptic matrix shown in Fig. A.2.8 (where x indicates a damaged synapse which has no effect, but was previously 1), and now present the second CS, the retrieval is as follows:

CS

$1 \rightarrow$	1	2	0	1
$1 \rightarrow$	0	1	0	x
$0 \rightarrow$	1	1	0	0
$0 \rightarrow$	0	0	0	0
$0 \rightarrow$	1	x	0	0
$1 \rightarrow$	0	1	0	1
	$\downarrow$	$\downarrow$	$\downarrow$	$\downarrow$

1	4	0	2	Activation h_i
0	1	0	1	Firing r_i

Fig. A.2.8

The binary output firings were again produced with the threshold set to 2. The recalled vector, 0101, is perfect. This illustration again shows the value of some threshold non-linearity in the activation function of the neurons. It is left as an exercise to the reader to verify that recall is still perfect to CS1, the vector 101010. (The output activation vector **h** is 3301, and the output firing vector **r** with the same threshold of 2 is 1100, which is perfect recall.)

A.2.4.3 The importance of distributed representations for pattern associators

A distributed representation is one in which the firing or activity of all the elements in the vector is used to encode a particular stimulus. For example, in the vector CS1 which has the value 101010, we need to know the state of all the elements to know which stimulus is being represented. Another stimulus, CS2, is represented by the vector 110001. We can represent many different events or stimuli with such overlapping sets of elements, and because in general any one element cannot be used to identify the stimulus, but instead the information about which stimulus is present is distributed over the population of elements or neurons, this is called a distributed representation. If, for binary neurons, half the neurons are in one state (e.g. 0), and the others are in the other state (e.g. 1), then the representation is described as *fully distributed*. The CS representations above are thus fully distributed. If only a smaller proportion of the neurons is active to represent a stimulus, as in the vector 100001, then this is a *sparse representation*. For binary representations, we can quantify the sparseness *a* by the proportion of neurons in the active (1) state.

In contrast, a *local representation* is one in which all the information that a particular stimulus or event has occurred is provided by the activity of one of the neurons, or elements in the vector. One stimulus might be represented by the vector 100000, another stimulus by the vector 010000, and a third stimulus by the vector 001000. The activity of neuron or element 1 would indicate that stimulus 1 was present, and of neuron 2, that stimulus 2 was present. The representation is local in that if a particular neuron is active, we know that the stimulus represented by that neuron is present. In neurophysiology, if such cells were present, they might be called 'grandmother cells' (cf. Barlow 1972, 1995), in that one neuron might represent a stimulus in the environment as complex and specific as one's grandmother. Where the activity of a number of cells must be taken into account in order to represent a stimulus (such as an individual taste), then the representation is sometimes described as using ensemble encoding.

Now, the properties just described for associative memories, generalization and graceful degradation, are only implemented if the representation of the CS or $\mathbf{r}'$ vector is distributed. This occurs because the recall operation involves computing the dot (inner) product of the input pattern vector $\mathbf{r}'_r$ with the synaptic weight vector $\mathbf{w}_i$. This allows the output activation h_i to reflect the similarity of the current input pattern to a previously learned input pattern $\mathbf{r}'$ only if several or many elements of the $\mathbf{r}'$ and $\mathbf{r}'_r$ vectors are in the active state to represent a pattern. If local encoding were used, e.g. 100 000, then if the first element of the vector (which might be the firing of axon 1, i.e. r'_1, or the strength of synapse $i1$, w_{i1}) is lost, then the resulting vector is not similar to any other CS vector, and the output activation is 0. In the case of local encoding, the important properties of associative memories, generalization, and graceful degradation, do not thus emerge. Graceful degradation and generalization are dependent on distributed representations, for then the dot product can reflect similarity even when some elements of the vectors involved are altered. If we think of the correlation between Y and X in a graph, then this correlation is affected only little if a few X,Y pairs of data are lost (see Appendix A1 of Rolls and Treves 1998).

A.2.4.4 Prototype extraction, extraction of central tendency, and noise reduction

If a set of similar conditioned stimulus vectors $\mathbf{r}'$ are paired with the same unconditioned stimulus e_i, the weight vector $\mathbf{w}_i$ becomes (or points towards) the sum (or with scaling the average) of the set of similar vectors $\mathbf{r}'$. This follows from the operation of the Hebb rule in eqn (A.2.2). When tested at recall, the output of the memory is then best to the average input pattern vector denoted $\langle \mathbf{r}' \rangle$. If the average is thought of as a prototype, then even though the prototype vector $\langle \mathbf{r}' \rangle$ itself might never have been seen, the best output of the neuron or network is to the prototype. This produces 'extraction of the prototype' or 'central tendency'. The same phenomenon is a feature of human memory performance (see McClelland and Rumelhart 1986 Chapter 17, and Rolls and Treves 1998, Section 3.4.4), and this simple process with distributed representations in a neural network accounts for the phenomenon.

If the different exemplars of the vector $\mathbf{r}'$ are thought of as noisy versions of the true input pattern vector $\langle \mathbf{r}' \rangle$ (with incorrect values for some of the elements), then the pattern associator has performed 'noise reduction', in that the output produced by any one of these vectors will represent the true, noiseless, average vector $\langle \mathbf{r}' \rangle$.

A.2.4.5 Speed

Recall is very fast in a real neuronal network, because the conditioned stimulus input firings r'_j ($j = 1, C$ axons) can be applied simultaneously to the synapses w_{ij}, and the activation h_i can be accumulated in one or two time constants of the dendrite (e.g. 10–20 ms). Whenever the threshold of the cell is exceeded, it fires. Thus, in effectively one step, which takes the brain no more than 10–20 ms, all the output neurons of the pattern associator can be firing with rates that reflect the input firing of every axon. This is very different from a conventional digital computer, in which computing h_i in eqn (A.2.2) would involve C multiplication and addition operations occurring one after another, or $2C$ time steps. The brain performs parallel computation in at least two senses in even a pattern associator. One is that for a single neuron, the separate contributions of the firing rate r'_j of each axon j multiplied by the synaptic weight w_{ij} are computed in parallel and added in the same time-step. The second is that this can be performed in parallel for all neurons $i = 1, N$ in the network, where there are N output neurons in the network. It is these types of parallel processing which enable these classes of neuronal network in the brain to operate so fast, in effectively so few steps.

Learning is also fast ('one-shot') in pattern associators, in that a single pairing of the conditioned stimulus $\mathbf{r}'$ and the unconditioned stimulus $\mathbf{e}$ which produces the unconditioned output firing $\mathbf{r}$ enables the association to be learned. There is no need to repeat the pairing in order to discover over many trials the appropriate mapping. This is extremely important for biological systems, in which a single co-occurrence of two events may lead to learning which could have life-saving consequences. (For example, the pairing of a visual stimulus with a potentially life-threatening aversive event may enable that event to be avoided in future.) Although repeated pairing with small variations of the vectors is used to obtain the useful properties of prototype extraction, extraction of central tendency, and noise reduction, the essential properties of generalization and graceful degradation are obtained with just one pairing. The actual time scales of the learning in the brain are indicated by studies of associative synaptic modification using long-term potentiation paradigms (LTP, see Section A.1). Co-occurrence or near simultaneity of the CS and UCS is required for periods of as little as 100 ms, with expression of the synaptic modification being present within typically a few seconds.

A.2.4.6 Local learning rule

The simplest learning rule used in pattern association neural networks, a version of the Hebb rule, is as in eqn (A.2.2) above

$$\delta w_{ij} = k r_i r'_j$$

This is a local learning rule in that the information required to specify the change in synaptic weight is available locally at the synapse, as it is dependent only on the presynaptic firing rate r'_j available at the synaptic terminal, and the postsynaptic activation or firing r_i available on the dendrite of the neuron receiving the synapse. This makes the learning rule biologically plausible, in that the information about how to change the synaptic weight does not have to be carried from a distant source, where it is computed, to every synapse. Such a non-local learning rule would not be biologically plausible, in that there are no appropriate connections known in most parts of the brain to bring in the synaptic training or teacher signal to every synapse.

Evidence that a learning rule with the general form of eqn (A.2.2) is implemented in at least some parts of the brain comes from studies of long-term potentiation, described in section A.1. Long-term potentiation (LTP) has the synaptic specificity defined by eqn (A.2.2), in that only synapses from active afferents, not those from inactive afferents, become strengthened. Synaptic specificity is important for a pattern associator, and most other types of neuronal network, to operate correctly.

Another useful property of real neurons in relation to eqn (A.2.2) is that the postsynaptic term, r_i, is available on much of the dendrite of a cell, because the electrotonic length of the dendrite is short. Thus if a neuron is strongly activated with a high value for r_i, then any active synapse on to the cell will be capable of being modified. This enables the cell to learn an association between the pattern of activity on all its axons and its postsynaptic activation, which is stored as an addition to its weight vector $\mathbf{w}_i$. Then later on, at recall, the output can be produced as a vector dot product operation between the input pattern vector $\mathbf{r}'$ and the weight vector $\mathbf{w}_i$, so that the output of the cell can reflect the correlation between the current input vector and what has previously been learned by the cell.

A.2.4.7 Capacity

The question of the storage capacity of a pattern associator is considered in detail in Appendix A3 of Rolls and Treves (1998). It is pointed out there that, for this type of associative network, the number of memories that it can hold simultaneously in storage has to be analysed together with the retrieval quality of each output representation, and then only for a given quality of the representation provided in the input. This is in contrast with autoassociative nets, in which a critical number of stored memories exists (as a function of various parameters of the network) beyond which attempting to store additional memories results in it becoming impossible to retrieve essentially anything. With a pattern associator, instead, one will always retrieve something, but this *something* will be very little (in information or correlation terms) if too many associations are simultaneously in storage and/or if too little is provided as input.

The conjoint quality–capacity–input analysis can be carried out, for any specific instance of a pattern associator, by using formal mathematical models and established analytical procedures (see, e.g., Treves 1995). This, however, has to be done case by case. It is anyway useful to develop some intuition for how a pattern associator operates, by considering what its capacity would be in certain well-defined simplified cases.

Linear associative neuronal networks

These networks are made up of units with a linear activation function, which appears to make them unsuitable to represent real neurons with their positive-only firing rates. However, even purely linear units have been considered as provisionally relevant models of real neurons, by assuming that the latter operate sometimes in the linear regime of their transfer function. (This implies a high level of spontaneous activity, and may be closer to conditions observed early on in sensory systems rather than in areas more specifically involved in memory.) As usual, the connections are trained by a Hebb (or similar) associative learning rule. The capacity of these networks can be defined as the total number of associations that can be learned independently of each other, given that the linear nature of these systems prevents anything more than a linear transform of the inputs. This implies that if input pattern C can be written as the weighted sum of input patterns A and B, the output to C will be just the same weighted sum of the outputs to A and B. If there are N' input axons, only at most N' input patterns are all mutually independent (i.e. none can be written as a weighted sum of the others), and therefore the capacity of linear networks, defined above, is just N', or equal to the number of input lines. In general, a random set of less than N' vectors (the CS input pattern vectors) will tend to be mutually independent but not mutually orthogonal (at 90° to each other). If they are not orthogonal (the normal situation), then their dot product is not 0, and the output pattern activated by one of the input vectors will be partially activated by other input pattern vectors, in accordance with how similar they are (see eqns (A.2.5) and (A.2.6)). This amounts to interference, which is therefore the more serious the less orthogonal, on the whole, is the set of input vectors.

Since input patterns are made of elements with positive values, if a simple Hebbian learning rule like the one of eqn (A.2.2) is used (in which the input pattern enters directly with no subtraction term), the output resulting from the application of a stored input vector will be the sum of contributions from all other input vectors that have a non-zero dot product with it (see Rolls and Treves 1998, Appendix A1), and interference will be disastrous. The only situation in which this would not occur is when different input patterns activate completely different input lines, but this is clearly an uninteresting circumstance for networks operating with distributed representations. A solution to this issue is to use a modified learning rule of the following form:

$$\delta w_{ij} = kr_i(r_j' - x) \qquad (A.2.7)$$

where x is a constant, approximately equal to the average value of r_j'. This learning rule includes (in proportion to r_i) increasing the synaptic weight if $(r_j' - x) > 0$ (long-term potentiation), and decreasing the synaptic weight if $(r_j' - x) < 0$ (heterosynaptic long-term depression). It is useful for x to be roughly the average activity of an input axon r_j' across patterns, because then the dot product between the various patterns stored on the weights and the input vector will tend to cancel out with the subtractive term, except for the pattern equal to (or correlated with) the input vector itself. Then up to N' input vectors can still be learned by the network, with only minor interference (provided of course that they are mutually independent, as they will in general tend to be).

This modified learning rule can also be described in terms of a contingency table (Table A.2.1) showing the synaptic strength modifications produced by different types of learning rule, where LTP indicates an increase in synaptic strength (called long-term potentiation in neurophysiology), and LTD indicates a decrease in synaptic strength (called long-term depression in neurophysiology). Heterosynaptic long-term depression is so-called because it is the decrease in synaptic strength that occurs to a synapse which is other than that through which the postsynaptic cell is being activated. This heterosynaptic long-term depression is the type of change of synaptic strength that is required (in addition to LTP) for effective subtraction of the average presynaptic firing rate, in order, as it were, to make

Table A.2.1
Effects of pre- and postsynaptic activity on synaptic modification

	Postsynaptic activation	
Presynaptic firing	**0**	**High**
0	No change	Heterosynaptic LTD
High	Homosynaptic LTD	LTP

the CS vectors appear more orthogonal to the pattern associator (see Rolls, 1996f). The rule is sometimes called the Singer–Stent rule, after work by Singer (1987) and Stent (1973), and was discovered in the brain by Levy (Levy 1985; Levy and Desmond 1985; see Brown *et al.* 1990). Homosynaptic long-term depression is so-called because it is the decrease in synaptic strength that occurs to a synapse which is (the same as that which is) active. For it to occur, the postsynaptic neuron must simultaneously be inactive, or have only low activity. (This rule is sometimes called the BCM rule after the paper of Bienenstock, Cooper and Munro 1982; see Rolls and Treves 1998, Chapter 4, on competitive networks.)

Associative neuronal networks with non-linear neurons

With non-linear neurons, that is with at least a threshold in the activation function so that the output firing r_i is 0 when the activation h_i is below the threshold, the capacity can be measured in terms of the number of different clusters of output pattern vectors that the network produces. This is because the non-linearities now present (one per output unit) result in some clustering of all possible (conditioned stimulus) input patterns $\mathbf{r}'$. Input patterns that are similar to a stored input vector can result due to the non-linearities in output patterns even closer to the stored output; and vice versa sufficiently dissimilar inputs can be assigned to different output clusters thereby increasing their mutual dissimilarity. As with the linear counterpart, in order to remove the correlation that would otherwise occur between the patterns because the elements can take only positive values, it is useful to use a modified Hebb rule

$$\delta w_{ij} = kr_i(r'_j - x)$$

With fully distributed output patterns the number p of associations that leads to different clusters is of order C, the number of input lines (axons) per output unit (that is, of order N' for a fully connected network), as shown in Appendix A3 of Rolls and Treves (1998). If sparse patterns are used in the output, or alternatively if the learning rule includes a non-linear postsynaptic factor that is effectively equivalent to using sparse output patterns, the coefficient of proportionality between p and C can be much higher than unity, that is many more patterns can be stored than inputs per neuron (see Appendix A3 of Rolls and Treves 1998). Indeed, the number of different patterns or prototypes p that can be stored can be derived, for example in the case of binary units (Gardner 1988) to be:

$$p \approx C/[a_0 \log(1/a_0)] \tag{A.2.8}$$

where a_0 is the sparseness of the *output* firing pattern **r** produced by the unconditioned stimulus (see eqn A.1.4). p can in this situation be much larger than C (see Rolls and Treves 1990 and Rolls and Treves 1998, Appendix A3). This is an important result for encoding in pattern associators, for it means that provided the activation functions are non-linear (which is the case with real neurons), there is a very great advantage to using sparse encoding, for then many more than C pattern associations can be stored. Sparse representations may well be present in brain regions involved in associative memory for this reason (see Chapters 6 and 7 of Rolls and Treves 1998).

A.2.4.8 Interference

Interference occurs in linear pattern associators if two vectors are not orthogonal, and is simply dependent on the angle between the originally learned vector and the recall cue or CS vector, for the activation of the output neuron depends simply on the dot product of the recall vector and the synaptic weight vector (eqn (A.2.5)). Also in non-linear pattern associators (the interesting case for all practical purposes), interference might occur if two CS patterns are not orthogonal, though the effect can be controlled with sparse encoding of the UCS patterns, effectively by setting high thresholds for the firing of output units. In other words the CS vectors need not be strictly orthogonal, but if they are too similar, some interference will still be likely to occur.

The fact that interference is a property of neural network pattern associator memories is of interest, for interference is a major property of human memory. Indeed, the fact that interference is a property of human memory and of network association memories is entirely consistent with the hypothesis that human memory is stored in associative memories of the type described here, or at least that network associative memories of the type described represent a useful exemplar of the class of parallel distributed storage network used in human memory. It may also be suggested that one reason that interference is tolerated in biological memory is that it is associated with the ability to generalize between stimuli, which is an invaluable feature of biological network associative memories, in that it allows the memory to cope with stimuli which will almost never on different occasions be identical, and in that it allows useful analogies which have survival value to be made.

A.2.4.9 Expansion recoding

If patterns are too similar to be stored in associative memories, then one solution which the brain seems to use repeatedly is to expand the encoding to a form in which the different stimuli are less correlated, that is more orthogonal, before they are presented as CS stimuli to a pattern associator. The problem can be highlighted by a non-linearly separable mapping (which captures part of the eXclusive OR (XOR) problem), in which the mapping that is desired is as follows. The neuron has two inputs, A and B (see Fig. A.2.9).

Input A	1	0	1
Input B	0	1	1
Required Output	1	1	0

Fig. A.2.9

This is a mapping of patterns that is impossible for a one-layer network, because the patterns are not linearly separable (see Appendix A1 of Rolls and Treves 1998. There is no set of synaptic weights in a one-layer net that could solve the problem shown in Fig. A.2.9. Two classes of patterns are not linearly separable if no hyperplane can be positioned in their *N*-dimensional space so as to separate them, see Appendix A1. The XOR problem has the additional constraint that A = 0, B = 0 must be mapped to Output = 0.) A solution is to re-map the two input lines A and B to three input lines 1–3, that is, to use expansion recoding, as shown in Fig. A.2.10. This can be performed by a

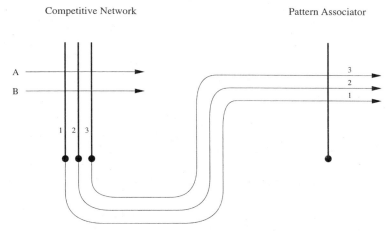

Fig. A.2.10   Expansion recoding. A competitive network followed by a pattern associator that can enable patterns that are not linearly separable to be learned correctly.

competitive network. The synaptic weights on the dendrite of the output neuron could then learn the following values using a simple Hebb rule, eqn (A.2.2), and the problem could be solved as in Fig. A.2.11.

	Synaptic weight
Input 1 (A = 1, B = 0)	1
Input 2 (A = 0, B = 1)	1
Input 3 (A = 1, B = 1)	0

Fig. A.2.11

The whole network would look like that shown in Fig. A.2.10.

Rolls and Treves (1998) show that competitive networks could help with this type of

Table A.2.2
Coding in associative memories*

	Local	Sparse distributed	Fully distributed
Generalization, completion, graceful degradation	No	Yes	Yes
Number of patterns that can be stored	N (large)	of order $C/[a_0 \log(1/a_0)]$ (can be larger)	of order C (usually smaller than N)
Amount of information in each pattern (values if binary)	Minimal ($\log(N)$ bits)	Intermediate ($Na_0 \log(1/a_0)$ bits)	Large (N bits)

*N refers here to the number of output units, and C to the average number of inputs to each output unit. a_0 is the sparseness of output patterns, or roughly the proportion of output units activated by a UCS pattern. Note: logs are to the base 2.

recoding, and could provide very useful preprocessing for a pattern associator in the brain. It is possible that the lateral nucleus of the amygdala performs this function, for it receives inputs from the temporal cortical visual areas, and may preprocess them before they become the inputs to associative networks at the next stage of amygdala processing (see Fig. 4.12).

A.2.4.10 Implications of different types of coding on storage in pattern associators

Throughout this section, we have made statements about how the properties of pattern associators, such as the number of patterns that can be stored, and whether generalization and graceful degradation occur, depend on the type of encoding of the patterns to be associated. (The types of encoding considered, local, sparse distributed, and fully distributed, are described in Section A.1.) We draw together these points in Table A.2.2. The amount of information that can be stored in each pattern in a pattern associator is considered in Rolls and Treves (1998), Appendix A3, and some of the relevant information theory itself is described in Appendix A2 of Rolls and Treves (1998).

A.3 Reinforcement learning

In **supervised networks**, an error signal is provided for each output neuron in the network, and whenever an input to the network is provided, the error signals specify the *magnitude and direction* of the error in the output produced by each neuron. These error signals are then used to correct the synaptic weights in the network in such a way that the output errors for each input pattern to be learned gradually diminish over trials. These networks have an architecture which might be similar to that of the pattern associator shown in Fig. A.2.1, except that instead of an unconditioned stimulus, there is an error input provided for each neuron. Such a network trained by an error-correcting (or delta) rule is known as a one-layer perceptron. The architecture is not very plausible for most brain regions, in that it is not clear how an individual error signal could be computed for each of thousands of neurons in a network, and fed into each neuron as its error signal and then used in a delta rule synaptic correction (see Rolls and Treves 1998, Chapter 5). The architecture can be generalized to a multilayer feedforward architecture with many layers between the input and output (Rumelhart, Hinton and Williams 1986), but the learning is very non-local and rather biologically implausible (see Rolls and Treves 1998, Chapter 5), in that an error term (magnitude and direction) for each neuron in the network must be computed from the errors and synaptic weights of all subsequent neurons in the network that any neuron influences, usually on a trial-by-trial basis, by a process known as error backpropagation. Thus although computationally powerful, an issue with perceptrons and multilayer perceptrons that makes them generally biologically implausible for many brain regions is that a separate error signal must be supplied for each output neuron, and that with multilayer perceptrons, computed error backpropagation must occur.

When operating in an environment, usually a simple binary or scalar signal representing success or failure of the whole network or organism is received. This is usually response-dependent feedback which provides a single evaluative measure of the success or failure. Evaluative feedback tells the learner whether or not, and possibly by how much, its behaviour has improved; or it provides a measure of the 'goodness' of the behaviour. Evaluative feedback does not directly tell the learner what it should have done, and although it may provide an index of the degree (i.e. magnitude) of success, it does not include directional information telling the learner how to change its behaviour towards a target, as does error-correction learning (see Barto 1995). Partly for this reason, there has been some interest in networks that can be taught with such a *single reinforcement signal*. In this section, one such approach to such networks is described. It is noted that such networks are classified as reinforcement networks in which there is a single teacher, and that these networks attempt to perform an optimal mapping between an input vector and an output neuron or set of neurons. They thus solve the same class of problems as single and (if multilayer) multilayer perceptrons. They should be distinguished from pattern-association networks in the brain, which might learn associations between previously neutral stimuli and primary reinforcers such as taste (signals which might be interpreted appropriately by a subsequent part of the brain), but do not attempt to produce arbitrary mappings between an input and an output, using a single reinforcement signal. A class of problems to which such reinforcement networks might be applied are motor-control problems. It was to such a problem that Barto and Sutton (Barto 1985; Sutton and Barto 1981) applied their reinforcement learning algorithm known as the associative reward-penalty algorithm.

A.3.1 Associative reward-penalty algorithm of Barto and Sutton

The terminology of Barto and Sutton is followed here (see Barto 1985).

A.3.1.1 Architecture

The architecture, shown in Fig. A.3.1, uses a single reinforcement signal, r, $= +1$ for

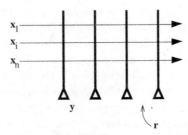

Fig. A.3.1 A network trained by a single reinforcement input r. The inputs to each neuron are in the terminology used by Barto and Sutton x_i, $i=1$, n; and y is the output of one of the output neurons.

reward, and -1 for penalty. The inputs x_i take real (continuous) values. The output of a neuron, y, is binary, $+1$ or -1. The weights on the output neuron are designated w_i.

A.3.1.2 Operation

1 An input vector is applied to the network, and produces output activation, s, in the normal way as follows:

$$s = \sum w_i x_i$$

where x_i is the firing of the input axon i.

2 The output is calculated from the activation with a noise term η included. The principle of the network is that if the added noise on a particular trial helps performance, then whatever change it leads to should be incorporated into the synaptic weights, in such a way that the next time that input occurs, the performance is improved.

$$\text{Output } y = +1 \text{ if } s + \eta > 0$$
$$= -1 \text{ else}$$

where $\eta =$ noise added on each trial.

3 Learning rule. The weights are changed as follows:

$$\delta w_i = \rho(y - E[y\,|\,s])x_i \qquad \text{if } r = +1$$
$$\delta w_i = \rho\lambda(-y - E[y\,|\,s])x_i \qquad \text{if } r = -1.$$

ρ and λ are learning rate-constants. (They are set so that the learning rate is higher when positive reinforcement is received than when negative reinforcement is received.) $E[y\,|\,s]$ is the expectation of y given s (usually a sigmoidal function of s with the range ± 1). $E[y\,|\,s]$ is a (continuously varying) indication of how the unit usually responds to the current input pattern, i.e. if the actual output y is larger than normally expected, by computing $s = \sum w_i x_i$, because of the noise term, and the reinforcement is $+1$, increase the weight from x_i; and vice versa. The expectation could be the prediction generated before the noise term is incorporated.

This network combines an associative capacity with its properties of generalization and graceful degradation, with a single 'critic' or error signal for the whole network (Barto 1985). The network can solve difficult problems (such as balancing a pole by moving a trolley which supports the pole from side to side, as the pole starts to topple). Although described for single-layer networks, the algorithm can be applied to multilayer networks. The learning rate is very slow, for there is a single reinforcement signal on each trial for the whole network, not a separate error signal for each neuron in the network.

An important advance in the area of reinforcement learning was the introduction of algorithms that allow for learning to occur when the reinforcement is delayed or received over a number of time steps. A solution to this problem is the addition of an **adaptive critic** that learns through a **time difference (TD) algorithm** how to predict the future value of the reinforcer. The time difference algorithm takes into account not only the current reinforcement just received, but also a temporally weighted average of errors in predicting future reinforcements. The temporal difference error is the error by which any two temporally adjacent error predictions are inconsistent (see Barto 1995). The output of the critic is used as an effective reinforcer instead of the instantaneous reinforcement being received (see Sutton and Barto 1990; Barto 1995). This is a solution to the temporal credit assignment problem. The algorithm has been applied to modelling the time course of classical conditioning (Sutton and Barto 1990). The algorithm effectively allows the future reinforcement predicted from past history to influence the responses made, and in this sense allows behaviour to be guided not just by immediate reinforcement, but also by 'anticipated' reinforcements.

The reinforcement-learning algorithm is certainly a move towards biological relevance, in that learning with a single reinforcer can be achieved. That single reinforcer might be broadcast throughout the system by a general projection system, such as the dopamine pathways in the brain, which distribute to large parts of the striatum and the prefrontal cortex. It is not clear yet how a biological system might store the expected output $E[y|s]$ for comparison with the actual output when noise has been added, and might take into account the sign and magnitude of the noise. Nevertheless, this is an interesting algorithm.

References

Abbott, L. F., Rolls, E. T., and Tovee, M. J. (1996). Representational capacity of face coding in monkeys. *Cerebral Cortex*, **6**, 498–505.

Abbott, L. F., Varela, J. A., Sen, K., and Nelson, S. B. (1997). Synaptic depression and cortical gain control. *Science*, **275**, 220–4.

Abercrombie, E. D., Keefe, K. A., DiFrischia, D. S., and Zigmond, M. J. (1989). Differential effect of stress on in vivo dopamine release in striatum, nucleus accumbens, and medial frontal cortex. *Journal of Neurochemistry*, **52**, 1655–8.

Adams, J. E. (1976). Naloxone reversal of analgesia produced by brain stimulation in the human. *Pain*, **2**, 161–6.

Adelmann, P. K. and Zajonc, R. B. (1989). Facial efference and the experience of emotion. *Annual Review of Psychology*, **40**, 249–80.

Adolphs, R., Tranel, D., Damasio, H., and Damasio, A. (1994). Impaired recognition of emotion in facial expressions following bilateral damage to the human amygdala. *Nature*, **372**, 669–72.

Adolphs, R., Tranel, D., Damasio, H., and Damasio, A. R. (1995). Fear and the human amygdala. *Journal of Neuroscience*, **15**, 5879–91.

Aggleton, J. P. (1992). The functional effects of amygdala lesions in humans, a comparison with findings from monkeys. In *The amygdala*, (ed. J. P. Aggleton), Chapter 19, pp. 485–503. Wiley–Liss, New York.

Aggleton, J. P. and Passingham, R. E. (1981). Syndrome produced by lesions of the amygdala in monkeys (*Macaca mulatta*). *Journal of Comparative Physiology and Psychology*, **95**, 961–77.

Aggleton, J. P. and Passingham, R. E. (1982). An assessment of the reinforcing properties of foods after amygdaloid lesions in rhesus monkeys. *Journal of Comparative Physiology and Psychology*, **96**, 71–7.

Aggleton, J. P., Burton, M. J., and Passingham, R. E. (1980). Cortical and subcortical afferents to the amygdala in the rhesus monkey (*Macaca mulatta*). *Brain Research*, **190**, 347–68.

Aigner, T. G., Mitchell, S. J., Aggleton, J. P., DeLong, M. R., Struble, R. G., Price, D. L., *et al.* (1991). Transient impairment of recognition memory following ibotenic acid lesions of the basal forebrain in macaques. *Experimental Brain Research*, **86**, 18–26.

Akert, K., Gruesen, R. A., Woolsey, C. N., and Meyer, D. R. (1961). Kluver–Bucy syndrome in monkeys with neocortical ablations of temporal lobe. *Brain*, **84**, 480–98.

Akil, H., Mayer, D. J., and Liebeskind, J. C. (1976). Antagonism of stimulation-produced analgesia by naloxone, a narcotic antagonist. *Science*, **191**, 961–2.

Alexander, G. E., Crutcher, M. D., and DeLong, M. R. (1990). Basal ganglia thalamo-cortical circuits: parallel substrates for motor, oculomotor, 'prefrontal' and 'limbic' functions. *Progress in Brain Research*, **85**, 119–46.

Alexander, R. D. (1975). The search for a general theory of behavior. *Behavioral Sciences*, **20**, 77–100.

Alexander, R. D. (1979). Darwinism and human affairs. University of Washington Press, Seattle.

Allport, A. (1988). What concept of consciousness? In *Consciousness in contemporary science* (ed. A. J. Marcel and E. Bisiach) pp. 159–82, Oxford University Press.

Amaral, D. G. and Price, J. L. (1984). Amygdalo-cortical projections in the monkey (*Macaca fascicularis*). *Journal of Comparative Neurology*, **230**, 465–96.

Amaral, D. G., Price, J. L., Pitkanen, A., and Carmichael, S. T. (1992). Anatomical organization of the primate amygdaloid complex. In *The Amygdala*, (ed. J. P. Aggleton), Chapter 1, pp. 1–66. Wiley–Liss, New York.

Amsel, A. (1958). The role of frustrative non-reward in non-continuous reward situations. *Psychological Bulletin*, **55**, 102–19.

Amsel, A. (1962). Frustrative non-reward in partial reinforcement and discrimination learning: some recent history and a theoretical extension. *Psychological Review*, **69**, 306–28.

Anderson, M.E. (1978). Discharge patterns of basal ganglia neurons during active maintenance of postural stability and adjustment to chair tilt. *Brain Research*, **143**, 325–38.

Anand, B. K. and Brobeck, J. R. (1951). Localization of a feeding center in the hypothalamus of the rat. *Proceedings of the Society for Experimental Biology and Medicine*, **77**, 323–4.

Antelman, S. M. and Szechtman, H. (1975). Tail pinch induces eating in sated rats which appears to depend on nigrostriatal dopamine. *Science*, **189**, 731–3.

Aou, S., Oomura, Y, Lenard, L., Nishino, H., Inokuchi, A., Minami, T., and *et al.* (1984). Behavioral significance of monkey hypothalamic glucose-sensitive neurons. *Brain Research*, **302**, 69–74.

Apanius, V., Penn, D., Slev, P. R., Ruff, L. R., and Potts, W. K. (1997). The nature of selection on the major histocompatibility complex. *Critical Reviews in Immunology*, **17**, 179–224.

Armstrong, D. M. and Malcolm, N. (1984). *Consciousness and causality*. Blackwell, Oxford.

Artola, A. and Singer, W. (1993). Long-term depression: related mechanisms in cerebellum, neocortex and hippocampus. In *Synaptic plasticity: molecular, cellular and functional aspects*, (ed. M. Baudry, R. F. Thompson, and J. L. Davis), Chapter 7, pp. 129–46. MIT Press, Cambridge, MA.

Baker, R. (1996). *Sperm wars*. Fourth Estate, London.

Baker, R. and Bellis, M. (1995). *Human sperm competition: copulation, competition and infidelity*. Chapman and Hall, London.

Balkenius, C. (1995). Natural intelligence in artificial creatures. Lund University Studies (37), Lund, Sweden.

Barbas, H. (1988). Anatomic organization of basoventral and mediodorsal visual recipient prefrontal regions in the rhesus monkey. *Journal of Comparative Neurology*, **276**, 313–42.

Barbas, H. (1993). Organization of cortical afferent input to the orbitofrontal area in the rhesus monkey. *Neuroscience*, **56**, 841–64.

Barbas, H. (1995). Anatomic basis of cognitive–emotional interactions in the primate prefrontal cortex. *Neuroscience and Biobehavioral Reviews*, **19**, 499–510.

Barbas, H. and Pandya, D. N. (1989). Architecture and intrinsic connections of the prefrontal cortex in the rhesus monkey. *Journal of Comparative Neurology*, **286**, 353–75.

Barlow, H. B. (1972). Single units and sensation: A neuron doctrine for perceptual psychology. *Perception*, **1**, 371–94.

Barlow, H. (1995). The neuron doctrine in perception. In *The cognitive neurosciences*, (ed. M. S. Gazzaniga), Chapter 26, pp. 415–35. MIT Press, Cambridge, MA.

Barlow, H. B. (1997). Single neurons, communal goals, and consciousness. In *Cognition, computation, and consciousness*, (ed. M. Ito, Y. Miyashita, and E. T. Rolls), Chapter 7, pp. 121–36. Oxford University Press.

Barto, A. G. (1985). Learning by statistical cooperation of self-interested neuron-like computing elements (COINS Tech. Rep. 85-11). University of Massachusetts, Department of Computer and Information Science, Amherst.

Barto, A. G. (1995). Adaptive critics and the basal ganglia. In *Models of information processing in the basal ganglia*, (ed. J. C. Houk, J. L. Davis, and D. G. Beiser), Chapter 11, pp. 215–32. MIT Press, Cambridge, MA.

Baum, M. J., Everitt, B. J., Herbert, J., and Keverne, E. B. (1977). Hormonal basis of proceptivity and receptivity in female primates. *Archives of Sexual Behavior*, **6**, 173–92.

Baylis, G. C., and Rolls, E. T. (1987). Responses of neurons in the inferior temporal cortex in short term and serial recognition memory tasks. *Experimental Brain Research*, **65**, 614–22.

Baylis, G. C., Rolls, E. T., and Leonard, C. M. (1985). Selectivity between faces in the responses of a population of neurons in the cortex in the superior temporal sulcus of the monkey. *Brain Research*, **342**, 91–102.

Baylis, G. C., Rolls, E. T., and Leonard, C. M. (1987). Functional subdivisions of temporal lobe neocortex. *Journal of Neuroscience*, **7**, 330–42.

Baylis, L. L. and Gaffan, D. (1991). Amygdalectomy and ventromedial prefrontal ablation produce similar deficits in food choice and in simple object discrimination learning for an unseen reward. *Experimental Brain Research*, **86**, 617–22.

Baylis, L. L. and Rolls, E. T. (1991). Responses of neurons in the primate taste cortex to glutamate. *Physiology and Behavior*, **49**, 973–9.

Baylis, L. L., Rolls, E. T., and Baylis, G. C. (1994). Afferent connections of the orbitofrontal cortex taste area of the primate. *Neuroscience*, **64**, 801–12.

Bear, M. F. and Singer, W. (1986). Modulation of visual cortical plasticity by acetylcholine and noradrenaline. *Nature*, **320**, 172–6.

Bechara, A., Damasio, A. R., Damasio, H., and Anderson, S. W. (1994). Insensitivity to future consequences following damage to human prefrontal cortex. *Cognition*, **50**, 7–15.

Bechara, A., Tranel, D., Damasio, H., and Damasio, A. R. (1996). Failure to respond autonomically to anticipated future outcomes following damage to prefrontal cortex. *Cerebral Cortex*, **6**, 215–25.

Bechara, A., Damasio, H., Tranel, D., and Damasio, A. R. (1997). Deciding advantageously before knowing the advantageous strategy. *Science*, **275**, 1293–5.

Beckstead, R. M. and Norgren, R. (1979). An autoradiographic examination of the central distribution of the trigeminal, facial, glossopharyngeal, and vagal nerves in the monkey. *Journal of Comparative Neurology*, **184**, 455–72.

Beckstead, R. M., Morse, J. R., and Norgren, R. (1980). The nucleus of the solitary tract in the monkey: projections to the thalamus and brainstem nuclei. *Journal of Comparative Neurology*, **190**, 259–82.

Beluzzi, J. D., Grant, N., Garsky, V., Sarantakis, D., Wise, C. D., and Stein, L. (1976). Analgesia induced in vivo by central administration of enkephalin in rat. *Nature*, **260**, 625–6.

Berliner, D. L., Monti-Bloch, L., Jennings-White, C., and Diaz-Sanchez, V. (1996). The functionality of the human vomeronasal organ (VNO): evidence for steroid receptors. *Journal of Steroid Biochemistry and Molecular Biology*, **58**, 259–65.

Bermond, B., Fasotti, L., Niewenhuyse, B., and Schuerman, J. (1991). Spinal cord lesions, peripheral feedback and intensities of emotional feelings. *Cognition and Emotion*, **5**, 201–20.

Berridge, K. C., Flynn, F. W., Schulkin, J. and Grill, H. J. (1984). Sodium depletion enhances salt palatability in rats. *Behavioral Neuroscience*, **98**, 652–60.

Betzig, L. (ed.) (1997). Human nature: a critical reader. Oxford University Press, New York.

Bienenstock, E. L., Cooper, L. N., and Munro, P. W. (1982). Theory for the development of neuron selectivity: orientation specificity and binocular interaction in visual cortex. *Journal of Neuroscience*, **2**, 32–48.

Birkhead, T. R. and Moller, A. P. (1992). Sperm competition in birds. Academic Press, London.

Bishop, M. P., Elder, S. T., and Heath, R. G. (1963). Intracranial self-stimulation in man. *Science*, **140**, 394–5.

Bjorklund, A. and Lindvall, O. (1986). Catecholaminergic brainstem regulatory systems. In *Handbook of physiology: the nervous system, Vol. 4, Intrinsic systems of the brain*, (ed. V. B. Mountcastle, F. E. Bloom, and S. R. Geiger), pp. 155–236. American Physiological Society, Bethesda.

Blaney, P. H. (1986). Affect and memory: a review. *Psychological Bulletin*, **99**, 229–46.

Blass, E. M. and Epstein, A. N. (1971). A lateral preoptic osmosensitive zone for thirst in the rat. *Journal of Comparative and Physiological Psychology*, **76**, 378–94.

Bliss, T. V. P. and Collingridge, G. L. (1993). A synaptic model of memory: long-term potentiation in the hippocampus. *Nature*, **361**, 31–9.

Block, N. (1995). On a confusion about a function of consciousness. *Behavioral and Brain Sciences*, **18**, 227–47.

Boden, M. A. (ed.) (1996). The Philosophy of Artificial Life. Oxford University Press.

Booth, D. A. (1985). Food-conditioned eating preferences and aversions with interoceptive elements: learned appetites and satieties. *Annals of the New York Academy of Sciences*, **443**, 22–37.

Booth, M. C. A. and Rolls, E. T. (1998). View-invariant representations of familiar objects by neurons in the inferior temporal visual cortex. *Cerebral Cortex*, in press.

Borsini, F. and Rolls, E. T. (1984). Role of noradrenaline and serotonin in the basolateral region of the amygdala in food preferences and learned taste aversions in the rat. *Physiology and Behavior*, **33**, 37–43.

Boussaoud, D., Desimone, R., and Ungerleider, L. G. (1991). Visual topography of area TEO in the macaque, *Journal of Computational Neurology*, **306**, 554–75.

Boyd, E. S. and Gardner, L. C. (1967). Effect of some brain lesions on intracranial self-stimulation in the rat. *American Journal of Physiology*, **213**, 1044–52.

Bray, G. A., Inoue, S., and Nishizawa, Y. (1981). Hypothalamic obesity: the autonomic hypothesis and the lateral hypothalamus. *Diabetologia*, **20** (Suppl.), 366–78.

Brothers, L. and Ring, B. (1993). Mesial temporal neurons in the macaque monkey with responses selective for aspects of social stimuli. *Behavioural Brain Research*, **57**, 53–61.

Brown, T. H., Kairiss, E. W., and Keenan, C. L. (1990). Hebbian synapses: biophysical mechanisms and algorithms. *Annual Review of Neuroscience*, **13**, 475–511.

Buck, L. and Axel, R. (1991). A novel multigene family may encode odorant receptors: a molecular basis for odor recognition. *Cell*, **65**, 175–87.

Buggy, J. and Johnson, A. (1977a). Anteroventral third ventricle periventricular ablation: temporary adipsia and persisting thirst deficits. *Neuroscience Letters*, **5**, 177–82.

Buggy, J. and Johnson, A. (1977b). Preoptic–hypothalamic periventricular lesions: thirst deficits and hypernatremia. *American Journal of Physiology*, **23**, R44–R52.

Bunney, B. S. and Aghajanian, G. K. (1976). Dopamine and norepinephrine innervated cells in the rat prefrontal cortex: pharmacological differentiation using micro-iontophoretic techniques. *Life Sciences*, **19**, 1783–92.

Burton, M. J., Rolls, E. T., and Mora, F. (1976a). Visual responses of hypothalamic neurones. *Brain Research*, **107**, 215–16.

Burton, M. J., Rolls, E. T., and Mora, F. (1976b). Effects of hunger on the responses of neurones in the lateral hypothalamus to the sight and taste of food. *Experimental Neurology*, **51**, 668–77.

Buss, D. M. (1989). Sex differences in human mate preferences: evolutionary hypotheses tested in 37 cultures. *Behavioural and Brain Sciences*, **12**, 1–14. (Reprinted in Betzig, L. (ed.) (1997). Human nature: a critical reader. Oxford University Press, New York.)

Butter, C. M. (1969). Perseveration in extinction and in discrimination reversal tasks following selective prefrontal ablations in *Macaca mulatta*. *Physiology and Behavior*, **4**, 163–71.

Butter, C. M. and Snyder, D. R. (1972). Alterations in aversive and aggressive behaviors following orbitofrontal lesions in rhesus monkeys. *Acta Neurobiologica Experimentalis*, **32**, 525–65.

Butter, C. M., McDonald, J. A., and Snyder, D. R. (1969). Orality, preference behavior, and reinforcement value of non-food objects in monkeys with orbital frontal lesions. *Science*, **164**, 1306–7.

Butter, C. M., Snyder, D. R., and McDonald, J. A. (1970). Effects of orbitofrontal lesions on aversive and aggressive behaviors in rhesus monkeys. *Journal of Comparative Physiology and Psychology*, **72**, 132–44.

Caan, W., Perrett, D. I., and Rolls, E. T. (1984). Responses of striatal neurons in the behaving monkey. 2. Visual processing in the caudal neostriatum. *Brain Research*, **290**, 53–65.

Cabanac, M. (1971). Physiological role of pleasure. *Science*, **173**, 1103–7.

Cabanac, M. and Duclaux, R. (1970). Specificity of internal signals in producing satiety for taste stimuli. *Nature*, **227**, 966–7.

Cabanac, M. and Fantino, M. (1977). Origin of olfacto–gustatory alliesthesia: Intestinal sensitivity to carbohydrate concentration? *Physiology and Behavior*, **10**, 1039–45.

Cacioppo, J. T., Klein, D. J., Berntson, G. C., and Hatfield, E. (1993). The psychophysiology of emotion. In *Handbook of Emotions*, (ed. M. Lewis and J. M. Hatfield), pp. 119–42. Guilford, New York.

Cador, M., Robbins, T. W., and Everitt, B. J. (1989). Involvement of the amygdala in stimulus–reward associations: interaction with the ventral striatum. *Neuroscience*, **30**, 77–86.

Caggiula, A. R. (1970). Analysis of the copulation–reward properties of posterior hypothalamic stimulation in male rats. *Journal of Comparative and Physiological Psychology*, **70**, 399–412.

Calabresi, P., Maj, R., Pisani, A., Mercuri, N. B., and Bernardi, G (1992). Long-term synaptic depression in the striatum: physiological and pharmacological characterization. *Journal of Neuroscience*, **12**, 4224–33.

Campfield, L. A. and Smith, F. J. (1990). Systemic factors in the control of food intake: evidence for patterns as signals. In *Handbook of Behavioral Neurobiology, Vol. 10. Neurobiology of Food and Fluid Intake*, (ed. E. M. Stricker). Plenum, New York.

Campfield, L. A., Smith, F. J., Guisez, Y., Devos, R., and Burn, P. (1995). Recombinant mouse OB protein: evidence for a peripheral signal linking adiposity and central neural networks. *Science*, **269**, 546–9.

Cannon, W. B. (1927). The James–Lange theory of emotion: a critical examination and an alternative theory. *American Journal of Psychology*, **39**, 106–24.

Cannon, W. B. (1929). *Bodily changes in pain, hunger, fear and rage*, (2nd edn). Appleton, New York.

Cannon, W. B. (1931). Again the James–Lange theory of emotion: a critical examination and an alternative theory. *Psychological Review*, **38**, 281–95.

Carlson, N. R. (1994). *Physiology of behavior*, (5th edn). Allyn and Bacon, Boston.

Carmichael, S. T. and Price, J. L. (1994). Architectonic subdivision of the orbital and medial prefrontal cortex in the macaque monkey. *Journal of Comparative Neurology*, **346**, 366–402.

Carmichael, S. T. and Price, J. L. (1995a). Limbic connections of the orbital and medial prefrontal cortex in macaque monkeys. *Journal of Comparative Neurology*, **363**, 615–41.

Carmichael, S. T. and Price, J. L. (1995b). Sensory and premotor connections of the orbital and medial prefrontal cortex of macaque monkeys. *Journal of Comparative Neurology*, **363**, 642–64.

Carmichael, S. T., Clugnet, M.-C., and Price, J. L. (1994). Central olfactory connections in the macaque monkey. *Journal of Comparative Neurology*, **346**, 403–34.

Carruthers, P (1996). *Language, thought and consciousness*. Cambridge University Press.

Chalmers, D. J. (1996). *The conscious mind*. Oxford University Press.

Chaudhari, N., Yang, H., Lamp, C., Delay, E., Cartford, C. Than, T., and Roper,S. (1996). The taste of monosodium glutamate: membrane receptors in taste buds. *Journal of Neuroscience*, **16**, 3817–26.

Cheney, D. L. and Seyfarth, R. M. (1990). *How monkeys see the world*. University of Chicago Press.

Christie, B. R. (1996). Long-term depression in the hippocampus. *Hippocampus*, **6**, 1–2.

Clark, J. M., Clark, A. J. M., Bartle, A., and Winn, P. (1991). The regulation of feeding and drinking in rats with lesions of the lateral hypothalamus made by N-methyl-D-aspartate. *Neuroscience*, **45**, 631–40.

Clavier, R. M. (1976). Brain stem self-stimulation: catecholamine or non-catecholamine mediation? In *Brain-stimulation reward*, (ed. A. Wauquier and E. T. Rolls), pp. 239–50. North-Holland, Amsterdam.

Clavier, R. M. and Routtenberg, A. (1976). Brain stem self-stimulation attenuated by lesions of medial forebrain bundle but not by lesions of locus coeruleus or the caudal ventral norepinephrine bundle. *Brain Research*, **101**, 251–71.

Coghill, R. C., Talbot, J. D., Evans, A. C., Meyer, E., Gjedde, A., Bushnell, M. C., *et al.* (1994) Distributed processing of pain and vibration by the human brain. *Journal of Neuroscience*, **14**, 4095–108.

Collingridge, G. L. and Bliss, T. V. P. (1987). NMDA receptors: their role in long-term potentiation. *Trends in Neurosciences*, **10**, 288–93.

Cooper, J. R., Bloom, F. E., and Roth, R. H. (1996). *The biochemical basis of neuropharmacology*, (7th edn). Oxford University Press.

Cowley, J. J. and Brooksbank, B. W. L. (1991). Human exposure to putative pheromones and changes in aspects of social behaviour. *Journal of Steroid Biochemistry and Molecular Biology*, **39**, 647–59.

Craig, A. D., Reiman, E. M., Evans, A., Bushnell, M. C. *et al.* (1996). Functional imaging of an illusion of pain. *Nature*, **384**, 258–60.

Crick, F. H. C. and Koch, C. (1990). Towards a neurobiological theory of consciousness. *Seminars in the Neurosciences*, **2**, 263–75.

Critchley, H. D. and Rolls, E. T. (1996a). Olfactory neuronal responses in the primate orbitofrontal cortex: analysis in an olfactory discrimination task. *Journal of Neurophysiology*, **75**, 1659–72.

Critchley, H. D. and Rolls, E. T. (1996b). Hunger and satiety modify the responses of olfactory and visual neurons in the primate orbitofrontal cortex. *Journal of Neurophysiology*, **75**, 1673–1686.

Critchley, H. D. and Rolls, E. T. (1996c). Responses of primate taste cortex neurons to the astringent tastant tannic acid. *Chemical Senses*, **21**, 135–45.

Crow, T. J. (1976). Specific monoamine systems as reward pathways. In *Brain-stimulation reward*, (ed. A. Wauquier and E. T. Rolls), pp. 211–38. North-Holland, Amsterdam.

Crow, T. J., Spear, P. J., and Arbuthnott, G. W. (1972). Intracranial self-stimulation with electrodes in the region of the locus coeruleus. *Brain Research*, **36**, 275–87.

Crutcher, M. D. and DeLong, M. R. (1984a). Single cell studies of the primate putamen. I. Functional organization. *Experimental Brain Research*, **53**, 233–43.

Crutcher, M. D. and DeLong, M. R. (1984b). Single cell studies of the primate putamen. II. Relations to direction of movements and pattern of muscular activity. *Experimental Brain Research*, **53**, 244–58.

Dahlström, A. and Fuxe, K. (1965). Evidence for the existence of monoamine-containing neurons in the central nervous system: I, Demonstration of monoamines in the cell bodies of brain stem neurons. *Acta Physiologia Scandinavica*, **62**, Suppl. 232, 1–55.

Damasio, A. R. (1994). *Descartes' error*. Putnam, New York.

Darwin, C. (1872). *The expression of the emotions in man and animals*. University of Chicago Press. [(1998) (3rd edn), (ed. P. Ekman). Harper Collins, Glasgow.]

Davidson, R. J. (1992). Anterior cerebral asymmetry and the nature of emotion. *Brain and Cognition*, **6**, 245–68.

Davidson, R. J., Ekman, P., Saron, C., Senulis, J., and Friesen, W. V. (1990). Approach/withdrawal and cerebral asymmetry. *Journal of Personality and Social Research*, **58**, 330–41.

Davis, M. (1992). The role of the amygdala in conditioned fear. In *The amygdala*, (ed. J. P. Aggleton), Chapter 9, pp. 255–305. Wiley–Liss, New York.

Davis, M. (1994). The role of the amygdala in emotional learning. *International Review of Neurobiology*, **36**, 225–66.

Davis, M., Campeau, S., Kim, M., and Falls, W. A. (1995). Neural systems and emotion: the amygdala's role in fear and anxiety. In *Brain and memory: modulation and mediation of neuroplasticity*, (ed. J. L. McGaugh, N. M. Weinberger, and G. Lynch). Oxford University Press, New York.

Dawkins, M. S. (1993). *Through our eyes only? The search for animal consciousness*. Freeman, Oxford.

Dawkins, M. S. (1986). *Unravelling animal behaviour*. Longman, Harlow.

Dawkins, M. S. (1995). *Unravelling animal behaviour*, (2nd edn). Longman, Harlow. (Optimality. Chapter 2, pp. 21–36; Inclusive fitness, Chapter 6.)

Dawkins, R. (1986). *The blind watchmaker*. Longman, Harlow.

Dawkins, R. (1989). *The selfish gene*, (2nd edn). Oxford University Press.

Delgado, J. M. R. (1976). New orientations in brain stimulation in man. In *Brain-stimulation reward*, (ed. A. Wauquier and E. T. Rolls), pp. 481–504. North-Holland, Amsterdam.

DeLong, M. R., Georgopoulos, A. P., Crutcher, M. D., Mitchell, S. J., Richardson, R. T., and Alexander, G. E. (1984). Functional organization of the basal ganglia: contributions of single-cell recording studies. In *Functions of the basal ganglia*, Ciba Foundation Symposium 107, pp. 64–78. Pitman, London.

Dennett, D. C. (1991). *Consciousness explained*. Penguin, London.

Derbyshire, S. W. G., Vogt, B. A., and Jones, A. K. P. (1998). Pain and Stroop interference tasks activate separate processing modules in anterior cingulate cortex. *Experimental Brain Research*, **118**, 52–60.

Deutsch, J. A. and Di Cara, L. (1967). Hunger and extinction in intracranial self-stimulation. *Journal of Comparative and Physiological Psychology*, **63**, 344–7.

DiChiara, G., Acquas, E., and Carboni, E. (1992). Drug motivation and abuse: a neurobiological perspective. *Annals of the New York Academy of Sciences*, **654**, 207–19.

Dickinson, A. (1980). *Contemporary animal learning theory*. Cambridge University Press.

Divac, I. (1975). Magnocellular nuclei of the basal forebrain project to neocortex, brain stem, and olfactory bulb. Review of some functional correlates. *Brain Research*, **93**, 385–98.

Divac, I. and Oberg, R. G. E. (1979). Current conceptions of neostriatal functions. In *The neostriatum*, (ed. I. Divac and R. G. E. Oberg), pp. 215–230. Pergamon, New York.

Divac, I., Rosvold, H. E., Szwarcbart, M. K. (1967). Behavioral effects of selective ablation of the caudate nucleus. *Journal of Comparative and Physiological Psychology*, **63**, 184–90.

Dolan, R. J. (1997). Mood disorders and abnormal cingulate cortex. *Trends in Cognitive Sciences*, **1**, 283–4.

Dolan, R. J., Bench, C. J., Brown, R. G., Scott, L. C., Friston, K. J. and Frackowiak, C. S. (1992). Regional cerebral blood flow abnormalities in depressed patients with cognitive impairment. *Journal of Neurology, Neurosurgery, and Psychiatry*, **55**, 768–73.

Drevets, W. C. and Raichle, M. E. (1992). Neuroanatomical circuits in depression: implications for treatment mechanisms. *Psychopharmacology Bulletin*, **28**, 261–74.

Drevets, W. C., Price, J. L., Simpson, J. R. Jr, Todd, R. D., Reich, T., Vannier, M., *et al.* (1997). Subgenual prefrontal cortex abnormalities in mood disorders. *Nature*, **386**, 824–7.

Dunbar, R. (1996). *Grooming, gossip, and the evolution of language*. Faber and Faber, London.

Dunn, L. T. and Everitt, B. J. (1988). Double dissociations of the effects of amygdala and insular cortex lesions on conditioned taste aversion, passive avoidance, and neophobia in the rat using the excitotoxin ibotenic acid. *Behavioral Neuroscience*, **102**, 3–23.

Dunnett, S. B. and Iversen, S. D. (1981). Learning impairments following selective kainic acid-induced lesions within the neostriatum of rats. *Behavioural Brain Research*, **2**, 189–209.

Dunnett, S. B. and Iversen, S. D. (1982a). Sensorimotor impairments following localised kainic acid and 6-hydroxydopamine lesions of the neostriatum. *Brain Research*, **248**, 121–7.

Dunnett, S. B. and Iversen, S. D. (1982b). Neurotoxic lesions of ventrolateral but not anteromedial neostriatum impair differential reinforcement of low rates (DRL) performance. *Behavioural Brain Research*, **6**, 213–26.

Dunnett, S. B., Lane, D. M., and Winn, P. (1985). Ibotenic acid lesions of the lateral hypothalamus: comparison with 6-hydroxydopamine-induced sensorimotor deficits. *Neuroscience*, **14**, 509–18.

Edmonds, D. E. and Gallistel, C. R. (1977). Reward vs. performance in self-stimulation: electrode-specific effects of AMPT on reward. *Journal of Comparative and Physiological Psychology*, **91**, 962–74.

Eggert, F., Holler, C., Luszyk, D., Muller-Ruchholtz, W., and Ferstl, R. (1996). MHC-associated and MHC-independent urinary chemosignals in mice. *Physiology and Behavior*, **59**, 57–62.

Ekman, P., Levenson, R. W., and Friesen, W. V. (1983). Autonomic nervous system activity distinguishes between the emotions. *Science*, **221**, 1208–10.

Elithorn, A., Piercy, M. F., and Crosskey, M. A. (1955). Prefrontal leucotomy and the anticipation of pain. *Journal of Neurology, Neurosurgery and Psychiatry*, **18**, 34–43.

Ellis, B. J. and Symons, D. (1990). Sex differences in sexual fantasy: an evolutionary psychological approach. *Journal of Sex Research*, **27**, 527–55. (Reprinted in Betzig, L. (ed.) (1997). *Human nature: a critical reader*. Oxford University Press, New York.)

Epstein, A. N. (1960). Water intake without the act of drinking. *Science*, **131**, 497–8.

Epstein, A. N., Fitzsimons, J. T., and Rolls, B. J. (1970). Drinking induced by injection of angiotensin into the brain of the rat. *Journal of Physiology* (London), **210**, 457–74.

Eslinger, P. and Damasio, A. (1985). Severe disturbance of higher cognition after bilateral frontal lobe ablation: patient EVR. *Neurology*, **35**, 1731–41.

Etcoff, N. L. (1989). Asymmetries in recognition of emotion. In *Handbook of psychology*, Vol. 3, (ed. F. Boller and F. Grafman), pp. 363–82. Elsevier, Amsterdam.

Evarts, E. V. and Wise, S. P. (1984). Basal ganglia outputs and motor control. *In Functions of the Basal Ganglia. Ciba Foundation Symposium*, **107**, 83–96. Pitman, London.

Everitt, B. J. (1990). Sexual motivation: a neural and behavioural analysis of the mechanisms underlying appetitive and copulatory responses of male rats. *Neuroscience and Biobehavioral Reviews*, **14**, 217–32.

Everitt, B. (1997). Craving cocaine cues: cognitive neuroscience meets drug addiction research. *Trends in Cognitive Sciences*, **1**, 1–2.

Everitt, B. J. and Robbins, T. W. (1992). Amygdala–ventral striatal interactions and reward-related processes. In *The amygdala*, (ed. J. P. Aggleton), pp. 401–29. Wiley, Chichester.

Everitt, B. J., Cador, M., and Robbins, T. W. (1989). Interactions between the amygdala and ventral striatum in stimulus–reward association: studies using a second order schedule of sexual reinforcement. *Neuroscience*, **30**, 63–75.

Everitt, B. J., Morris, K. A., O'Brien, A. and Robbins, T. W. (1991). The basolateral amygdala–ventral striatal system and conditioned place preference: further evidence of limbic–striatal interactions underlying reward–related processes. *Neuroscience*, **42**, 1–18.

Ewart, W. (1993). Hepatic and other parenteral visceral afferents affecting ingestive behaviour. In *The neurophysiology of ingestion*, (ed. D. A. Booth). Manchester University Press.

Eysenck, H. J. and Eysenck, S. B. G. (1968). *Personality structure and measurement*. R. R. Knapp, San Diego.

Fazeli, M. S. and Collingridge, G. L. (ed.) (1996). *Cortical plasticity: LTP and LTD*. Bios, Oxford.

Fibiger, H. C. (1978). Drugs and reinforcement mechanisms: a critical review of the catecholamine theory. *Annual Review of Pharmacology and Toxicology*, **18**, 37–56.

Fibiger, H. C., LePiane, F. G., Jakubovic, A., and Phillips, A. G. (1987). The role of dopamine in intracranial self-stimulation of the ventral tegmental area. *Journal of Neuroscience*, **7**, 3888–96.

File, S. E. (1987). The contribution of behavioural studies to the neuropharmacology of anxiety. *Neuropharmacology*, **26**, 877–86.

Fiorino, D. F., Coury, A., Fibiger, H. C., and Phillips, A. G. (1993). Electrical stimulation of reward sites in the ventral tegmental area increases dopamine transmission in the nucleus accumbens of the rat. *Behavioural Brain Research*, **55**, 131–41.

Fiorino, D. F., Coury, A., and Phillips, A. G. (1997). Dynamic changes in nucleus accumbens dopamine efflux during the Coolidge effect in male rats. *Journal of Neuroscience*, **17**, 4849-4855.

Fitzsimons, J. T. (1992). Physiology and pathophysiology of thirst and sodium appetite. In *The kidney: physiology and pathophysiology*, (2nd edn), (ed. D. W. Seldin and G. Giebisch), Chapter 44, pp. 1615–48. Raven, New York.

Fitzsimons, J. T. and Moore-Gillon, M. J. (1980). Drinking and antidiuresis in response to reductions in venous return in the dog: neural and endocrine mechanisms. *Journal of Physiology*, **308**, 403–16.

Fitzsimons, J. T. and Simons, B. J. (1969). The effects on drinking in the rat of intravenous infusion of angiotensin, given alone or in combination with other stimuli of thirst. *Journal of Physiology*, **203**, 45–57.

Freeman, W. J. and Watts, J. W. (1950). *Psychosurgery in the treatment of mental disorders and intractable pain*, (2nd edn). Thomas, Springfield, Illinois.

Friedman, D. P, Murray, E. A., O'Neill, J. B., and Mishkin, M. (1986). Cortical connections of the somatosensory fields of the lateral sulcus of macaques: evidence for a corticolimbic pathway for touch. *Journal of Comparative Neurology*, **252**, 323–47.

Frijda, N. H. (1986). The Emotions. Cambridge University Press.

Friston, K. J., Holmes, A. P., Poline, J. B., Grasby, P. J., Williams, S. C. R., and Frakowiak, R. S. J. (1995). Analysis of fMRI time-series revisited. *Neuroimage*, **2**, 45–53.

Fulton, J. F. (1951). *Frontal lobotomy and affective behavior. A neurophysiological analysis*. W. W. Norton, New York.

Fuster, J. M. (1973). Unit activity in prefrontal cortex during delayed-response performance: neuronal correlates of transient memory. *Journal of Neurophysiology*, **36**, 61–78.

Fuster, J. M. (1996). *The prefrontal cortex*, (3rd edn). Raven Press, New York.

Fuster, J. M. and Jervey, J. P. (1982). Neuronal firing in the inferotemporal cortex of the monkey in a visual memory task. *Journal of Neuroscience,* **2**, 361–75.

Gaffan, D. (1992). Amygdala and the memory of reward. In *The amygdala*, (ed. J. P. Aggleton), Chapter 18, pp. 471–83. Wiley–Liss, New York.

Gaffan, D. and Gaffan, E. A. (1991). Amnesia in man following transection of the fornix. A review. *Brain*, **114**, 2611–8.

Gaffan, D. and Harrison, S. (1987). Amygdalectomy and disconnection in visual learning for auditory secondary reinforcement by monkeys. *Journal of Neuroscience*, **7**, 2285–92.

Gaffan, D., Saunders, R. C., Gaffan, E. A., Harrison, S., Shields, C., and Owen, M. J. (1984). Effects of fornix section upon associative memory in monkeys: role of the hippocampus in learned action. *Quarterly Journal of Experimental Psychology*, **36B**, 173–221.

Gaffan, D., Gaffan, E. A., and Harrison, S. (1989). Visual–visual associative learning and reward–associative learning in monkeys; the role of the amygdala. *Journal of Neuroscience*, **9**, 558–64.

Gaffan, E. A., Gaffan, D., and Harrison, S. (1988). Disconnection of the amygdala from visual association cortex impairs visual reward–association learning in monkeys. *Journal of Neuroscience*, **8**, 3144–50.

Gallagher, M. and Holland, P. C. (1994). The amygdala complex: multiple roles in associative learning and attention. *Proceedings of the National Academy of Sciences USA*, **91**, 11771–6.

Gallistel, C. R. (1969a). The incentive of brain-stimulation reward. *Journal of Comparative and Physiological Psychology*, **69**, 713–21.

Gallistel, C. R. (1969b). Self-stimulation: failure of pretrial stimulation to affect rats' electrode preference. *Journal of Comparative and Physiological Psychology*, **69**, 722–9.

Gallistel, C. R. (1973). Self-stimulation: the neurophysiology of reward and motivation. In *The physiological basis of memory*, (ed. J. A. Deutsch), Chapter 7, pp. 175–267. Academic Press, New York.

Gallistel, C. R. and Beagley, G. (1971). Specificity of brain-stimulation reward in the rat. *Journal of Comparative and Physiological Psychology*, **76**, 199–205.

Gardner, E. (1988). The space of interactions in neural network models. *Journal of Physics A*, **21**, 257–70.

Gazzaniga, M. S. (1988). Brain modularity: towards a philosophy of conscious experience. In *Consciousness in contemporary science*, (ed. A. J. Marcel and E. Bisiach), Chapter 10, pp. 218–38. Oxford University Press.

Gazzaniga, M. S. (1995). Consciousness and the cerebral hemispheres. In *The cognitive neurosciences*, (ed. M. S. Gazzaniga), Chapter 92, pp. 1392–400. MIT Press, Cambridge, MA.

Gazzaniga, M. S. and LeDoux, J. (1978). *The integrated mind*. Plenum, New York.

George, M. S., Ketter, T. A., Parekh, P. I., Herscovitch, P., and Post, R. M. (1996). Gender differences in regional cerebral blood flow during transient self-induced sadness or happiness. *Biological Psychiatry*, **40**, 859–71.

Gibbs, J., Fauser, D. J., Rowe, E. A., Rolls, B. J., Rolls, E. T., and Maddison, S. P. (1979). Bombesin suppresses feeding in rats. *Nature*, **282**, 208–10.

Gibbs, J., Maddison, S. P., and Rolls, E. T. (1981). The satiety role of the small intestine in sham feeding rhesus monkeys. *Journal of Comparative and Physiological Psychology*, **95**, 1003–15.

Gibbs, J., Rolls, B. J., and Rolls, E. T. (1986). Preabsorptive and postabsorptive factors in the termination of drinking in the rhesus monkey. In *Physiology of thirst and sodium appetite*, (ed. G. De Caro, A. N. Epstein, and M. Massi), pp. 287–94. Plenum, New York.

Gibson, W. E., Reid, L. D., Sakai, M., and Porter, P. B. (1965). Intracranial reinforcement compared with sugar–water reinforcement. *Science*, **148**, 1357–9.

Glickman, S. E. and Schiff, B. B. (1967). A biological theory of reinforcement. *Psychological Review*, **74**, 81–109.

Goldman, P. S. and Nauta, W. J. H. (1977). An intricately patterned prefronto-caudate projection in the rhesus monkey. *Journal of Comparative Neurology*, **171**, 369–86.

Goldman, P. S., Rosvold, H. E., Vest, B., and Galkin, T. W. (1971). Analysis of the delayed–alternation deficit produced by dorso–lateral pre-frontal lesions in the rhesus monkey. *Journal of Comparative and Physiological Psychology*, **77**, 212–20.

Goldman-Rakic, P. S. (1996). The prefrontal landscape: implications of functional architecture for understanding human mentation and the central executive. *Philosophical Transactions of the Royal Society B*, **351**, 1445–53.

Goleman, D. (1996). *Emotional intelligence*. Bloomsbury, London.

Goodglass, H. and Kaplan, E. (1979). Assessment of cognitive deficit in brain-injured patient. In *Handbook of behavioral neurobiology. Vol. 2, Neuropsychology*, (ed. M. S. Gazzaniga), pp. 3–22. Plenum, New York.

Graham, H. N. (1992). Green tea composition, consumption and polyphenol chemistry. *Preventative Medicine*, **21**, 334–50.

Gray, J. A. (1970). The psychophysiological basis of introversion–extraversion. *Behaviour Research and Therapy*, **8**, 249–66.

Gray, J. A. (1975). *Elements of a two-process theory of learning*. Academic Press, London.

Gray, J. A. (1981). Anxiety as a paradigm case of emotion. *British Medical Bulletin*, **37**, 193–7.

Gray, J. A. (1987). *The psychology of fear and stress*, (2nd edn). Cambridge University Press.

Gray, J. A., Young, A. M. J. and Joseph, M. H. (1997). Dopamine's role. *Science*, **278**, 1548–9.

Gray, T. S., Piechowski, R. A., Yracheta, J. M., Rittenhouse, P. A., Betha, C. L., and Van der Kar, L. D. (1993). Ibotenic acid lesions in the bed nucleus of the stria terminalis attenuate conditioned stress-induced increases in prolactin, ACTH and corticosterone. *Neuroendocrinology*, **57**, 517–24.

Graybiel, A. M. and Kimura, M. (1995). Adaptive neural networks in the basal ganglia. In *Models of information processing in the basal ganglia*, (ed. J. C. Houk, J. L. Davis, and D. G. Beiser), Chapter 5, pp. 103–16. MIT Press, Cambridge, MA.

Green, A. R. and Costain, D. W. (1981). *Pharmacology and biochemistry of psychiatric disorders*. Chichester, Wiley.

Greenberg, D., Smith, G. P., and Gibbs, J. (1990). Intraduodenal infusions of fats elicit satiety in sham-feeding rats. *American Journal of Physiology*, **259**, R110–18.

Griffin, D. R. (1992). *Animal minds*. University of Chicago Press.

Grill, H. J. and Norgren, R. (1978). Chronically decerebrate rats demonstrate satiation but not bait shyness. *Science*, **201**, 267–9.

Groenewegen, H. J., Berendse, H. W., Meredith, G. E., Haber, S. N., Voorn, P., Wolters, J. G., *et al.* (1991). Functional anatomy of the ventral, limbic system-innervated striatum. In *The mesolimbic dopamine system: from motivation to action*, (ed. P. Willner and J. Scheel-Kruger), pp. 19–60. Wiley, Chichester.

Gross, C. G., Bender, D. B., and Gerstein, G. L. (1979). Activity of inferior temporal neurons in behaving monkeys. *Neuropsychologia*, **17**, 215–29.

Gross, C. G., Desimone, R., Albright, T. D., and Schwartz, E. L. (1985). Inferior temporal cortex and pattern recognition. *Experimental Brain Research*, Suppl. **11**, 179–201.

Grossman, S. P. (1967). *A textbook of physiological psychology*. Wiley, New York.

Grossman, S. P. (1973). *Essentials of physiological psychology*. Wiley, New York.

Grossman, S. P. (1990). *Thirst and sodium appetite*. Academic Press, London.

Groves, P. M. (1983). A theory of the functional organization of the neostriatum and the neostriatal control of voluntary movement. *Brain Research Reviews*, **5**, 109–32.

Groves, P. M., Garcia-Munoz, M., Linder, J. C., Manley, M. S., Martone, M. E., and Young, S. J. (1995). Elements of the intrinsic organization and information processing in the neostriatum. In *Models of information processing in the basal ganglia*, (ed. J. C. Houk, J. L. Davis, and D. G. Beiser), Chapter 4, pp. 51–96. MIT Press, Cambridge, MA.

Grueninger, W. E., Kimble, D. P., Grueninger, J., and Levine, S. (1965). GSR and corticosteroid response in monkeys with frontal ablations. *Neuropsychologia*, **3**, 205–16.

Halgren, E. (1992). Emotional neurophysiology of the amygdala within the context of human cognition. In *The amygdala*, (ed. J. P. Aggleton), Chapter 7, pp. 191–228. Wiley–Liss, New York.

Hamer, D. (1998). D4 dopamine receptor genes and promiscuity. Paper presented to the American Association for the Advancement of Science, Philadelphia, February 1998.

Hamilton, W. (1964). The genetical evolution of social behaviour. *Journal of Theoretical Biology*, **7**, 1–52.

Harlow, H. F. and Stagner, R. (1933). Psychology of feelings and emotion. *Psychological Review*, **40**, 84–194.

Hasselmo, M. E. and Bower, J. M. (1993). Acetylcholine and memory. *Trends in Neurosciences*, **16**, 218–22.

Hasselmo, M. E., Rolls, E. T., and Baylis, G. C. (1989). The role of expression and identity in the face-selective responses of neurons in the temporal visual cortex of the monkey. *Behavioural Brain Research*, **32**, 203–18.

Hasselmo, M. E., Rolls, E. T., Baylis, G. C., and Nalwa, V. (1989). Object-centered encoding by face-selective neurons in the cortex in the superior temporal sulcus of the monkey. *Experimental Brain Research*, **75**, 417–29.

Hasselmo, M. E., Schnell, E., and Barkai, E. (1995). Learning and recall at excitatory recurrent synapses and cholinergic modulation in hippocampal region CA3. *Journal of Neuroscience*, **15**, 5249–62.

Hatfield, T., Han, J. S., Conley, M., Gallagher, M., and Holland, P. (1996). Neurotoxic lesions of basolateral, but not central, amygdala interfere with Pavlovian second-order conditioning and reinforcer devaluation effects. *Journal of Neuroscience*, **16**, 5256–65.

Heath, R. G. (1954). *Studies in schizophrenia. A multidisciplinary approach to mind–brain relationship*. Harvard University Press, Cambridge, MA.

Heath, R. G. (1963). Electrical self-stimulation of the brain in man. *American Journal of Psychiatry*, **120**, 571–7.

Heath, R. G. (1972). Pleasure and brain activity: deep and surface encephalograms during orgasm. *Journal of Nervous and Mental Disorders*, **154**, 3–18.

Hebb, D. O. (1949). *The organization of behavior: a neuropsychological theory*. Wiley, New York.

Hebert, M. A., Ardid, D., Henrie, J. A., Tamashiro, K., Yim, J., Tringali, A., *et al.* (1997). The Fakir test, an ethological approach to the biology of pain: evidence for analgesia following amygdala lesions. *Society for Neuroscience Abstracts*, **23**, 69. 6.

Hecaen, H. and Albert, M. L. (1978). *Human neuropsychology*. Wiley, New York.

Heimer, L. and Alheid, G. F. (1990). Piecing together the puzzle of basal forebrain anatomy. In *The basal forebrain: anatomy to function*, (ed. T. C. Napier, P. W. Kalivas, and I. Hanin). Plenum, New York.

Heimer, L., Switzer, R. D., and Van Hoesen, G. W. (1982). Ventral striatum and ventral pallidum. Components of the motor system? *Trends in Neurosciences*, **5**, 83–7.

Herzog, A. G. and Van Hoesen, G. W. (1976). Temporal neocortical afferent connections to the amygdala in the rhesus monkey, *Brain Research*, **115**, 57–69.

Hladik, C. M. (1978) Adaptive strategies of primates in relation to leaf-eating. In *The ecology of arboreal folivores*, (ed. G. G. Montgomery), pp. 373–95. Smithsonian Institute Press, Washington, DC.

Hoebel, B. G. (1969). Feeding and self-stimulation. *Annals of the New York Academy of Sciences*, **157**, 757–78.

Hoebel, B. G. (1976). Brain-stimulation reward and aversion in relation to behavior. In *Brain-stimulation reward*, (ed. A. Wauquier and E. T. Rolls), pp. 335–372. North-Holland, Amsterdam.

Hoebel, B. G. (1997). Neuroscience, and appetitive behavior research: 25 years. *Appetite*, **29**, 119–33.

Hoebel, B. G., Rada, P., Mark, G. P., Parada, M., Puig de Parada, M., Pothos, E. and Hernandez, L. (1996). Hypothalamic control of accumbens dopamine: a system for feeding reinforcement. In *Molecular and Genetic Aspects of Obesity*, (ed. G. Bray and D. Ryan), Vol. 5, pp. 263–280. Louisiana State University Press.

Hohmann, G. W. (1966). Some effects of spinal cord lesions on experienced emotional feelings. *Psychophysiology*, **3**, 143–56.

Hornak, J., Rolls, E. T., and Wade, D. (1996). Face and voice expression identification in patients with emotional and behavioural changes following ventral frontal lobe damage. *Neuropsychologia*, **34**, 247–61.

Hornykiewicz, O. (1973). Dopamine in the basal ganglia: its role and therapeutic implications including the use of L-Dopa). *British Medical Bulletin*, **29**, 172–8.

Houk, J. C., Adams, J. L., and Barto, A. C. (1995). A model of how the basal ganglia generates and uses neural signals that predict reinforcement. In *Models of information processing in the basal ganglia*, (ed. J. C. Houk, J. L. Davies, and D. G. Beiser), Chapter 13, pp. 249–270. MIT Press, Cambridge, MA.

Howarth, C. I. and Deutsch, J. A. (1962). Drive decay: the cause of fast 'extinction' of habits learned for brain stimulation. *Science*, **137**, 35–6.

Huang, Y. H. and Mogenson, G. J. (1972). Neural pathways mediating drinking and feeding in rats. *Experimental Neurology*, **37**, 269–86.

Hughes, J. (1975). Isolation of an endogenous compound from the brain with pharmacological properties similar to morphine. *Brain Research*, **88**, 293–308.

Hughes, J., Smith, T. W., Kosterlitz, H. W., Fothergill, L. A., Morgan, B. A., and Morris, H. R. (1975). Identification of two related pentapeptides from the brain with potent opiate antagonist activity. *Nature*, **258**, 577–9.

Humphrey, N. K. (1980). Nature's psychologists. In *Consciousness and the physical world*, (ed. B. D. Josephson and V. S. Ramachandran), pp. 57–80. Pergamon, Oxford.

Humphrey, N. K. (1986). *The inner eye*. Faber, London.

Huston, J. P. and Borbely, A. A. (1973). Operant conditioning in forebrain ablated rats by use of rewarding hypothalamic stimulation. *Brain Research*, **50**, 467–72.

Ikeda, K. (1909). On a new seasoning, *Journal of the Tokyo Chemistry Society*, **30**, 820–36.

Imamura, K., Mataga, N., and Mori, K. (1992). Coding of odor molecules by mitral/tufted cells in rabbit olfactory bulb. I. Aliphatic compounds. *Journal of Neurophysiology*, **68**, 1986–2002.

Insausti, R., Amaral, D. G., and Cowan, W. M. (1987). The entorhinal cortex of the monkey. II. Cortical afferents. *Journal of Comparative Neurology*, **264**, 356–95.

Ishizuka, N., Weber, J., and Amaral, D. G. (1990). Organization of intrahippocampal projections originating from CA3 pyramidal cells in the rat. *Journal of Comparative Neurology*, **295**, 580–623.

Ito, M. (1976). Mapping unit responses to rewarding stimulation. In *Brain-stimulation reward*, (ed. A. Wauquier and E. T. Rolls), pp. 89–96. North-Holland, Amsterdam.

Ito, M. (1984). *The cerebellum and neural control*. Chapter 10, Neuronal network model, pp. 115–30. Raven Press, New York.

Ito, M. (1989). Long-term depression. *Annual Review of Neuroscience*, **12**, 85–102.

Ito, M. (1993a). Synaptic plasticity in the cerebellar cortex and its role in motor learning. *Canadian Journal of Neurological Science, Suppl. 3*, S70–74.

Ito, M. (1993b). Cerebellar mechamisms of long-term depression. In *Synaptic Plasticity: Molecular, Cellular and Functional Aspects*, (ed. M. Baudry, R. F. Thompson and J. L. Davis) Ch. 6, pp. 117–128. MIT Press, Cambridge, Mass.

Iversen, S. D. (1979). Behaviour after neostriatal lesions in animals. In *The neostriatum*, (ed. I. Divac and R. G. E. Oberg), pp. 195–210. Pergamon, Oxford.

Iversen, S. D. (1984). Behavioural effects of manipulation of basal ganglia neurotransmitters. In *Functions of the basal ganglia*, Ciba Symposium 107, pp. 183–95. Pitman, London.

Iversen, S. D. and Mishkin, M. (1970). Perseverative interference in monkey following selective lesions of the inferior prefrontal convexity. *Experimental Brain Research*, **11**, 376–86.

Izard (1993). Four systems for emotion activation: cognitive and non-cognitive processes. *Psychological Review*, **100**, 68–90.

Jacobsen, C. F. (1936). The functions of the frontal association areas in monkeys. *Comparative Psychology Monographs*, **13**, 1–60.

James, W. (1884). What is an emotion? *Mind*, **9**, 188–205.

Jarvis, C. D. and Mishkin, M. (1977). Responses of cells in the inferior temporal cortex of monkeys during visual discrimination reversals. *Society for Neuroscience Abstracts*, **3**, 1794.

Johns, T. and Duquette, M. (1991). Detoxification and mineral supplementation as functions of geophagy. *American Journal of Clinical Nutrition*, **53**, 448–56.

Johnson, T. N., Rosvold, H. E., and Mishkin, M. (1968). Projections from behaviorally defined sectors of the prefrontal cortex to the basal ganglia, septum and diencephalon of the monkey. *Experimental Neurology*, **21**, 20–34.

Johnstone, S. and Rolls, E. T. (1990). Delay, discriminatory, and modality specific neurons in striatum and pallidum during short-term memory tasks. *Brain Research*, **522**, 147–51.

Jones, B. and Mishkin, M. (1972). Limbic lesions and the problem of stimulus–reinforcement associations. *Experimental Neurology*, **36**, 362–77.

Jones, E. G. and Powell, T. P. S. (1970). An anatomical study of converging sensory pathways within the cerebral cortex of the monkey. *Brain*, **93**, 793–820.

Jones-Gotman, M. and Zatorre, R. J. (1988). Olfactory identification in patients with focal cerebral excision. *Neuropsychologia*, **26**, 387–400.

Jouandet, M. and Gazzaniga, M. S. (1979). The frontal lobes. In *Handbook of behavioral neurobiology. Vol. 2 Neuropsychology*, (ed. M. S. Gazzaniga), pp. 25–59. Plenum, New York.

Kandel, E. R., Schwartz, J. H., and Jessel, T. H. (ed.) (1998). *Principles of neural science*, (4th edn). Elsevier, Amsterdam.

Kapp, B. S., Whalen, P. J., Supple, W. F., and Pascoe, J. P. (1992). Amygdaloid contributions to conditioned arousal and sensory information processing. In *The amygdala*, (ed. J. P. Aggleton), pp. 229–45. Wiley–Liss, New York.

Karadi, Z., Oomura, Y., Nishino, H., Scott, T. R., Lenard, L., and Aou, S. (1990). Complex attributes of lateral hypothalamic neurons in the regulation of feeding of alert monkeys. *Brain Research Bulletin*, **25**, 933–9.

Karadi, Z., Oomura, Y., Nishino, H., Scott, T. R., Lenard, L., and Aou, S. (1992). Responses of lateral hypothalamic glucose-sensitive and glucose-insensitive neurons to chemical stimuli in behaving rhesus monkeys. *Journal of Neurophysiology*, **67**, 389–400.

Kawamura, Y. and Kare, M. R. (ed.) (1987). *Umami: a basic taste*. Dekker, New York.

Keesey, R. E. (1964). Intracranial reward delay and the acquisition rate of a brightness discrimination. *Science*, **143**, 702–3.

Kemp, J. M. and Powell, T. P. S. (1970). The cortico-striate projections in the monkey. *Brain*, **93**, 525–46.

Kenrick, D. T., DaSadalla, E. K., Groth, G. and Trost, M. R. (1990). Evolution, traits, and the stages of human courtship: qualifying the parental investment model. *Journal of Personality*, **58**, 97–116. (Reprinted in Betzig, L. (ed.) (1997) Human nature: a critical reader. Oxford University Press, New York.)

Kent, R. and Grossman, S. P. (1969). Evidence for a conflict interpretation of anomalous effects of rewarding brain stimulation. *Journal of Comparative and Physiological Psychology*, **69**, 381–90.

Kievit, J. and Kuypers, H. G. J. M. (1975). Subcortical afferents to the frontal lobe in the rhesus monkey studied by means of retrograde horseradish peroxidase transport. *Brain Research*, **85**, 261–6.

Killcross, S., Robbins, T. W., and Everitt, B. J. (1997). Different types of fear-conditioned behaviour mediated by separate nuclei within amygdala. *Nature*, **388**, 377–80.

Kling, A. and Steklis, H. D. (1976). A neural substrate for affiliative behavior in nonhuman primates. *Brain, Behavior, and Evolution*, **13**, 216–38.

Kling, A. S. and Brothers, L. A. (1992). The amygdala and social behavior. In *The amygdala*, (ed. J. P. Aggleton), Chapter 13, pp. 353–377. Wiley–Liss, New York.

Kluver, H. and Bucy, P. C. (1939). Preliminary analysis of functions of the temporal lobes in monkeys. *Archives of Neurology and Psychiatry*, **42**, 979–1000.

Kolb, B. and Whishaw, I. Q. (1990). *Fundamentals of human neuropsychology*. (3rd edn). Freeman, New York.

Koob, G. F. (1992). Dopamine, addiction and reward. *Seminars in the Neurosciences*, **4**, 139–48.

Koob, J. F. (1996). Hedonic valence, dopamine and motivation. *Molecular Psychiatry*, **1**, 186–9.

Koob, G. F. and Le Moal, M. (1997). Drug abuse: hedonic homeostatic dysregulation. *Science*, **278**, 52–8.

Kowalska, D.-M., Bachevalier, J., and Mishkin, M. (1991). The role of the inferior prefrontal convexity in performance of delayed nonmatching-to-sample. *Neuropsychologia*, **29**, 583–600.

Kraut, R. E. and Johnson, R. E. (1979). Social and emotional messages of smiling: an ethological approach. *Journal of Personality and Social Psychology*, **37**, 1539–53.

Krebs, J. R. and Kacelnik, A. (1991). Decision making. In *Behavioural ecology*, (3rd edn) (ed. J. R. Krebs and N. B. Davies), Chapter 4, pp. 105–36. Blackwell, Oxford.

Krettek, J. E. and Price, J. L. (1974). A direct input from the amygdala to the thalamus and the cerebral cortex. *Brain Research*, **67**, 169–74.

Krettek, J. E. and Price, J. L. (1977). The cortical projections of the mediodorsal nucleus and adjacent thalamic nuclei in the rat. *Journal of Comparative Neurology*, **171**, 157–92.

Kuhar, M. J., Pert, C. B., and Snyder, S. H. (1973). Regional distribution of opiate receptor binding in monkey and human brain. *Nature*, **245**, 447–50.

Lane, R. D., Fink, G. R., Chau, P. M.-L., and Dolan, R. J. (1997). Neural activation during selective attention to subjective emotional responses. *Neuroreport*, **8**, 3969–72.

Lange, C. (1885). The emotions. In *The emotions*, (1922 edn) (ed. E. Dunlap). Williams and Wilkins, Baltimore.

Lazarus, R. S. (1991). *Emotion and adaptation*. Oxford University Press, New York.

Leak, G. K. and Christopher, S. B. (1982). Freudian psychoanalysis and sociobiology: a synthesis. *American Psychologist*, **37**, 313–22.

LeDoux, J. E. (1987). Emotion. In Handbook of physiology the nervous system V. Higher function, (ed. F. Plum and V. B. Mouncastle), pp. 419–59. American Physiological Society, Washington, DC.

LeDoux, J. E. (1992). Emotion and the amygdala. In *The amygdala*, (ed. J. P. Aggleton), pp. 339–51. Wiley–Liss, New York.

LeDoux, J. E. (1994). Emotion, memory and the brain. *Scientific American*, **270**, 32–9.

LeDoux, J. E. (1995). Emotion: clues from the brain. *Annual Review of Psychology*, **46**, 209–35.

LeDoux, J. E. (1996). *The emotional brain*. Simon and Schuster, New York.

LeDoux, J. E., Iwata, J., Cicchetti, P., and Reis, D. J. (1988). Different projections of the central amygdaloid nucleus mediate autonomic and behavioral correlates of conditioned fear. *Journal of Neuroscience*, **8**, 2517–29.

Lehrman, D. S. (1965). Reproductive behavior in the ring dove. *Scientific American*, **211**, 48–54.

Leibowitz, S. F. and Hoebel, B. G. (1998). Behavioral neuroscience and obesity. In *The handbook of obesity*, (ed. G. A. Bray, C. Bouchard, and P. T. James), Chapter 15, pp. 313–58. Dekker, New York.

LeMagnen, J. (1956). Hyperphagia produced in the white rat by alteration of the peripheral satiety mechanism. *C. R. Soc. Biol.* **150**, 32–50. (In French)

LeMagnen, J. (1971). Advances in studies on the physiological control and regulation of food intake. In *Progress in physiological psychology*, Vol. 4, (ed. E. Stellar and J. M. Sprague), pp. 204–61. Academic Press, New York.

LeMagnen, J. (1992). *Neurobiology of feeding and nutrition*. Academic Press, San Diego.

Leonard, C. M., Rolls, E. T., Wilson, F. A. W., and Baylis, G. C. (1985). Neurons in the amygdala of the monkey with responses selective for faces. *Behavioural Brain Research*, **15**, 159–76.

Lestang, I., Cardo, B., Roy, M. T., and Velley, L. (1985). Electrical self-stimulation deficits in the anterior and posterior parts of the medial forebrain bundle after ibotenic acid lesion of the middle lateral hypothalamus. *Neuroscience*, **15**, 379–88.

Levenson, R. W., Ekman, P., and Friesen, W. V. (1990). Voluntary facial action generates emotion-specific autonomic nervous system activity. *Psychophysiology*, **27**, 363–84.

Levy, W. B. (1985). Associative changes in the synapse: LTP in the hippocampus. In *Synaptic modification, neuron selectivity, and nervous system organization*, (ed. W. B. Levy, J. A. Anderson, and S. Lehmkuhle), Chapter 1, pp. 5–33. Erlbaum, Hillsdale, NJ.

Levy, W. B. and Desmond, N. L. (1985). The rules of elemental synaptic plasticity. In *Synaptic modification, neuron selectivity, and nervous system organization*, (ed. W. B. Levy, J. A. Anderson, and S. Lehmkuhle), Chapter 6, pp. 105–121. Erlbaum, Hillsdale, NJ.

Liebeskind, J. C. and Paul, L. A. (1977). Psychological and physiological mechanisms of pain. *Annual Review of Psychology*, **88**, 41–60.

Liebeskind, J. C., Giesler, G. J., and Urca, G. (1976). Evidence pertaining to an endogenous mechanism of pain inhibition in the central nervous system. In *Sensory functions of the skin*, (ed. Y. Zotterman). Pergamon, Oxford.

Liebman, J. M. and Cooper, S. J. (ed.) (1989). *Neuropharmacological basis of reward*. Oxford University Press.

Lyness, W. H., Friedle, N. M., and Moore, K. E. (1980). Destruction of dopaminergic nerve terminals in nucleus accumbens: effect on d-amphetamine self-administration. *Pharmacology, Biochemistry, and Behavior*, **11**, 553–6.

Mackintosh, N. J. (1974). *The psychology of animal learning*. Academic Press, London.

Mackintosh, N. J. (1983). *Conditioning and associative learning*. Oxford University Press.

Mackintosh, N. J. and Dickinson, A. (1979). Instrumental (type II) conditioning. In *Mechanisms of learning and motivation*, (ed. A. Dickinson and A. Boakes), pp. 143–69. Erlbaum, Hillsdale, NJ.

Maddison, S., Wood, R. J., Rolls, E. T., Rolls, B. J., and Gibbs, J. (1980). Drinking in the rhesus monkey: peripheral factors. *Journal of Comparative and Physiological Psychology*, **94**, 365–74.

Malkova, L. Gaffan, D., and Murray, E. A. (1997). Excitotoxic lesions of the amygdala fail to produce impairment in visual learning for auditory secondary reinforcement but interfere with reinforcer devaluation effects in rhesus monkeys. *Journal of Neuroscience*, **17**, 6011–20.

Malsburg, C. von der (1990). A neural architecture for the representation of scenes. In *Brain organization and memory: cells, systems and circuits*, (ed. J. L. McGaugh, N. M. Weinberger, and G. Lynch), Chapter 18, pp. 356–372. Oxford University Press, New York.

Markram, H and Siegel, M. (1992). The inositol 1,4,5-triphosphate pathway mediates cholinergic potentiation of rat hippocampal neuronal responses to NMDA. *Journal of Physiology*, **447**, 513–33.

Markram, H. and Tsodyks, M. (1996). Redistribution of synaptic efficacy between neocortical pyramidal neurons. *Nature*, **382**, 807–10.

Marshall, J. (1951). Sensory disturbances in cortical wounds with special reference to pain. *Journal of Neurology, Neurosurgery and Psychiatry*, **14**, 187–204.

Marshall, J. F., Richardson, J. S., and Teitelbaum, P. (1974). Nigrostriatal bundle damage and the lateral hypothalamic syndrome. *Journal of Comparative and Physiological Psychology*, **87**, 808–30.

Mayberg, H. S. (1997). Limbic–cortical dysregulation: a proposed model of depression. *Journal of Neuropsychiatry*, **9**, 471–81.

Mayberg, H. S., Brannan, S. K., Mahurin, R. K., Jerobek, P. A., Brickman, J. S., Tekell, J. L. *et al.* (1997). Cingulate function in depression: a potential predictor of treatment response. *Neuroreport*, **8**, 1057–61.

Maynard Smith, J. (1984). Game theory and the evolution of behaviour. *Behavioral and Brain Sciences*, **7**, 95–125.

McClelland, J. L. and Rumelhart, D. E. (1986). A distributed model of human learning and memory. In *Parallel distributed processing*, Vol. 2, (ed. J. L. McClelland and D. E. Rumelhart), Chapter 17, pp. 170–215. MIT Press, Cambridge, MA.

McDonald, A. J. (1992). Cell types and intrinsic connections of the amygdala. In *The amygdala*, (ed. J. P. Aggleton), Chapter 2, pp. 67–96. Wiley–Liss, New York.

McGinty, D. and Szymusiak, R. (1988). Neuronal unit activity patterns in behaving animals: brainstem and limbic system. *Annual Review of Psychology*, **39**, 135–68.

McLeod, P., Plunkett, K., and Rolls, E. T. (1998). *Introduction to connectionist modelling of cognitive processes*. Oxford University Press.

Melzack, R. (1973). *The puzzle of pain*. Basic Books, New York.

Melzack, R. and Wall, P. D. (1996). *The challenge of pain*. Penguin, Harmondsworth, UK.

Mei, N. (1993). Gastrointestinal chemoreception and its behavioural role. In *The neurophysiology of ingestion*, (ed. D. A. Booth), Chapter 4, pp. 47–56. Manchester University Press.

Mei, N. (1994). Role of digestive afferents in food intake regulation. In *Appetite. Neural and Behavioural Bases*, (ed. C. R. Legg and D. A. Booth), Chapter 4, pp. 86–97. Oxford University Press.

Mesulam, M.-M. (1990). Human brain cholinergic pathways. *Progress in Brain Research*, **84**, 231–41.

Mesulam, M.-M. and Mufson, E. J. (1982a). Insula of the old world monkey. I: Architectonics in the insulo–orbito–temporal component of the paralimbic brain. *Journal of Comparative Neurology*, **212**, 1–22.

Mesulam, M.-M. and Mufson, E. J. (1982b). Insula of the old world monkey. III. Efferent cortical output and comments on function. *Journal of Comparative Neurology*, **212**, 38–52.

Meunier, M., Bachevalier, J., and Mishkin, M. (1997). Effects of orbital frontal and anterior cingulate lesions on object and spatial memory in rhesus monkeys. *Neuropsychologia*, **35**, 999–1015.

Middleton, F. A. and Strick, P. L. (1994). Anatomical evidence for cerebellar and basal ganglia involvement in higher cognitive function. *Science*, **266**, 458–61.

Middleton, F. A. and Strick, P. L. (1996a). The temporal lobe is a target of output from the basal ganglia. *Proceedings of the National Academy of Sciences of the USA*, **93**, 8683–7.

Middleton, F. A. and Strick, P. L. (1996b). New concepts about the organization of the basal ganglia. In *Advances in neurology: the basal ganglia and the surgical treatment for Parkinson's disease*, (ed. J. A. Obeso). Raven, New York.

Millenson, J. R. (1967). *Principles of behavioral analysis*. MacMillan, New York (Collier–Macmillan, London).

Miller, G. F. (1992). Sexual selection for protean expressiveness: a new model of hominid encephalization. (see Ridley, 1993).

Millhouse, O. E. (1986). The intercalated cells of the amygdala. *Journal of Comparative Neurology*, **247**, 246–71.

Millhouse, O. E. and DeOlmos, J. (1983). Neuronal configuration in lateral and basolateral amygdala. *Neuroscience*, **10**, 1269–1300.

Milner, B. (1963). Effects of different brain lesions on card sorting. *Archives of Neurology*, **9**, 90–100.

Milner, B. (1982). Some cognitive effects of frontal-lobe lesions in man. *Philosophical Transactions of the Royal Society B*, **298**, 211–26.

Milner, A. D. and Goodale, M. A. (1995). *The visual brain in action*. Oxford University Press.

Mirenowicz, J and Schultz, W. (1996). Preferential activation of midbrain dopamine neurons by appetitive rather than aversive stimuli. *Nature*, **279**, 449–51.

Miselis, R. R., Shapiro, R. E., and Hand, P. J. (1979). Subfornical organ efferents to neural systems for control of body water. *Science*, **205**, 1022–5.

Mishkin, M. and Aggleton, J. (1981). Multiple functional contributions of the amygdala in the monkey. In *The amygdaloid complex*, (ed. Y. Ben-Ari), pp. 409–20. Elsevier, Amsterdam.

Mishkin, M. and Manning, F. J. (1978). Non-spatial memory after selective prefrontal lesions in monkeys. *Brain Research*, **143**, 313–24.

Miyashita, Y. and Chang, H. S. (1988). Neuronal correlate of pictorial short-term memory in the primate temporal cortex. *Nature*, **331**, 68–70.

Mogenson, G., Takigawa, M., Robertson, A., and Wu, M. (1979). Self-stimulation of the nucleus accumbens and ventral tegmental area of Tsai attenuated by microinjections of spiroperidol into the nucleus accumbens. *Brain Research*, **171**, 247–59.

Mogenson, G. J., Jones, D. L., and Yim, C. Y. (1980). From motivation to action: functional interface between the limbic system and the motor system. *Progress in Neurobiology*, **14**, 69–97.

Moniz, E. (1936). *Tentatives opératoires dans le traitement de certaines psychoses*. Masson, Paris.

Monti-Bloch, L., Jennings-White, C., Dolberg, D. S., and Berliner, D. L. (1994). The human vomeronasal system. *Psychoneuroendocrinology*, **19**, 673–86.

Monti-Bloch, L., Jennings-White, C. and Berliner, D. L. (1998). The human vomeronasal system: a review. In *Olfaction and Taste*, Vol XII, (ed. C. Murphy.) *Annals of the New York Academy of Sciences*, in press.

Mora, F. and Myers, R. (1977). Brain self-stimulation: direct evidence for the involvement of dopamine in the prefrontal cortex. *Science*, **197**, 1387–9.

Mora, F., Sanguinetti, A. M., Rolls, E. T., and Shaw, S. G. (1975). Differential effects on self-stimulation and motor behaviour produced by micro-intracranial injections of a dopamine-receptor blocking agent. *Neuroscience Letters*, **1**, 179–84.

Mora, F., Phillips, A. G., Koolhaas, J. M., and Rolls, E. T. (1976a). Prefrontal cortex and neostriatum. Self-stimulation in the rat: differential effects produced by apomorphine. *Brain Research Bulletin*, **1**, 421–4.

Mora, F., Rolls, E. T., and Burton, M. J. (1976b). Modulation during learning of the responses of neurons in the hypothalamus to the sight of food. *Experimental Neurology*, **53**, 508–19.

Mora, F., Rolls, E. T., Burton, M. J., and Shaw, S. G. (1976c). Effects of dopamine-receptor blockade on self-stimulation in the monkey. *Pharmacology, Biochemistry, and Behavior*, **4**, 211–16.

Mora, F., Sweeney, K. F., Rolls, E. T., and Sanguinetti, A. M. (1976d). Spontaneous firing rate of neurones in the prefrontal cortex of the rat: evidence for a dopaminergic inhibition. *Brain Research*, **116**, 516–522.

Mora, F., Mogenson, G. J., and Rolls, E. T. (1977). Activity of neurones in the region of the substantia nigra during feeding. *Brain Research*, **133**, 267–76.

Mora, F., Avrith, D. B., Phillips, A, G., and Rolls, E. T. (1979). Effects of satiety on self-stimulation of the orbitofrontal cortex in the monkey. *Neuroscience Letters*, **13**, 141–5.

Mora, F., Avrith, D. B., and Rolls, E. T. (1980). An electrophysiological and behavioural study of self-stimulation in the orbitofrontal cortex of the rhesus monkey. *Brain Research Bulletin*, **5**, 111–5.

Morecraft, R. J., Geula, C., and Mesulam, M.-M. (1992). Cytoarchitecture and neural afferents of orbitofrontal cortex in the brain of the monkey. *Journal of Comparative Neurology*, **323**, 341–58.

Mori, K., Mataga, N., and Imamura, K. (1992). Differential specificities of single mitral cells in rabbit olfactory bulb for a homologous series of fatty acid odor molecules. *Journal of Neurophysiology*, **67**, 786–9.

Morris, R. G. M. (1989). Does synaptic plasticity play a role in information storage in the vertebrate brain? In *Parallel distributed processing: implications for psychology and neurobiology*, (ed. R. G. M. Morris), Chapter 11, pp. 248–85. Oxford University Press.

Morris, R. G. M. (1996). Spatial memory and the hippocampus: the need for psychological analyses to identify the information processing underlying spatial learning. In *Perception, memory, and emotion: frontiers in neuroscience*, (ed. T. Ono, B. L. McNaughton, S. Molotchnikoff, E. T. Rolls, and H. Nishijo), Chapter 22, pp. 319–42. Elsevier, Amsterdam.

Morris, J. S., Frith, C. D., Perrett, D. I., Rowland, D., Young, A. W., Calder, A. J., *et al.* (1996). A differential neural response in the human amygdala to fearful and happy facial expressions. *Nature*, **383**, 812–5.

Muir, J. L, Everitt, B. J., and Robbins, T. W. (1994). AMPA-induced excitotoxic lesions of the basal forebrain: a significant role for the cortical cholinergic system in attentional function. *Journal of Neuroscience*, **14**, 2313–26.

Murray, E. A., Gaffan, E. A. and Flint, R. W. (1996). Anterior rhinal cortex and amygdala: dissociation of their contributions to memory and food preference in rhesus monkeys. *Behavioral Neuroscience*, **110**, 30–42.

Nauta, W. J. H. (1961). Fiber degeneration following lesions of the amygdaloid complex in the monkey. *Journal of Anatomy*, **95**, 515–31.

Nauta, W. J. H. (1964). Some efferent connections of the prefrontal cortex in the monkey. In *The frontal granular cortex and behavior*, (eds. J. M. Warren and K. Akert), pp. 397–407. McGraw Hill, New York.

Nauta, W. J. H. (1972). Neural associations of the frontal cortex. *Acta Neurobiologica Experimentalis*, **32**, 125–40.

Nauta, W. J. H. and Domesick, V. B. (1978). Crossroads of limbic and striatal circuitry: hypothalamonigral connections. In *Limbic mechanisms*, (ed. K. E. Livingston and O. Hornykiewicz), pp. 75–93. Plenum, New York.

Nesse, R. M. and Lloyd, A. T. (1992). The evolution of psychodynamic mechanisms. In *The adapted mind*, (ed. J. H. Barkow, L. Cosmides, and J. Tooby), Chapter 17, pp. 601–24. Oxford University Press, New York.

Nicolaidis, S. and Rowland, N. (1974). Long-term self-intravenous 'drinking' in the rat. *Journal of Comparative and Physiological Psychology*, **87**, 1–15.

Nicolaidis, S. and Rowland, N. (1975). Systemic vs oral and gastro-intestinal metering of fluid intake. In *Control mechanisms of drinking*, (ed. G. Peters and J. T. Fitzsimons). Springer, Berlin.

Nicolaidis, S. and Rowland, N. (1976). Metering of intravenous versus oral nutrients and regulation of energy balance. *American Journal of Physiology*, **231**, 661–9.

Nicolaidis, S. and Rowland, N. (1977). Intravenous self-feeding: long-term regulation of energy balance in rats. *Science*, **195**, 589–91.

Nicoll, R. A. and Malenka, R. C. (1995). Contrasting properties of two forms of long-term potentiation in the hippocampus. *Nature*, **377**, 115–8.

Nishijo, H., Ono, T., and Nishino, H. (1988). Single neuron responses in amygdala of alert monkey during complex sensory stimulation with affective significance. *Journal of Neuroscience*, **8**, 3570–83.

Norgren, R. (1984). Central neural mechanisms of taste. In *Handbook of physiology—the nervous system III, Sensory processes 1*, (ed. I. Darien-Smith; section ed. J. Brookhart and V. B. Mountcastle), pp. 1087–128. American Physiological Society, Washington, DC.

Oatley, K. and Jenkins, J. M. (1996). *Understanding emotions*. Blackwell, Oxford.

Oatley, K. and Johnson-Laird, P. N. (1987). Towards a cognitive theory of emotions. *Cognition and Emotion*, **1**, 29–50.

Oberg, R. G. E. and Divac, I. (1979). 'Cognitive' functions of the striatum. In *The neostriatum*, (ed. I. Divac and R. G. E. Oberg). Pergamon, New York.

Olds,J. (1956). Pleasure centers in the brain. *Scientific American*, **195**, 105–16.

Olds, J. (1958). Effects of hunger and male sex hormone on self-stimulation of the brain. *Journal of Comparative and Physiological Psychology*, **51**, 320–4.

Olds, J. (1961). Differential effects of drive and drugs on self-stimulation at different brain sites. In *Electrical stimulation of the brain*, (ed. D. E. Sheer). University of Texas Press, Austin.

Olds, J. (1977). *Drives and reinforcements: behavioral studies of hypothalamic functions*. Raven Press, New York.

Olds, J. and Milner, P. (1954). Positive reinforcement produced by electrical stimulation of septal area and other regions of the rat brain. *Journal of Comparative and Physiological Psychology*, **47**, 419–27.

Olds, J. and Olds, M. (1965). Drives, rewards, and the brain. In *New directions in psychology*, Vol. II (ed. F. Barron and W. C. Dement), pp. 327–410. Holt, Rinehart and Winston, New York.

Olds, J., Allan, W. S., and Briese, A. E. (1971). Differentiation of hypothalamic drive and reward centres. *American Journal of Physiology*, **221**, 368–75.

Olds, M. E. and Olds, J. (1969). Effects of lesions in medial forebrain bundle on self-stimulation behaviour. *American Journal of Physiology*, **217**, 1253–64.

Ono, T. and Nishijo, H. (1992). Neurophysiological basis of the Kluver–Bucy syndrome: responses of monkey amygdaloid neurons to biologically significant objects. In *The amygdala*, (ed. J. P. Aggleton), Chapter 6, pp. 167–90. Wiley–Liss, New York.

Ono, T., Nishino, H., Sasaki, K., Fukuda, M., and Muramoto, K. (1980). Role of the lateral hypothalamus and amygdala in feeding behavior. *Brain Research Bulletin*, **5**, Suppl. 4, 143–9.

Ono, T., Tamura, R., Nishijo, H., Nakamura, K., and Tabuchi, E. (1989). Contribution of amygdala and LH neurons to the visual information processing of food and non-food in the monkey. *Physiology and Behavior*, **45**, 411–21.

Oomura, Y and Yoshimatsu, H. (1984). Neural network of glucose monitoring system. *Journal of the Autonomic Nervous System*, **10**, 359–72.

Oomura, Y., Aou, S., Koyama, Y., Fujita, I., and Yoshimatsu, H. (1988). Central control of sexual behavior. *Brain Research Bulletin*, **20**, 863–70.

Oomura, Y., Nishino, H., Karadi, Z., Aou, S., and Scott, T. R. (1991). Taste and olfactory modulation of feeding related neurons in the behaving monkey. *Physiology and Behavior*, **49**, 943–50.

Pager, J. (1974). A selective modulation of the olfactory bulb electrical activity in relation to the learning of palatability in hungry and satiated rats. *Physiology and Behavior*, **12**, 189–96.

Pager, J., Giachetti, I., Holley, A., and LeMagnen, J. (1972). A selective control of olfactory bulb electrical activity in relation to food deprivation and satiety in rats. *Physiology and Behavior*, **9**, 573–80.

Pandya, D. N. (1996). Comparison of prefrontal architecture and connections. *Philosophical Transactions of the Royal Society B*, **351**, 1423–32.

Panksepp, J. and Trowill, J. A. (1967a). Intraoral self-injection: I, Effects of delay of reinforcement on resistance to extinction and implications for self-stimulation. *Psychonomic Science*, **9**, 405–6.

Panksepp, J. and Trowill, J. A. (1967b). Intraoral self-injection: II, The simulation of self-stimulation phenomena with a conventional reward. *Psychonomic Science*, **9**, 407–8.

Papez, J. W. (1937). A proposed mechanism for emotion. *Archives of Neurology, and Psychiatry*, **38**, 725–43.

Parga, N. and Rolls, E. T. (1998). Transform invariant recognition by association in a recurrent network. *Neural Computation*, in press.

Passingham, R. (1975). Delayed matching after selective prefrontal lesions in monkeys (*Macaca mulatta*). *Brain Research*, **92**, 89–102.

Pearce, J. M. (1996). *Animal learning and cognition*, (2nd edn). Psychology Press, Hove.

Peck, J. W. and Novin, D. (1971). Evidence that osmoreceptors mediating drinking in rabbits are in the lateral preoptic area. *Journal of Comparative and Physiological Psychology*, **74**, 134–47.

Pennartz, C. M., Ameerun, R. F., Groenewegen, H. J., and Lopes da Silva, F. H. (1993). Synaptic plasticity in an in vitro slice preparation of the rat nucleus accumbens. *European Journal of Neuroscience*, **5**, 107–17.

Percheron, G., Yelnik, J., and François, C. (1984a). A Golgi analysis of the primate globus pallidus. III. Spatial organization of the striato–pallidal complex. *Journal of Comparative Neurology*, **227**, 214–27.

Percheron, G., Yelnik, J., and François, C. (1984b). The primate striato–pallido–nigral system: an integrative system for cortical information. In *The basal ganglia: structure and function*, (ed. J. S. McKenzie, R. E. Kemm, and L. N. Wilcox), pp. 87–105. Plenum, New York.

Percheron, G., Yelnik, J., François, C., Fenelon, G., and Talbi, B. (1994). Informational neurology of the basal ganglia related system. *Revue Neurologique (Paris)*, **150**, 614–26.

Perl, E. R. and Kruger, L. (1996). Nociception and pain: evolution of concepts and observations. In *Pain and touch*, (ed. L. Kruger), Chapter 4, pp. 180–211. Academic Press, San Diego.

Perrett, D. I. and Rolls, E. T. (1983). Neural mechanisms underlying the visual analysis of faces. In *Advances in vertebrate neuroethology*, (ed. J.-P. Ewert, R. R. Capranica, and D. J. Ingle), pp. 543–66. Plenum Press, New York.

Perrett, D. I., Rolls, E. T., and Caan, W. (1982). Visual neurons responsive to faces in the monkey temporal cortex. *Experimental Brain Research*, **47**, 329–42.

Perrett, D. I., Smith, P. A. J., Potter, D. D., Mistlin, A. J., Head, A. S., Milner, D., *et al.* (1985). Visual cells in temporal cortex sensitive to face view and gaze direction. *Proceedings of the Royal Society of London, Series B*, **223**, 293–317.

Petri, H. L. and Mishkin, M. (1994). Behaviorism, cognitivism, and the neuropsychology of memory. *American Scientist*, **82**, 30–7.

Petrides, M. (1996). Specialized systems for the processing of mnemonic information within the primate frontal cortex. *Philosophical Transactions of the Royal Society B*, **351**, 1455–62.

Petrides, M. and Pandya, D. N. (1988). Association fiber pathways to the frontal cortex from the superior temporal region in the rhesus monkey. *Journal of Comparative Neurology*, **273**, 52–66.

Petrides, M. and Pandya, D. N. (1995). Comparative architectonic analysis of the human and macaque frontal cortex. In *Handbook of neuropsychology*, (ed. J. Grafman and F. Boller). Elsevier, Amsterdam.

Pfaff, D. W. (1980). *Estrogens and brain function*. Springer, New York.

Pfaff, D. W. (1982). Neurobiological mechanisms of sexual behavior. In *The physiological mechanisms of motivation*, (ed. D. W. Pfaff), pp. 287–317. Springer, New York.

Pfaus, J. G., Damsma, G., Nomikos, G. G., Wenkstern, D., Blaha, C. D., Phillips, A. G., *et al.* (1990). Sexual behavior enhances central dopamine transmission in the male rat. *Brain Research*, **530**, 345–8.

Phillips, M. I. (1978). Angiotensin in the brain. *Neuroendocrinology*, **25**, 354–77.

Phillips, M. I. and Felix, D. (1976). Specific angiotensin II receptive neurones in the cat subfornical organ. *Brain Research*, **109**, 531–40.

Phillips, A. G. and Fibiger, H. C. (1976). Long-term deficits in stimulation-induced behaviors and self-stimulation after 6-hydroxydopamine administration in rats. *Behavioral Biology*, **16**, 127–43.

Phillips, A. G. and Fibiger, H. C. (1978). The role of dopamine in mediating self-stimulation in the ventral tegmentum, nucleus accumbens and medial prefrontal cortex. *Canadian Journal of Psychology*, **32**, 58–66.

Phillips, A. G. and Fibiger, H. C. (1989). Neuroanatomical bases of intracranial self-stimulation: untying the Gordian knot. In *The neuropharmacological basis of reward*, (ed. J. M. Liebman and S. J. Cooper), pp. 66–105. Oxford University Press.

Phillips, A. G. and Fibiger, H. C. (1990). Role of reward and enhancement of conditioned reward in persistence of responding for cocaine. *Behavioral Pharmacology*, **1**, 269–82.

Phillips, A. G., Mora, F., and Rolls, E. T. (1979). Intracranial self-stimulation in the orbitofrontal cortex and caudate nucleus of the alert monkey: effects of apomorphine, pimozide and spiroperidol. *Psychopharmacology*, **62**, 79–82.

Phillips, A. G., Mora, F., and Rolls, E. T. (1981). Intra-cerebral self-administration of amphetamine by rhesus monkeys. *Neuroscience Letters*, **24**, 81–6.

Phillips, A. G., LePiane, F. G., and Fibiger, H. C. (1982). Effects of kainic acid lesions of the striatum on self-stimulation in the substantia nigra and ventral tegmental area. *Behavioural Brain Research*, **5**, 297–310.

Phillips, A. G., Blaha, C. D., and Fibiger, H. C. (1989). Neurochemical correlates of brain-stimulation reward measured by ex vivo and in vivo analyses. *Neuroscience and Biobehavioral Reviews*, **13**, 99–104.

Phillips, A. G., Pfaus, J. G., and Blaha, C. D. (1991). Dopamine and motivated behavior: insights provided by in vivo analysis. In *The mesolimbic dopamine system: from motivation to action*, (ed. P. Willner and J. Scheel-Kruger), Chapter 8, pp. 199–224. Wiley, New York

Phillips, P., Rolls, B. J., Ledingham, J., and Morton, J. (1984). Body fluid changes, thirst and drinking in man during free access to water. *Physiology and Behavior*, **33**, 357–63.

Phillips, P., Rolls, B. J., Ledingham, J., Morton, J., and Forsling, M. (1985). Angiotensin-II induced thirst and vasopressin release in man. *Clinical Science*, **68**, 669–74.

Phillips, R. R., Malamut, B. L., Bachevalier, J., and Mishkin, M. (1988). Dissociation of the effects of inferior temporal and limbic lesions on object discrimination learning with 24-h intertrial intervals. *Behavioural Brain Research*, **27**, 99–107.

Pinker, S. and Bloom, P. (1992). Natural language and natural selection. In *The adapted mind*, (ed. J. H. Barkow, L. Cosmides, and J. Tooby), Chapter 12, pp. 451–93. Oxford University Press, New York.

Preuss, T. M. and Goldman-Rakic, P. S. (1989). Connections of the ventral granular frontal cortex of macaques with perisylvian premotor and somatosensory areas: anatomical evidence for somatic representation in primate frontal association cortex. *Journal of Comparative Neurology*, **282**, 293–316.

Price, J. L., Carmichael, S. T., Carnes, K. M., Clugnet, M.-C., and Kuroda, M. (1991). Olfactory input to the prefrontal cortex. In *Olfaction: a model system for computational neuroscience*, (ed. J. L. Davis and H. Eichenbaum), pp. 101–120. MIT Press, Cambridge, MA.

Price, J. L., Carmichael, S. T., and Drevets, W. C. (1996). Networks related to the orbital and medial prefrontal cortex; a substrate for emotional behavior? *Progress in Brain Research*, **107**, 523–36.

Priest, C. A. and Pfaff, D. W. (1995). Actions of sex steroids on behaviours beyond reproductive reflexes. Ciba Foundation Symposia, **191**, 74–84.

Quartermain, D. and Webster, D. (1968). Extinction following intracranial reward: the effect of delay between acquisition and extinction. *Science*, **159**, 1259–60.

Quirk, G. J., Armony, J. L., Repa, J. C., Li, X.-F., and LeDoux, J. E. (1996). Emotional memory: a search for sites of plasticity. Cold Spring Harbor Symposia on Quantitative Biology, **61**, 247–57.

Rada, P., Mark, G. P., and Hoebel, B. G. (1998). Dopamine in the nucleus accumbens released by hypothalamic stimulation-escape behavior. *Brain Research*, in press.

Rainville, P., Duncan, G. H., Price, D. D., Carrier, B., and Bushnell, M. C. (1997). Pain affect encoded in human anterior cingulate but not somatosensory cortex. *Science*, **277**, 968–71.

Ramsay, D. J., Rolls, B. J., and Wood, R. J. (1975). The relationship between elevated water intake and oedema associated with congestive cardiac failure in the dog. *Journal of Physiology, (London)*, **244**, 303–12.

Rawlins, J. N., Winocur, G., and Gray, J. A. (1983). The hippocampus, collateral behavior, and timing. *Behavioral Neuroscience*, **97**, 857–72.

Reid, L. D., Hunsicker, J. P., Kent, E. W., Lindsay, J. L., and Gallistel, C. E. (1973). Incidence and magnitude of the 'priming effect' in self-stimulating rats. *Journal of Comparative and Physiological Psychology*, **82**, 286–93.

Reisenzein, R. (1983). The Schachter theory of emotion: two decades later. *Psychological Bulletin*, **94**, 239–64.

Ridley, M. (1993). *The red queen: sex and the evolution of human nature*. Penguin, London.

Ridley, M. (1996). *The origins of virtue*. Viking, London.

Ridley, R. M., Hester, N. S., and Ettlinger, G. (1977). Stimulus- and response-dependent units from the occipital and temporal lobes of the unanaesthetized monkey performing learnt visual tasks. *Experimental Brain Research*, **27**, 539–52.

Ritter, S. (1986). Glucoprivation and the glucoprivic control of food intake. In *Feeding behavior: neural and humoral controls*, (ed. R. C. Ritter, S. Ritter, and C. D. Barnes), Chapter 9, pp. 271–313. Academic Press, New York.

Robbins, T. W. and Everitt, B. J. (1992). Functions of dopamine in the dorsal and ventral striatum. *Seminars in the Neurosciences*, **4**, 119–28.

Robbins, T. W., Cador, M., Taylor, J. R., and Everitt, B. J. (1989). Limbic-striatal interactions in reward-related processes. *Neuroscience and Biobehavioral Reviews*, **13**, 155–62.

Roberts, D. C. S., Koob, G. F., Klonoff, P., and Fibiger, H. C. (1980). Extinction and recovery of cocaine self-administration following 6-hydroxydopamine lesions of the nucleus accumbens. *Pharmacology, Biochemistry and Behavior*, **12**, 781–7.

Rogan, M. T., Staubli, U. V., and LeDoux, J. E. (1997). Fear conditioning induces associative long-term potentiation in the amygdala. *Nature*, **390**, 604–7.

Rolls, B. J. (1990). The role of sensory-specific satiety in food intake and food selection. In *Taste, experience, and feeding*, (ed. E. D. Capaldi and T. L. Powley), Chapter 14, pp. 197–209. American Psychological Association, Washington, DC.

Rolls, B. J. and Hetherington, M. (1989). The role of variety in eating and body weight regulation. In *Handbook of the psychophysiology of human eating*, (ed. R. Shepherd), Chapter 3, pp. 57–84. Wiley, Chichester.

Rolls, B. J. and Rolls, E. T. (1973). Effects of lesions in the basolateral amygdala on fluid intake in the rat. *Journal of Comparative and Physiological Psychology*, **83**, 240–7.

Rolls, B. J. and Rolls, E. T. (1982). *Thirst*. Cambridge University Press.

Rolls, B. J., Wood, R. J., and Rolls, E. T. (1980a). Thirst: the initiation, maintenance, and termination of drinking. *Progress in Psychobiology and Physiological Psychology*, **9**, 263–321.

Rolls, B. J., Wood, R. J., Rolls, E. T., Lind, H., Lind, R., and Ledingham, J. (1980b). Thirst following water deprivation in humans. *American Journal of Physiology*, **239**, R476–82.

Rolls, B. J., Rolls, E. T., Rowe, E. A., and Sweeney, K. (1981a). Sensory-specific satiety in man. *Physiology and Behavior*, **27**, 137–42.

Rolls, B. J., Rowe, E. A., Rolls, E. T., Kingston, B., Megson, A., and Gunary, R. (1981b). Variety in a meal enhances food intake in man. *Physiology and Behavior*, **26**, 215–21.

Rolls, B. J., Rowe, E. A., and Rolls, E. T. (1982a). How sensory properties of foods affect human feeding behavior. *Physiology and Behavior*, **29**, 409–17.

Rolls, B. J., Rowe, E. A., and Rolls, E. T. (1982b). How flavour and appearance affect human feeding. *Proceedings of the Nutrition Society*, **41**, 109–17.

Rolls, B. J., Van Duijenvoorde, P. M., and Rowe, E. A. (1983). Variety in the diet enhances intake in a meal and contributes to the development of obesity in the rat. *Physiology and Behavior*, **31**, 21–7.

Rolls, B. J., Van Duijenvoorde, P. M., and Rolls, E. T. (1984). Pleasantness changes and food intake in a varied four course meal. *Appetite*, **5**, 337–48.

Rolls, E. T. (1971a). Involvement of brainstem units in medial forebrain bundle self-stimulation. *Physiology and Behavior*, **7**, 297–310.

Rolls, E. T. (1971b). Absolute refractory period of neurons involved in MFB self-stimulation. *Physiology and Behavior*, **7**, 311–15.

Rolls, E. T. (1971c). Contrasting effects of hypothalamic and nucleus accumbens septi self-stimulation on brain stem single unit activity and cortical arousal. *Brain Research*, **31**, 275–85.

Rolls, E. T. (1974). The neural basis of brain-stimulation reward. *Progress in Neurobiology*, **3**, 71–160.

Rolls, E. T. (1975). *The brain and reward*. Pergamon, Oxford.

Rolls, E. T. (1976a). The neurophysiological basis of brain-stimulation reward. In *Brain-stimulation reward*, (ed. A. Wauquier and E. T. Rolls), pp. 65–87. North-Holland, Amsterdam.

Rolls, E. T. (1976b). Neurophysiology of feeding. *Life Sciences Research Report* (Dahlem Konferenzen) **2**, 21–42.

Rolls, E. T. (1979). Effects of electrical stimulation of the brain on behavior. In *Psychology surveys*, Vol. 2, (ed. K. Connolly), pp. 151–69. George Allen, and Unwin, Hemel Hempstead, UK.

Rolls, E. T. (1980). Activity of hypothalamic and related neurons in the alert animal. In *Handbook of the hypothalamus*, Vol. 3A, (ed. P. J. Morgane and J. Panksepp), pp. 439–66. Dekker, New York.

Rolls, E. T. (1981a). Processing beyond the inferior temporal visual cortex related to feeding, memory, and striatal function. In *Brain mechanisms of sensation*, (ed. Y. Katsuki, R. Norgren, and M. Sato), pp. 241–69. Wiley, New York.

Rolls, E. T. (1981b). Responses of amygdaloid neurons in the primate. In *The amygdaloid complex*, (ed. Y. Ben-Ari), pp. 383–93. Elsevier, Amsterdam.

Rolls, E. T. (1981c). Central nervous mechanisms related to feeding and appetite. *British Medical Bulletin*, **37**, 131–4.

Rolls, E. T. (1982). Feeding and reward. In *The neural basis of feeding and reward*, (ed. B. G. Hoebel and D. Novin), pp. 323–37. Haer Institute for Electrophysiological Research, Brunswick, Maine.

Rolls, E. T. (1984a). Neurons in the cortex of the temporal lobe and in the amygdala of the monkey with responses selective for faces. *Human Neurobiology*, **3**, 209–22.

Rolls, E. T. (1984b). Activity of neurons in different regions of the striatum of the monkey. In *The basal ganglia: structure and function*, (ed. J. S. McKenzie, R. E. Kemm, and L. N. Wilcox), pp. 467–93. New York, Plenum.

Rolls, E. T. (1985). Connections, functions and dysfunctions of limbic structures, the prefrontal cortex, and hypothalamus. In *The scientific basis of clinical neurology*, (ed. M. Swash and C. Kennard), pp. 201–13. London, Churchill Livingstone.

Rolls, E. T. (1986a). A theory of emotion, and its application to understanding the neural basis of emotion. In *Emotions. Neural and chemical control*, (ed. Y. Oomura), pp. 325–44. Japan Scientific Societies Press, Tokyo and Karger, Basel.

Rolls, E. T. (1986b). Neural systems involved in emotion in primates. In *Emotion: theory, research, and experience*. Vol. 3: Biological foundations of emotion, (ed. R. Plutchik and H. Kellerman), Chapter 5, pp. 125–43. Academic Press, New York.

Rolls, E. T. (1986c). Neuronal activity related to the control of feeding. In *Feeding behavior: neural and humoral controls*, (ed. R. C. Ritter, S. Ritter, and C. D. Barnes), Chapter 6, pp. 163–90. Academic Press, New York.

Rolls, E. T. (1987). Information representation, processing and storage in the brain: analysis at the single neuron level. In *The neural and molecular bases of learning*, (ed. J.-P. Changeux and M. Konishi), pp. 503–40. Wiley, Chichester.

Rolls, E. T. (1989a). Functions of neuronal networks in the hippocampus and neocortex in memory. In *Neural models of plasticity: experimental and theoretical approaches*, (ed. J. H. Byrne and W. O. Berry), Chapter 13, pp. 240–65. Academic Press, San Diego.

Rolls, E. T. (1989b). Information processing in the taste system of primates. *Journal of Experimental Biology*, **146**, 141–64.

Rolls, E. T. (1989c). The representation and storage of information in neuronal networks in the primate cerebral cortex and hippocampus. In *The computing neuron*, (ed. R. Durbin, C. Miall, and G. Mitchison), Chapter 8, pp. 125–59. Addison–Wesley, Wokingham, UK.

Rolls, E. T. (1989d). Functions of neuronal networks in the hippocampus and cerebral cortex in memory. In *Models of brain function*, (ed. R. M. J. Cotterill), pp. 15–33. Cambridge University Press.

Rolls, E. T. (1990a). Functions of different regions of the basal ganglia. In *Parkinson's disease*, (ed. G. M. Stern), Chapter 5, pp. 151–84. Chapman and Hall, London.

Rolls, E. T. (1990b). A theory of emotion, and its application to understanding the neural basis of emotion. *Cognition and Emotion*, **4**, 161–90.

Rolls, E. T. (1990c). Functions of the primate hippocampus in spatial processing and memory. In *Neurobiology of comparative cognition*, (ed. D. S. Olton and R. P. Kesner), Chapter 12, pp. 339–62. L. Erlbaum, Hillsdale, NJ.

Rolls, E. T. (1991). Neural organisation of higher visual functions. *Current Opinion in Neurobiology*, **1**, 274–78.

Rolls, E. T. (1992a). Neurophysiological mechanisms underlying face processing within and beyond the temporal cortical visual areas. *Philosophical Transactions of the Royal Society*, **335**, 11–21.

Rolls, E. T. (1992b). Neurophysiology and functions of the primate amygdala. In *The amygdala*, (ed. J. P. Aggleton), Chapter 5, pp. 143–65. Wiley–Liss, New York.

Rolls, E. T. (1992c). The processing of face information in the primate temporal lobe. In *Processing images of faces*, (ed. V. Bruce and M. Burton), Chapter 3, pp. 41–68. Ablex, Norwood, New Jersey.

Rolls, E. T. (1993a). The neural control of feeding in primates. In *Neurophysiology of ingestion* (ed. D. A. Booth), Chapter 9, pp. 137–69. Pergamon, Oxford.

Rolls, E. T. (1994a). Neurophysiology and cognitive functions of the striatum. *Revue Neurologique (Paris)* **150**, 648–60.

Rolls, E. T. (1994b). Brain mechanisms for invariant visual recognition and learning. *Behavioural Processes*, **33**, 113–38.

Rolls, E. T. (1994c). Neural processing related to feeding in primates. In *Appetite: neural and behavioural bases*, (ed. C. R. Legg and D. A. Booth), Chapter 2, pp. 11–53. Oxford University Press.

Rolls, E. T. (1995a). Central taste anatomy and neurophysiology. In *Handbook of olfaction and gustation*, (ed. R. L. Doty), Chapter 24, pp. 549–73. Dekker, New York.

Rolls, E. T. (1995b). Learning mechanisms in the temporal lobe visual cortex. *Behavioural Brain Research*, **66**, 177–85.

Rolls, E. T. (1995c). A theory of emotion and consciousness, and its application to understanding the neural basis of emotion. In *The cognitive neurosciences*, (ed. M. S. Gazzaniga), Chapter 72, pp. 1091–1106. MIT Press, Cambridge, MA.

Rolls, E. T. (1996a). A theory of hippocampal function in memory. *Hippocampus*, **6**, 601–20.

Rolls, E. T. (1996b). A neurophysiological and computational approach to the functions of the temporal lobe cortical visual areas in invariant object recognition. In *Computational and biological mechanisms of visual coding*, (ed. L. Harris and M. Jenkin). Cambridge University Press.

Rolls, E. T. (1996c). The representation of space in the primate hippocampus, and episodic memory. In *Perception, memory and emotion: frontier in neuroscience*, (ed. T. Ono, B. L. McNaughton, S. Molotchnikoff, E. T. Rolls, and H. Nishijo), pp. 375–400. Elsevier, Amsterdam.

Rolls, E. T. (1996d). The orbitofrontal cortex. *Philosophical Transactions of the Royal Society*, B, **351**, 1433–44.

Rolls, E. T. (1996e). The representation of space in the primate hippocampus, and its relation to memory. In *Brain processes and memory*, (ed. K. Ishikawa, J. L. McGaugh, and H. Sakata), pp. 203–27. Elsevier, Amsterdam.

Rolls, E. T. (1996f). Roles of long term potentiation and long term depression in neuronal network operations in the brain. In *Cortical plasticity: LTP and LTD*, (ed. M. S. Fazeli and G. L. Collingridge), Chapter 11, pp. 223–50. Bios, Oxford.

Rolls, E. T. (1997a). Brain mechanisms of vision, memory, and consciousness. In: *Cognition, computation, and consciousness*, (ed. M. Ito, Y. Miyashita, and E. T. Rolls), Chapter 6, pp. 81–120. Oxford University Press.

Rolls, E. T. (1997b). Taste and olfactory processing in the brain. *Critical Reviews in Neurobiology*, **11**, 263–87.

Rolls, E. T. (1997c). A theory of emotion and its brain mechanisms. In *A century of psychology* (ed. R. Fuller, P. N. Walsh, and P. McGinley), Chapter 18, pp. 296–318. Routledge, London.

Rolls, E. T. (1997d). Consciousness in neural networks? *Neural Networks*, **10**, 1227–40.

Rolls, E. T. (1997e). A neurophysiological and computational approach to the functions of the temporal lobe cortical visual areas in invariant object recognition. In *Computational and psychophysical mechanisms of visual coding*, (ed. M. Jenkin and L. Harris), pp. 184–220. Cambridge University Press.

Rolls, E. T. (1998). Motivation. In *European introductory psychology*, (ed. M. Eysenck). Addison Wesley Longman, London.

Rolls, E. T. and Baylis, G. C. (1986). Size and contrast have only small effects on the responses to faces of neurons in the cortex of the superior temporal sulcus of the monkey. *Experimental Brain Research*, **65**, 38–48.

Rolls, E. T. and Baylis, L. L. (1994). Gustatory, olfactory and visual convergence within the primate orbitofrontal cortex. *Journal of Neuroscience*, **14**, 5437–52.

Rolls, E. T. and Cooper, S. J. (1973). Activation of neurones in the prefrontal cortex by brain-stimulation reward in the rat. *Brain Research*, **60**, 351–68.

Rolls, E. T. and Cooper, S. J. (1974). Connection between the prefrontal cortex and pontine brain-stimulation reward sites in the rat. *Experimental Neurology*, **42**, 687–99.

Rolls, E. T. and Johnstone, S. (1992). Neurophysiological analysis of striatal function. In *Neuropsychological disorders associated with subcortical lesions*, (ed. G. Vallar, S. F. Cappa, and C. Wallesch), Chapter 3, pp. 61–97. Oxford University Press.

Rolls, E. T. and Kelly, P. H. (1972). Neural basis of stimulus-bound locomotor activity in the rat. *Journal of Comparative and Physiological Psychology*, **81**, 173–82.

Rolls, E. T. and Mogenson, G. J. (1977). Brain self-stimulation behavior. In *The neurobiology of motivation*, (ed. G. J. Mogenson), Chapter 8, pp. 212–36. Erlbaum, Hillsdale, NJ.

Rolls, E. T. and Rolls, B. J. (1973). Altered food preferences after lesions in the basolateral region of the amygdala in the rat. *Journal of Comparative and Physiological Psychology*, **83**, 248–59.

Rolls, E. T. and Rolls, B. J. (1977). Activity of neurones in sensory, hypothalamic, and motor areas during feeding in the monkey. In *Food intake and chemical senses*, (ed. Y. Katsuki, M. Sato, S. F. Takagi, and Y. Oomura), pp. 525–49. University of Tokyo Press.

Rolls, E. T. and Rolls, B. J. (1982). Brain mechanisms involved in feeding. In *Psychobiology of human food selection*, (ed. L. M. Barker), Chapter 3, pp. 33–62. AVI, Westport, CT.

Rolls, E. T. and Rolls, J. H. (1997). Olfactory sensory-specific satiety in humans. *Physiology and Behavior*, **61**, 461–73.

Rolls, E. T. and Tovee, M. J. (1994). Processing speed in the cerebral cortex and the neurophysiology of visual masking. *Proceedings of the Royal Society B*, **257**, 9–15.

Rolls, E. T. and Tovee, M. J. (1995a). Sparseness of the neuronal representation of stimuli in the primate temporal visual cortex. *Journal of Neurophysiology*, **73**, 713–26.

Rolls, E. T. and Tovee, M. J. (1995b). The responses of single neurons in the temporal visual cortical areas of the macaque when more than one stimulus is present in the visual field. *Experimental Brain Research*, **103**, 409–20.

Rolls, E. T. and Treves, A. (1990). The relative advantages of sparse versus distributed encoding for associative neuronal networks in the brain. *Network*, **1**, 407–21.

Rolls, E. T. and Treves, A. (1998). *Neural networks and brain function*. Oxford University Press.

Rolls, E. T. and de Waal, A. W. L. (1985). Long-term sensory-specific satiety: evidence from an Ethiopian refugee camp. *Physiology and Behavior*, **34**, 1017–20.

Rolls, E. T. and Williams, G. V. (1987a). Sensory and movement-related neuronal activity in different regions of the primate striatum. In *Basal ganglia and behavior: sensory aspects and motor functioning*, (ed. J. S. Schneider and T. I. Lidsky), pp. 37–59. Hans Huber, Bern.

Rolls, E. T. and Williams, G. V. (1987b). Neuronal activity in the ventral striatum of the primate. In *The basal ganglia II—structure and function—current concepts*. (ed. M. B. Carpenter and A. Jayamaran), pp. 349–56. Plenum, New York.

Rolls, E. T., Kelly, P. H., and Shaw, S. G. (1974a). Noradrenaline, dopamine and brain-stimulation reward. *Pharmacology, Biochemistry, and Behavior*, **2**, 735–40.

Rolls, E. T., Rolls, B. J., Kelly, P. H., Shaw, S. G., and Dale, R. (1974b). The relative attenuation of self-stimulation, eating and drinking produced by dopamine-receptor blockade. *Psychopharmacologia (Berlin)*, **38**, 219–310.

Rolls, E. T., Burton, M. J., and Mora, F. (1976). Hypothalamic neuronal responses associated with the sight of food. *Brain Research*, **111**, 53–66.

Rolls, E. T., Judge, S. J., and Sanghera, M. (1977). Activity of neurones in the inferotemporal cortex of the alert monkey. *Brain Research*, **130**, 229–38.

Rolls, E. T., Perrett, D., Thorpe, S. J., Puerto, A., Roper-Hall, A., and Maddison, S. (1979a). Responses of neurons in area 7 of the parietal cortex to objects of different significance. *Brain Research*, **169**, 194–8.

Rolls, E. T., Sanghera, M. K., and Roper-Hall, A. (1979b). The latency of activation of neurons in the lateral hypothalamus and substantia innominata during feeding in the monkey. *Brain Research*, **164**, 121–35.

Rolls, E. T., Thorpe, S. J., Maddison, S., Roper-Hall, A., Puerto, A. and Perrett, D. (1979c). Activity of neurones in the neostriatum and related structures in the alert animal. In *The Neostriatum*, (eds I. Divac and R. G. E. Oberg), pp 163–182. Pergamon Press: Oxford.

Rolls, E. T., Burton, M. J., and Mora, F. (1980). Neurophysiological analysis of brain-stimulation reward in the monkey. *Brain Research*, **194**, 339–57.

Rolls, E. T., Rolls, B. J., and Rowe, E. A. (1983a). Sensory-specific and motivation-specific satiety for the sight and taste of food and water in man. *Physiology and Behavior*, **30**, 185–92.

Rolls, E. T., Thorpe, S. J., and Maddison, S. P. (1983b). Responses of striatal neurons in the behaving monkey. 1. Head of the caudate nucleus. *Behavioural Brain Research*, 7, 179–210.

Rolls, E. T., Thorpe, S. J., Boytim, M., Szabo, I., and Perrett, D. I. (1984). Responses of striatal neurons in the behaving monkey. 3. Effects of iontophoretically applied dopamine on normal responsiveness. *Neuroscience*, 12, 1201–12.

Rolls, E. T., Baylis, G. C., and Leonard, C. M. (1985). Role of low and high spatial frequencies in the face-selective responses of neurons in the cortex in the superior temporal sulcus. *Vision Research*, 25, 1021–35.

Rolls, E. T., Murzi, E., Yaxley, S., Thorpe, S. J., and Simpson, S. J. (1986). Sensory-specific satiety: food-specific reduction in responsiveness of ventral forebrain neurons after feeding in the monkey. *Brain Research*, 368, 79–86.

Rolls, E. T., Scott, T. R., Sienkiewicz, Z. J., and Yaxley, S. (1988). The responsiveness of neurones in the frontal opercular gustatory cortex of the macaque monkey is independent of hunger. *Journal of Physiology*, 397, 1–12.

Rolls, E. T., Baylis, G. C., Hasselmo, M. E., and Nalwa, V. (1989a). The effect of learning on the face-selective responses of neurons in the cortex in the superior temporal sulcus of the monkey. *Experimental Brain Research*, 76, 153–64.

Rolls, E. T., Sienkiewicz, Z. J., and Yaxley, S. (1989b). Hunger modulates the responses to gustatory stimuli of single neurons in the caudolateral orbitofrontal cortex of the macaque monkey. *European Journal of Neuroscience*, 1, 53–60.

Rolls, E. T., Yaxley, S., and Sienkiewicz, Z. J. (1990). Gustatory responses of single neurons in the orbitofrontal cortex of the macaque monkey. *Journal of Neurophysiology*, 64, 1055–66.

Rolls, E. T., Cahusac, P. M. B., Feigenbaum, J. D. and Miyashita, Y. (1993) Responses of single neurons in the hippocampus of the macaque related to recognition memory. *Experimental Brain Research*, 93, 299–306.

Rolls, E. T., Hornak, J., Wade, D., and McGrath, J. (1994a). Emotion-related learning in patients with social and emotional changes associated with frontal lobe damage. *Journal of Neurology, Neurosurgery, and Psychiatry*, 57, 1518–24.

Rolls, E. T., Tovee, M. J., Purcell, D. G., Stewart, A. L., and Azzopardi, P. (1994b). The responses of neurons in the temporal cortex of primates, and face identification and detection. *Experimental Brain Research*, 101, 474–84.

Rolls, E. T., Critchley, H., Mason, R., and Wakeman, E. A. (1996b). Orbitofrontal cortex neurons: role in olfactory and visual association learning. *Journal of Neurophysiology*, 75, 1970–81.

Rolls, E. T., Critchley, H. D., and Treves, A. (1996c). The representation of olfactory information in the primate orbitofrontal cortex. *Journal of Neurophysiology*, 75, 1982–96.

Rolls, E. T., Critchley, H., Wakeman, E. A., and Mason, R. (1996d). Responses of neurons in the primate taste cortex to the glutamate ion and to inosine 5'-monophosphate. *Physiology and Behavior*, 59, 991–1000.

Rolls, E. T., Francis, S., Bowtell, R., Browning, D., Clare, S., Smith, E., *et al.* (1997a). Pleasant touch activates the orbitofrontal cortex. *Neuroimage*, 5, S17.

Rolls, E. T., Francis, S., Bowtell, R., Browning, D., Clare, S., Smith, E., *et al.* (1997b). Taste and olfactory activation of the orbitofrontal cortex. *Neuroimage*, **5**, S199.

Rolls, E. T., Treves, A., and Tovee, M. J. (1997c). The representational capacity of the distributed encoding of information provided by populations of neurons in the primate temporal visual cortex. *Experimental Brain Research*, **114**, 149–62.

Rolls, E. T., Treves, A., Tovee, M., and Panzeri, S. (1997d). Information in the neuronal representation of individual stimuli in the primate temporal visual cortex. *Journal of Computational Neuroscience*, **4**, 309–33.

Rolls, E. T., Critchley, H. D., Browning, A., and Hernadi, I. (1998a). The neurophysiology of taste and olfaction in primates, and Umami flavor. In *Olfaction and taste, Vol. XII*, (ed. C. Murphy). *Annals of the New York Academy of Sciences*, in press.

Rolls, E. T., Treves, A., Robertson, R. G., Georges-François, P., and Panzeri, S. (1998b). Information about spatial view in an ensemble of primate hippocampal cells. *Journal of Neurophysiology*, **79**, 1797–1813.

Roper, S. (1998). Glutamate taste receptors. *Annals of the New York Academy of Sciences*, in press.

Rosenkilde, C. E. (1979). Functional heterogeneity of the prefrontal cortex in the monkey: a review. *Behavioral and Neural Biology*, **25**, 301–45.

Rosenkilde, C. E., Bauer, R. H., and Fuster, J. M. (1981). Single unit activity in ventral prefrontal cortex in behaving monkeys. *Brain Research*, **209**, 375–94.

Rosenthal, D. M. (1986). Two concepts of consciousness. *Philosophical Studies*, **49**, 329–59. Reprinted (1991) in *The Nature, of Mind*, (ed. D. M. Rosenthal), pp. 462–77. Oxford University Press, New York.

Rosenthal, D. (1990). A theory of consciousness. *ZIF Report No. 40*. Zentrum für Interdisziplinaire Forschung, Bielefeld, Germany.

Rosenthal, D. M. (1993). Thinking that one thinks. In *Consciousness*, (ed. M. Davies and G. W. Humphreys), Chapter 10, pp. 197–223. Blackwell, Oxford.

Routtenberg, A., Gardner, E. I., and Huang, Y. H. (1971). Self-stimulation pathways in the monkey, *Mucaca mulatta. Experimental Neurology*, **33**, 213–24.

Rozin, P. and Kalat, J. W. (1971). Specific hungers and poison avoidance as adaptive specializations of learning. *Psychological Review*, **78**, 459–86.

Rumelhart, D. E., Hinton, G. E., and Williams, R. J. (1986). Learning internal representations by error propagation. In *Parallel distributed processing: explorations in the microstructure of cognition*, Vol. 1, (ed. D. E. Rumelhart, J. L. McClelland, and the PDP Research Group), Chapter 8. MIT Press, Cambridge, MA.

Russchen, F. T., Amaral, D. G., and Price, J. L. (1985). The afferent connections of the substantia innominata in the monkey, *Macaca fascicularis. Journal of Comparative Neurology*, **242**, 1–27.

Rylander, G. (1948). Personality analysis before and after frontal lobotomy. *Association for Research into Nervous and Mental Disorders*, **27** (The Frontal Lobes), 691–705.

Saint-Cyr, J. A., Ungerleider, L. G., and Desimone, R. (1990). Organization of visual cortical inputs to the striatum and subsequent outputs to the pallido–nigral complex in the monkey. *Journal of Comparative Neurology*, **298**, 129–56.

Sanghera, M. K., Rolls, E. T., and Roper-Hall, A. (1979). Visual responses of neurons in the dorsolateral amygdala of the alert monkey. *Experimental Neurology*, **63**, 610–26.

Saper, C. B., Loewy, A. D., Swanson, L. W., and Cowan, W. M. (1976). Direct hypothalamo–autonomic connections. *Brain Research*, **117**, 305–12.

Saper, C. B., Swanson, L. W., and Cowan, W. M. (1979). An autoradiographic study of the efferent connections of the lateral hypothalamic area in the rat. *Journal of Comparative Neurology*, **183**, 689–706.

Sato, T., Kawamura, T., and Iwai, E. (1980). Responsiveness of inferotemporal single units to visual pattern stimuli in monkeys performing discrimination. *Experimental Brain Research*, **38**, 313–19.

Schachter, S. and Singer, J. (1962). Cognitive, social and physiological determinants of emotional state. *Psychological Review*, **69**, 378–99.

Schacter, G. B., Yang, C. R., Innis, N. K. and Mogenson, G. J. (1989). The role of the hippocampal-nucleus accumbens pathway in radial-arm maze performance. *Brain Research*, **494**, 339–49.

Schoenbaum, G. and Eichenbaum, H. (1995). Information encoding in the rodent prefrontal cortex. I. Single-neuron activity in orbitofrontal cortex compared with that in pyriform cortex. *Journal of Neurophysiology*, **74**, 733–50.

Schultz, W., Apicella, P., Scarnati, E., and Ljungberg, T. (1992). Neuronal activity in the ventral striatum related to the expectation of reward. *Journal of Neuroscience*, **12**, 4595–610.

Schultz, W., Apicella, P., Romo, R., and Scarnati, E. (1995a). Context-dependent activity in primate striatum reflecting past and future behavioral events. In *Models of information processing in the basal ganglia*, (ed. J. C. Houk, J. L. Davis, and D. G. Beiser), Chapter 2, pp. 11–27. MIT Press, Cambridge, MA.

Schultz, W., Romo, R., Ljunberg, T. Mirenowicz, J., Hollerman, J. R., and Dickinson, A. (1995b). Reward-related signals carried by dopamine neurons. In *Models of information processing in the basal ganglia*, (ed. J. C. Houk, J. L. Davis, and D. G. Beiser), Chapter 12, pp. 233–48. MIT Press, Cambridge, MA.

Schwaber, J. S., Kapp, B. S., Higgins, G. A., and Rapp, P. R. (1982). Amygdaloid and basal forebrain direct connections with the nucleus of the solitary tract and the dorsal motor nucleus. *Journal of Neuroscience*, **2**, 1424–38.

Scott, S. K., Young, A. W., Calder, A. J., Hellawell, D. J., Aggleton, J. P., and Johnson, M. (1997). Impaired auditory recognition of fear and anger following bilateral amygdala lesions. *Nature*, **385**, 254–7.

Scott, T. R., Yaxley, S., Sienkiewicz, Z. J., and Rolls, E. T. (1986a). Taste responses in the nucleus tractus solitarius of the behaving monkey. *Journal of Neurophysiology*, **55**, 182–200.

Scott, T. R., Yaxley, S., Sienkiewicz, Z. J., and Rolls, E. T. (1986b). Gustatory responses in the frontal opercular cortex of the alert cynomolgus monkey. *Journal of Neurophysiology*, **56**, 876–90.

Scott, T. R. and Giza, B. K. (1992). Gustatory control of ingestion. In *The neurophysiology of ingestion*, (ed. D. A. Booth). Manchester University Press.

Scott, T. R., Yan, J., and Rolls, E. T. (1995). Brain mechanisms of satiety and taste in macaques. *Neurobiology*, **3**, 281–92.

Seleman, L. D. and Goldman-Rakic, P. S. (1985). Longitudinal topography and interdigitation of corticostriatal projections in the rhesus monkey. *Journal of Neuroscience*, **5**, 776–94.

Seltzer, B. and Pandya, D. N. (1978). Afferent cortical connections and architectonics of the superior temporal sulcus and surrounding cortex in the rhesus monkey. *Brain Research*, **149**, 1–24.

Seltzer, B. and Pandya, D. N. (1989). Frontal lobe connections of the superior temporal sulcus in the rhesus monkey. *Journal of Comparative Neurology*, **281**, 97–113.

Sem-Jacobsen, C. W. (1968). Depth-electrographic stimulation of the human brain and behavior: from fourteen years of studies and treatment of Parkinson's Disease and mental disorders with implanted electrodes. C. C. Thomas, Springfield, IL.

Sem-Jacobsen, C. W. (1976). Electrical stimulation and self-stimulation in man with chronic implanted electrodes. Interpretation and pitfalls of results. In *Brain-stimulation reward*, (ed. A. Wauquier and E. T. Rolls), pp. 505–20. North-Holland, Amsterdam.

Seward, J. P., Uyeda, A. A., and Olds, J. (1959). Resistance to extinction following cranial self-stimulation. *Journal of Comparative and Physiological Psychology*, **52**, 294–9.

Shallice, T. and Burgess, P. (1996). The domain of supervisory processes and temporal organization of behaviour. *Philosophical Transactions of the Royal Society*, B, **351**, 1405–11.

Shaw, S. G. and Rolls, E. T. (1976). Is the release of noradrenaline necessary for self-stimulation? *Pharmacology, Biochemistry, and Behavior*, **4**, 375–79.

Shimura, T. and Shimokochi, M. (1990). Involvement of the lateral mesencephalic tegmentum in copulatory behavior of male rats: neuron activity in freely moving animals. *Neuroscience Research*, **9**, 173–83.

Shizgal, P. and Murray (1989). Neuronal basis of intracranial self-stimulation. In *The neuropharmacological basis of reward*, (ed. J. M. Liebman and S. J. Cooper). Oxford University Press.

Siegel, M. and Auerbach, J. M. (1996). Neuromodulators of synaptic strength. In *Cortical plasticity: LTP and LTD*, (ed. M. S. Fazeli and G. L. Collingridge), Chapter 7, pp. 137–148. Bios, Oxford.

Simpson, J. B., Epstein, A. N., and Camardo, J. S. (1977). The localization of receptors for the dipsogenic action of angiotensin II in the subfornical organ. *Journal of Comparative and Physiological Psychology*, **91**, 1220–31.

Singer, P. (1981). *The expanding circle: ethics and sociobiology*. Oxford University Press.

Singer, W. (1987). Activity-dependent self-organization of synaptic connections as a substrate for learning. In *The neural and molecular bases of learning*, (ed. J.-P. Changeux and M. Konishi), pp. 301–35. Wiley, Chichester.

Singer, W. (1995). Development and plasticity of cortical processing architectures. *Science*, **270**, 758–64.

Solomon, R. L. (1980). The opponent-process theory of acquired motivation: the costs of pleasure and the benefits of pain. *American Psychologist*, **35**, 691–712.

Solomon, R. L and Corbit, J. D. (1974). An opponent process theory of motivation. I. The temporal dynamics of affect. *Psychological Review*, **81**, 119–45.

Spiegler, B. J. and Mishkin, M. (1981). Evidence for the sequential participation of inferior temporal cortex and amygdala in the acquisition of stimulus–reward associations. *Behavioural Brain Research*, **3**, 303–17.

Squire, L. R. (1992). Memory and the hippocampus: A synthesis from findings with rats, monkeys and humans. *Psychological Review*, **99**, 195–231.

Squire, L. R. and Knowlton, B. J. (1995). Memory, hippocampus, and brain systems. In *The cognitive neurosciences*, (ed. M. S. Gazzaniga), Chapter 53, pp. 825–37. MIT Press, Cambridge, MA.

Starkstein, S. E. and Robinson, R. G. (1991). The role of the frontal lobe in affective disorder following stroke. In *Frontal lobe function and dysfunction*. (ed. H. S. Levin, H. M. Eisenberg, and A. L. Benton), pp. 288–303. Oxford University Press, New York.

Stein, L. (1967). Psychopharmacological substrates of mental depression. In *Anti-depressant drugs*, (ed. S. Garattini and M. N. G. Dukes). Excerpta Medica Foundation, Amsterdam.

Stein, L. (1969). Chemistry of purposive behavior. In *Reinforcement and behavior*, (ed. J. Tapp), pp. 328–35. Academic Press, New York.

Stein, N. L., Trabasso, T., and Liwag, M. (1994). The Rashomon phenomenon: personal frames and future-oriented appraisals in memory for emotional events. In *Future oriented processes*. (ed. M. M. Haith, J. B. Benson, R. J. Roberts, and B. F. Pennington). University of Chicago Press.

Stellar, E. (1954). The physiology of motivation. *Psychological Review*, **61**, 5–22.

Stellar, J. R. and Rice, M. B. (1989). In *The neuropharmacological basis of reward*, (ed. J. M. Liebman and S. J. Cooper), pp. 14–65. Oxford University Press.

Stellar, J. R. and Stellar, E. (1985). *The neurobiology of motivation and reward*. Springer, New York.

Stemmler, D. G. (1989). The autonomic differentiation of emotions revisited: convergent and discriminant validation. *Psychophysiology*, **26**, 617–32.

Stent, G. S. (1973). A psychological mechanism for Hebb's postulate of learning. *Proceedings of the National Academy of Sciences of the USA*, **70**, 997–1001.

Stern, C. E. and Passingham, R. E. (1995). The nucleus accumbens in monkeys (*Macaca fascicularis*): III. Reversal learning. *Experimental Brain Research*, **106**, 239–47.

Stern, C. E. and Passingham, R. E. (1996). The nucleus accumbens in monkeys (*Macaca fascicularis*): II. Emotion and motivation. *Behavioural Brain Research*, **75**, 179–93.

Stevens, J. R., Mark, V. H., Ervin, F., Pacheco, P., and Suematsu, K. (1969). Deep temporal stimulation in man. *Archives of Neurology*, **21**, 157–69.

Strauss, E. and Moscowitsch, M. (1981). Perception of facial expressions. *Brain and Language*, **13**, 308–32.

Strick, P. L., Dum, R. P., and Picard, N. (1995). Macro-organization of the circuits connecting the basal ganglia with the cortical motor areas. In *Models of information processing in the basal ganglia*. (ed. J. C. Houk, J. L. Davis, and D. G. Beiser), Chapter 6, pp. 117–30. MIT Press, Cambridge, MA.

Stricker, E. M. (1984). Brain catecholamines and the central control of food intake. *International Journal of Obesity*, **8**, Suppl. 1, 39–50.

Stricker, E. M. and Zigmond, M. J. (1976). Recovery of function after damage to central catecholamine-containing neurons: a neurochemical model for the lateral hypothalamic syndrome. *Progress in Psychobiology and Physiological Psychology*, **6**, 121–88.

Strongman, K. T. (1996). *The psychology of emotion*, (4th edn). Wiley, New York.

Sutton, R. S. and Barto, A. G. (1981). Towards a modern theory of adaptive networks: expectation and prediction. *Psychological Review*, **88**, 135–70.

Sutton, R. S. and Barto, A. G. (1990). Time-derivative models of Pavlovian reinforcement. In *Learning and Computational Neuroscience*, (ed. M. Gabriel and J. Moore), pp. 497–537. MIT Press, Cambridge, MA.

Swash, M. (1989). John Hughlings Jackson: a historical introduction. In *Hierarchies in neurology: a reappraisal of a Jacksonian concept*, (ed. C. Kennard and M. Swash), Chapter 1, pp. 3–10. Springer, London.

Taira, K. and Rolls, E. T. (1996). Receiving grooming as a reinforcer for the monkey. *Physiology and Behavior*, **59**, 1189–92.

Takagi, S. F. (1991). Olfactory frontal cortex and multiple olfactory processing in primates. In *Cerebral Cortex. 9*, (ed. A. Peters and E. G. Jones), pp. 133–52. Plenum Press, New York.

Tanabe, T., Yarita, H., Iino, M. Ooshima, Y., and Takagi, S. F. (1975a). An olfactory projection area in orbitofrontal cortex of the monkey. *Journal of Neurophysiology*, **38**, 1269–83.

Tanabe, T., Iino, M., and Takagi, S. F. (1975b). Discrimination of odors in olfactory bulb, pyriform–amygdaloid areas, and orbitofrontal cortex of the monkey. *Journal of Neurophysiology*, **38**, 1284–96.

Tanaka, D. (1973). Effects of selective prefrontal decortication on escape behavior in the monkey. *Brain Research*, **53**, 161–73.

Tanaka, K., Saito, C., Fukada, Y., and Moriya, M. (1990). Integration of form, texture, and color information in the inferotemporal cortex of the macaque. In *Vision, memory and the temporal lobe*, (ed. E. Iwai and M. Mishkin), Chapter 10, pp. 101–9. Elsevier, New York.

Thierry, A. M., Tassin, J. P., Blanc, G., and Glowinski, J. (1976). Selective activation of mesocortical DA system by stress. *Nature*, **263**, 242–244.

Thornhill, R. and Gangestad, S. W. (1996). The evolution of human sexuality. *Trends in Ecology and Evolution*, **11**, 98–102.

Thorpe, S. J., Rolls, E. T., and Maddison, S. (1983). Neuronal activity in the orbitofrontal cortex of the behaving monkey. *Experimental Brain Research*, **49**, 93–115.

Thrasher, T. N., Brown, C. J., Keil, L. C., and Ramsay, D. J. (1980a). Thirst and vasopressin release in the dog: an osmoreceptor or sodium receptor mechanism? *American Journal of Physiology*, **238**, R333–9.

Thrasher, T. N., Jones, R. G., Keil, L. C., Brown, C. J., and Ramsay, D. J. (1980b). Drinking and vasopressin release during ventricular infusions of hypertonic solutions. *American Journal of Physiology*, **238**, R340–5.

Tiihonen, J., Kuikka, J., Kupila, J., Partanen, K., Vainio, P., Airaksinen, J., *et al.* (1994). Increase in cerebral blood flow of right prefrontal cortex in man during orgasm. *Neuroscience Letters*, **170**, 241–3.

Tovee, M. J. and Rolls, E. T. (1992). Oscillatory activity is not evident in the primate temporal visual cortex with static stimuli. *Neuroreport*, **3**, 369–72.

Tovee, M. J. and Rolls, E. T. (1995). Information encoding in short firing rate epochs by single neurons in the primate temporal visual cortex. *Visual Cognition*, **2**, 35–58.

Tovee, M. J., Rolls, E. T., Treves, A., and Bellis, R. P. (1993). Information encoding and the responses of single neurons in the primate temporal visual cortex. *Journal of Neurophysiology*, **70**, 640–54.

Tovee, M. J., Rolls, E. T., and Azzopardi, P. (1994). Translation invariance and the responses of neurons in the temporal visual cortical areas of primates. *Journal of Neurophysiology*, **72**, 1049–60.

Towbin, E. J. (1949). Gastric distension as a factor in the satiation of thirst in esophagostomized dogs. *American Journal of Physiology*, **159**, 533–41.

Treves, A. (1995). Quantitative estimate of the information relayed by the Schaffer collaterals. *Journal of Computational Neuroscience*, **2**, 259–72.

Treves, A. and Rolls, E. T. (1991). What determines the capacity of autoassociative memories in the brain? *Network*, **2**, 371–97.

Treves, A. and Rolls, E. T. (1992). Computational constraints suggest the need for two distinct input systems to the hippocampal CA3 network. *Hippocampus*, **2**, 189–99.

Treves, A. and Rolls, E. T. (1994). A computational analysis of the role of the hippocampus in memory. *Hippocampus*, **4**, 374–91.

Treves, A., Rolls, E. T., and Simmen, M. (1997). Time for retrieval in recurrent associative memories. *Physica D*, **107**, 392–400.

Trivers, R. L. (1976). Foreword, In R. Dawkins, *The Selfish Gene*. Oxford University Press.

Trivers, R. L. (1985). *Social evolution*. Benjamin/Cummings, CA.

Uma-Pradeep, K., Geervani, P. and Eggum, B. O. (1993). Common Indian spices: nutrient composition, consumption and contribution to dietary value. Plant Foods Hum. Nutr. **44**, 138–48.

Ungerstedt, U. (1971). Adipsia and aphagia after 6-hydroxydopamine induced degeneration of the nigrostriatal dopamine system. *Acta Physiologia Scandinavica*, **81** (Suppl. 367), 95–122.

Valenstein, E. S. (1964). Problems of measurement and interpretation with reinforcing brain stimulation. *Psychological Review*, **71**, 415–37.

Valenstein, E. S. (1974). *Brain control. A critical examination of brain stimulation and psychosurgery*. Wiley, New York.

Valenstein, E. S., Cox, V. C., and Kakolewski, J. W. (1970). A re-examination of the role of the hypothalamus in motivation. *Psychological Review*, **77**, 16–31.

Van der Kooy, D., Koda, L. Y., McGinty, J. F. Gerfen, C. R., and Bloom, F. E. (1984). The organization of projections from the cortex, amygdala, and hypothalamus to the nucleus of the solitary tract in rat. *Journal of Comparative Neurology*, **224**, 1–24.

Van Hoesen, G. W. (1981). The differential distribution, diversity and sprouting of cortical projections to the amygdala in the rhesus monkey. In *The amygdaloid complex*, (ed. Y. Ben-Ari), pp. 77–90. Elsevier, Amsterdam.

Van Hoesen, G. W., Yeterian, E. H. and Lavizzo-Mourey, R. (1981). Widespread corticostriate projections from temporal cortex of the rhesus monkey. *Journal of Comparative Neurology*, **199**, 205–19.

Van Hoesen, G. W., Morecraft, R. J., and Vogt, B. A. (1993). Connections of the monkey cingulate cortex. In *The neurobiology of the cingulate cortex and limbic thalamus: a comprehensive handbook*. (ed. B. A. Vogt and M. Gabriel), pp. 249–84. Birkhauser, Boston.

Vogt, B. A. and Pandya, D. N. (1987). Cingulate cortex of the rhesus monkey: II. Cortical afferents. *Journal of Comparative Neurology*, **262**, 271–89.

Vogt, B. A., Pandya, D. N., and Rosene, D. L. (1987). Cingulate cortex of the rhesus monkey: I. Cytoarchitecture and thalamic afferents. *Journal of Comparative Neurology*, **262**, 256–70.

Vogt, B. A., Derbyshire, S., and Jones, A. K. P. (1996). Pain processing in four regions of human cingulate cortex localized with co-registered PET and MR imaging. *European Journal of Neuroscience*, **8**, 1461–73.

Wagner, H. (1989). The peripheral physiological differentiation of emotions. In *Handbook of social psychophysiology*, (ed. H. Wagner and A. Manstead), pp. 77–98. Wiley, Chichester.

Wallis, G. and Rolls, E. T. (1997). Invariant face and object recognition in the visual system. *Progress in Neurobiology*, **51**, 167–94.

Wallis, G., Rolls, E. T., and Foldiak, P. (1993). Learning invariant responses to the natural transformations of objects. *International Joint Conference on Neural Networks*, **2**, 1087–90.

Watson, J. B. (1929). *Psychology. From the standpoint of a behaviorist*. (3rd edn). Lippincott, Philadelphia.

Watson, J. B. (1930). *Behaviorism*, (revised edn). University of Chicago Press.

Wauquier, A. and Niemegeers, C. J. E. (1972). Intra-cranial self-stimulation in rats as a function of various stimulus parameters: II, influence of haloperidol, pimozide and pipamperone on medial forebrain stimulation with monopolar electrodes. *Psychopharmacology*, **27**, 191–202.

Weiskrantz, L. (1956). Behavioral changes associated with ablation of the amygdaloid complex in monkeys. *Journal of Comparative and Physiological Psychology*, **49**, 381–91.

Weiskrantz, L., (1968). Emotion. In *Analysis of behavioral change*, (ed. L. Weiskrantz), pp. 50–90. Harper and Row, New York.

Weiskrantz, L. (1997). *Consciousness lost and found*. Oxford University Press.

Weiskrantz, L. and Saunders, R. C. (1984). Impairments of visual object transforms in monkeys. *Brain*, **107**, 1033–72.

Whitelaw, R. B., Markou, A., Robbins, T. W. and Everitt, B. J. (1996). Excitotoxic lesions of the basolateral amygdala impair the acquisition of cocaine-seeking behaviour under a second-order schedule of reinforcement. *Psychopharmacology*, **127**, 213–24.

Wickens, J. and Kotter, R. (1995). Cellular models of reinforcement. In *Models of information processing in the basal ganglia*, (ed. J. C. Houk, J. L. Davis, and D. G. Beiser), Chapter 10, pp. 187–214. MIT Press, Cambridge, MA.

Wickens, J. R., Begg, A. J., and Arbuthnott, G. W. (1996). Dopamine reverses the depression of rat corticostriatal synapses which normally follows high-frequency stimulation of cortex in vitro. *Neuroscience*, **70**, 1–5.

Williams, G. V., Rolls, E. T., Leonard, C. M., and Stern, C. (1993). Neuronal responses in the ventral striatum of the behaving macaque. *Behavioural Brain Research*, **55**, 243–52.

Wilson, C. J. (1995). The contribution of cortical neurons to the firing pattern of striatal spiny neurons. In *Models of Information Processing in the Basal Ganglia*, (ed. J.C.Houk, J.L.Davis and D.G.Beiser) Ch. 3, pp. 29–50. MIT Press, Cambridge, Mass.

Wilson, F. A. W. and Rolls, E. T. (1990a). Neuronal responses related to reinforcement in the primate basal forebrain. *Brain Research*, **509**, 213–31.

Wilson, F. A. W. and Rolls, E. T. (1990b). Neuronal responses related to the novelty and familiarity of visual stimuli in the substantia innominata, diagonal band of Broca and periventricular region of the primate. *Experimental Brain Research*, **80**, 104–20.

Wilson, F. A. W. and Rolls, E. T. (1990c). Learning and memory are reflected in the responses of reinforcement-related neurons in the primate basal forebrain. *Journal of Neuroscience*, **10**, 1254–67.

Wilson, F. A. W. and Rolls, E. T. (1993). The effects of stimulus novelty and familiarity on neuronal activity in the amygdala of monkeys performing recognition memory tasks. *Experimental Brain Research*, **93**, 367–82.

Wilson, F. A. W. and Rolls, E. T. (1999). The primate amygdala and reinforcement: a dissociation between rule-based and associatively-mediated memory revealed in amygdala neuronal activity. In preparation.

Wilson, F. A. W., Scalaidhe, S. P. O., and Goldman-Rakic, P. S. (1993). Dissociation of object and spatial processing domains in primate prefrontal cortex. *Science*, **260**, 1955–8.

Winn, P., Tarbuck, A., and Dunnett, S. B. (1984). Ibotenic acid lesions of the lateral hypothalamus: comparison with electrolytic lesion syndrome. *Neuroscience*, **12**, 225–40.

Winn, P., Clark, A., Hastings, M., Clark, J., Latimer, M., Rugg, E., *et al.* (1990). Excitotoxic lesions of the lateral hypothalamus made by N-methyl-d-aspartate in the rat: behavioural, histological and biochemical analyses. *Experimental Brain Research*, **82**, 628–36.

Wise, R. A. (1989). Opiate reward: sites and substrates. *Neuroscience and Biobehavioral Reviews*, **13**, 129–33.

Wise, R. A. (1994). A brief history of the anhedonia hypothesis. In *Appetite: neural and behavioural bases*, (ed. C. R. Legg and D. A. Booth), Chapter 10, pp. 243–63. Oxford University Press.

Wise, R. A. and Rompre, P.-P. (1989). Brain dopamine and reward. *Annual Review of Psychology*, **40**, 191–225.

Wood, R. J., Rolls, B. J., and Ramsay, D. J. (1977). Drinking following intracarotid infusions of hypertonic solutions in dogs. *American Journal of Physiology*, **232**, R88–R92.

Wood, R. J., Maddison, S., Rolls, E. T., Rolls, B. J., and Gibbs, J. (1980). Drinking in rhesus monkeys: roles of pre-systemic and systemic factors in control of drinking. *Journal of Comparative and Physiological Psychology*, **94**, 1135–48.

Wood, R. J., Rolls, E. T., and Rolls, B. J. (1982). Physiological mechanisms for thirst in the nonhuman primate. *American Journal of Physiology*, **242**, R423–8.

Yamaguchi, S. (1967). The synergistic taste effect of monosodium glutamate and disodium 5'-inosinate, *Journal of Food Science*, **32**, 473–8.

Yamaguchi, S. and Kimizuka, A. (1979). Psychometric studies on the taste of monosodium glutamate. In *Glutamic acid: advances in biochemistry and physiology*, (ed. L. J. Filer, S. Garattini, M. R. Kare, A. R. Reynolds, and R. J. Wurtman), pp. 35–54 Raven Press, New York.

Yaxley, S., Rolls, E. T., Sienkiewicz, Z. J., and Scott, T. R. (1985). Satiety does not affect gustatory activity in the nucleus of the solitary tract of the alert monkey. *Brain Research*, **347**, 85–93.

Yaxley, S., Rolls, E. T., and Sienkiewicz, Z. J. (1988). The responsiveness of neurones in the insular gustatory cortex of the macaque monkey is independent of hunger. *Physiology and Behavior*, **42**, 223–9.

Yaxley, S., Rolls, E. T., and Sienkiewicz, Z. J. (1990). Gustatory responses of single neurons in the insula of the macaque monkey. *Journal of Neurophysiology*, **63**, 689–700.

Yeomans, J. S. (1990). *Principles of brain stimulation*. Oxford University Press, New York.

Yokel, R. A. and Wise, R. A. (1975). Increased lever pressing for amphetamine after pimozide in rats: implications for a dopamine theory of reinforcement. *Science*, **187**, 547–9.

Young, A. W., Aggleton, J. P., Hellawell, D. J., Johnson, M., Broks, P., and Hanley, J. R. (1995). Face processing impairments after amygdalotomy. *Brain*, **118**, 15–24.

Young, A. W., Hellawell, D. J., Van de Wal, C., and Johnson, M. (1996). Facial expression processing after amygdalotomy. *Neuropsychologia*, **34**, 31–9.

Zatorre, R. J. and Jones-Gotman, M. (1991). Human olfactory discrimination after unilateral frontal or temporal lobectomy. *Brain*, **114**, 71–84.

Zatorre, R. J., Jones-Gotman, M., Evans, A. C., and Meyer, E. (1992). Functional localization of human olfactory cortex. *Nature*, **360**, 339–40.

Index

acetyl choline   101, 140–3
action   138–40, 178–204, 245–65
action potential   288–9
activation h of a neuron   289–91
activation function of a neuron   290–1
addiction   168–78, 197–200
altruism   69, 273, 278–81
amphetamine   168–78, 197–200
amygdala   94–112, 47–9
  and brain-stimulation reward   158–9
  connections   96–8
  face representation   106–11
  and fear   100–2
  human   108–11
  lesions   44–5, 94–102
  neurophysiology   47–9, 102–12
  and novelty   48, 105–6
  and punishment   98–105
  and reward   98–103, 47–9
  role in feeding   44–9
  and sexual behaviour   221–3
  and stimulus-reinforcement association
    learning   98–112, 47–9
analgesia   159–60, 200–1
angiotensin   209–10
anxiety   202, 63–7
arousal   141–3, 163–4
associative reward–penalty algorithm
   316–19
astringency   30–1
autonomic response   4, 70–3, 98–102,
  138–9
avoidance   5, 62, 268–70

backprojections   245–6
  from the amygdala   144–5
basal forebrain   17–26, 140–3

basal forebrain cholinergic neurons   25,
  101, 141–3
basal ganglia   178–200
  and emotion   139–41
  and feeding   53–8
brain design   266–76
brain-stimulation reward   148–78
  effects of lesions   153–4
  nature of the reward   148–51
  neurophysiology of   154–60
  pharmacology   168–78
  properties of   160–4
  sites   151–3

capacity, of pattern associator   311–14
central gray of the midbrain   79, 159–60,
  200–1
cingulate cortex   134–6,
  and pain   79, 135–6
cholinergic neurons   140–3
classical conditioning   3, 101–2, 138–9,
  268–70
caudate nucleus   56–8, 178–98
cocaine   168–78
coding of information   43–4, 81–94,
  295–309
common currency   68, 267–76
communication   69, 106–11, 131–3, 260–1,
  272–3
conditioned appetite and satiety   17
conditioned response   4
conditioned stimulus   4
conditioning, classical   3, 101–2, 138–9,
  268–70
conditioning, instrumental   3, 67–8,
  268–70
confabulation   247–8